Nutrition Science: Macronutrients and Micronutrients

Nutrition Science: Macronutrients and Micronutrients

Edited by
Franklin Jackson

Larsen & Keller
www.larsen-keller.com

Nutrition Science: Macronutrients and Micronutrients
Edited by Franklin Jackson
ISBN: 978-1-63549-700-7 (Hardback)

Larsen & Keller
Published by Larsen and Keller Education,
5 Penn Plaza,
19th Floor,
New York, NY 10001, USA

Cataloging-in-Publication Data

Nutrition science : macronutrients and micronutrients / edited by Franklin Jackson.
p. cm.
Includes bibliographical references and index.
ISBN 978-1-63549-700-7
1. Nutrition. 2. Trace elements in nutrition. 3. Trace elements.
I. Jackson, Franklin.
RA784 .N87 2018
613.2--dc23

Printed and bound in China.

For more information regarding Larsen and Keller Education and its products, please visit the publisher's website www.larsen-keller.com

Table of Contents

Preface VII

Chapter 1 **An Introduction to Nutrient and Nutrition** 1
a. Nutrient 1
b. Essential Nutrient 5
c. Nutrition 16
d. Sports Nutrition 50
e. Prenatal Nutrition 54

Chapter 2 **Macronutrients: An Integrated Study** 67
a. Protein 67
b. Amino Acid 83
c. Fat 98
d. Fatty Acid 113
e. Carbohydrate 122
f. Dietary Fiber 132

Chapter 3 **An Overview of Micronutrients** 153
a. Micronutrient 153
b. Vitamin 156
c. Mineral (Nutrient) 200

Chapter 4 **Nutrition from Diet: A Comprehensive Study** 205
a. Diet (Nutrition) 205
b. Dietary Supplement 207
c. Nootropic 213
d. Raw Foodism 218

Permissions

Index

Preface

Nutrition science is the study of the interaction of nutrients with the other food substances and their importance in the growth, maintenance, development, reproduction, health, and disease control in a living organism. It also includes the study of the processes like biosynthesis, excretion, absorption, catabolism, assimilation, etc. This book elucidates the concepts and innovative models around prospective developments with respect to nutrition science. The topics included in it are of utmost significance and bound to provide incredible insights to readers. This textbook aims to serve as a resource guide for students and experts alike and contribute to the growth of the discipline.

A foreword of all Chapters of the book is provided below:

Chapter 1 - Nutrients are the building blocks of any organism. Essential nutrients are nutrients required for the normal functioning of a body. There are nine amino acids, thirteen vitamins, fifteen minerals and two fatty that are essential nutrients for humans. This chapter has been carefully written to provide an easy understanding of the varied facets of nutrition science; **Chapter 2 -** Proteins are made up of one or more amino acids. They have a number of functions to perform like DNA replication, responding to stimuli, catalyzing metabolic reactions, etc. The other macronutrients explained are amino acid, fat, fatty acid, dietary fiber and carbohydrate. The major categories of macronutrients are dealt with great details in the chapter; **Chapter 3 -** Micronutrients are essential elements that are necessarily required in small amounts by organisms. Some of the essential micronutrients are vitamins, minerals, etc. Both plants and animals can develop deficiencies in micronutrients. The chapter serves as a source to understand the major categories related to micronutrients; **Chapter 4 -** Diet plays an important role in the health and longevity of an organism. A complete diet consists of vitamins, proteins, fats and minerals. Dietary supplement, nootropic and raw foodism are some of the topics discussed in the following chapter. This chapter discusses the methods of nutrition science in a critical manner providing key analysis to the subject matter.

I would like to thank the entire editorial team who made sincere efforts for this book and my family who supported me in my efforts of working on this book. I take this opportunity to thank all those who have been a guiding force throughout my life.

Editor

1

An Introduction to Nutrient and Nutrition

Nutrients are the building blocks of any organism. Essential nutrients are nutrients required for the normal functioning of a body. There are nine amino acids, thirteen vitamins, fifteen minerals and two fatty acids that are essential nutrients for humans. This chapter has been carefully written to provide an easy understanding of the varied facets of nutrition science.

Nutrient

A nutrient is a component in foods that an organism uses to survive and grow. Macronutrients provide the bulk energy an organism's metabolic system needs to function while micronutrients provide the necessary cofactors for metabolism to be carried out. Both types of nutrients can be acquired from the environment. Micronutrients are used to build and repair tissues and to regulate body processes while macronutrients are converted to, and used for, energy. Methods of nutrient intake are different for plants and animals. Plants take in nutrients directly from the soil through their roots and from the atmosphere through their leaves. Animals and protists have specialized digestive systems that work to break down macronutrients for energy and utilize micronutrients for both metabolism and anabolism (constructive synthesis) in the body.

Organic nutrients consist of carbohydrates, fats, proteins (or their building blocks, amino acids), and vitamins. Inorganic chemical compounds such as dietary minerals, water (H2O), and oxygen may also be considered nutrients. A nutrient is considered essential if it must be obtained from an external source either because the organism cannot synthesize it or because insufficient quantities are produced. Nutrients needed in very small amounts are called micronutrients while those needed in large quantities are called macronutrients. The effects of nutrients are dose-dependent; shortages are called deficiencies.

Types of Nutrient

Macronutrients are defined in several different ways.

- The chemical elements humans consume in the largest quantities are carbon, hydrogen, nitrogen, oxygen, phosphorus, and sulphur, or CHNOPS.

- The classes of chemical compounds humans consume in the largest quantities and which provide bulk energy are carbohydrates, proteins, and fats. Water and atmospheric oxygen also must be consumed in large quantities, but are not always considered "food" or "nutrients".
- Calcium, salt (sodium and chloride), magnesium, and potassium (along with phosphorus and sulfur) are sometimes added to the list of macronutrients because they are required in large quantities compared to other vitamins and minerals. They are sometimes referred to as the macrominerals.

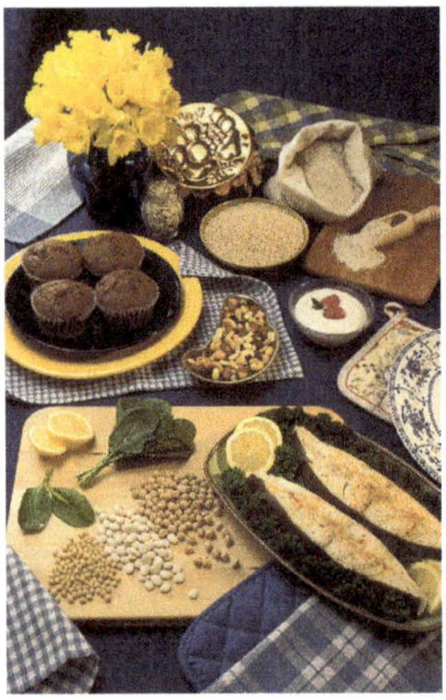

Good sources of magnesium: bran muffins, pumpkin seeds, barley, buckwheat flour, low-fat vanilla yogurt, trail mix, halibut steaks, garbanzo beans, lima beans, soybeans, and spinach.

Substances that Provide Energy

- Carbohydrates are compounds made up of types of sugars. Carbohydrates are classified by their number of sugar units: monosaccharides (such as glucose and fructose), disaccharides (such as sucrose and lactose), oligosaccharides, and polysaccharides (such as starch, glycogen, and cellulose).
- Proteins are organic compounds that consist of amino acids joined by peptide bonds. The body cannot manufacture some of the amino acids (termed essential amino acids); the diet must supply them. Proteins, in nutrition, are broken down through digestion by proteases back into free amino acids.
- Fats consist of a glycerin molecule with three fatty acids attached. Fatty acids are unbranched hydrocarbon chains,1 connected by single bonds alone (saturated fatty acids) or by both double and single bonds (unsaturated fatty acids). Fats are needed to keep cell membranes functioning properly, to insulate body organs against shock, to keep body temperature stable, and to maintain healthy skin and hair. The body does not manufacture certain fatty acids (termed essential fatty acids) and the diet must supply them.

Although alcohol provides energy, and can thus be compared to macronutrients, it is not a substance that is essential for normal function. The acetic acid in vinegar also provides a similar amount of energy per gram, but again, it is not a nutrient because it is not essential for normal function.

Fat has an energy content of 9 kcal/g (~37.7 kJ/g); proteins and carbohydrates 4 kcal/g (~16.7 kJ/g). Ethanol (grain alcohol) has an energy content of 7 kcal/g (~29.3 kJ/g).

Substances that Support Metabolism

- Dietary minerals are generally trace elements, salts, or ions such as copper and iron. Some of these minerals are essential to human metabolism.
- Vitamins are organic compounds essential to the body. They usually act as coenzymes or cofactors for various proteins in the body.
- Water is an essential nutrient and is the solvent in which all the chemical reactions of life take place.

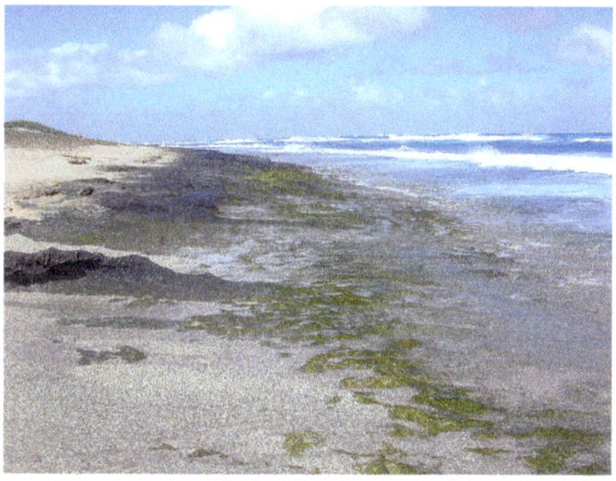

The strip of a green alga (*Enteromorpha*) along this shore indicates that there is a nearby source of nutrients (probably nitrates or ammonia from a small estuary).

Plants absorb nutrients from the soil or the atmosphere, or from water (mainly aquatic plants). An exception are the carnivorous plants, which externally digest nutrients from animals before ingesting them.

The chemical elements consumed in the greatest quantities by plants are carbon, hydrogen, and oxygen. These are present in the environment in the form of water and carbon dioxide; energy is provided by sunlight. Nitrogen, phosphorus, and sulfur are also needed in relatively large quantities. Together, the "Big Six" are the elemental macronutrients for all organisms, often represented by the acronym CHNOPS. Usually they are sourced from inorganic (e.g. carbon dioxide, water, nitrate, phosphate, sulfate) or organic (e.g. carbohydrates, lipids, proteins) compounds, although elemental diatomic molecules of nitrogen and (especially) oxygen are often used.

Other chemical elements are also necessary to carry out various life processes and build structures.

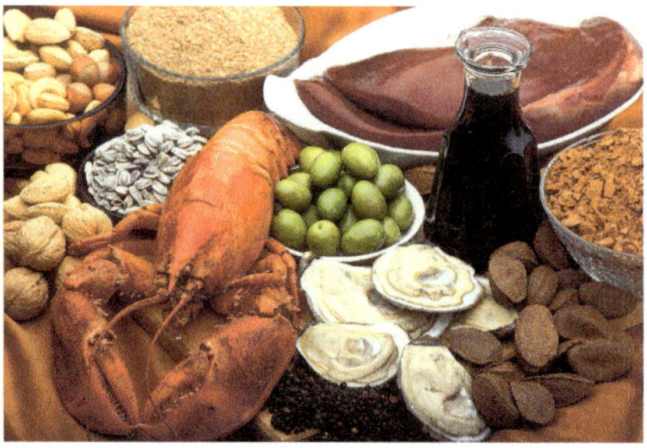

Rich sources of copper: oysters, beef or lamb liver, Brazil nuts, blackstrap molasses, cocoa, and black pepper. Good sources: lobster, nuts and sunflower seeds, green olives, and wheat bran.

Some of these are considered micronutrients in certain organisms. The mnemonic C. HOPKN'S CaFe Mg (to be used as C. Hopkins coffee mug) is used by some students to remember the list as: carbon, hydrogen, oxygen, phosphorus, potassium, nitrogen, sulfur, calcium, iron, and magnesium. Silicon, chloride, sodium, copper, zinc, and molybdenum are sometimes also included, but are in other cases considered micronutrients.

Essential and Non-Essential Nutrients

Nutrients are frequently categorized as essential and nonessential.

Essential Nutrients

Essential nutrients are unable to be synthesized internally (either at all, or in sufficient quantities), and so must be consumed by an organism from its environment.

For humans, these include essential fatty acids, essential amino acids, vitamins, and certain dietary minerals. Oxygen and water are also essential for human survival, but are generally not considered "food" when consumed in isolation. There are no "essential carbohydrates", animals can synthesize all the types of carbohydrates needed for growth.

Humans can derive energy from a wide variety of fats, carbohydrates, proteins, and simple chemicals such as ethanol and acetic acid.

Non-essential Nutrients

Non-essential nutrients are substances within foods can still have a significant impact on health, whether beneficial or toxic. For example, dietary fiber is not absorbed by the human digestive tract, but is important in maintaining the bulk of a bowel movement to avoid constipation. A subset, known as soluble fiber, can be metabolized by bacteria residing in the large intestine. Soluble fiber is marketed as serving a Probiotic (nutrition) function - promoting 'healthy' intestinal bacteria - even though there is not yet a scientific consensus on benefits of probiotics. Bacterial metabolism of soluble fiber is also thought to product short-chain fatty acids, which may be absorbed into intestinal cells as sources of calories.

Nonessential nutrients are those nutrients that can be made by the body; they may often also be absorbed from consumed food. The majority of animals ultimately derive their essential nutrients from plants, though some animals may consume mineral-based soils to supplement their diet.

Interest has recently increased in phytochemicals, which include many non-essential substances which may or may not have health benefits. These are not nutrients (or non-essential nutrients) by a strict definition, but labeling and marketing of dietary supplements can conflate these substances into a nutrients category.

Deficiencies and Toxicity

An inadequate amount of a nutrient is a deficiency. Deficiencies can be due to a number of causes including inadequacy in nutrient intake called dietary deficiency, or conditions that interfere with the utilization of a nutrient within an organism. Some of the conditions that can interfere with nutrient utilization include problems with nutrient absorption, substances that cause a greater than normal need for a nutrient, conditions that cause nutrient destruction, and conditions that cause greater nutrient excretion.

Nutrient toxicity occurs when an excess of a nutrient does harm to an organism.

Essential Nutrient

An essential nutrient is a nutrient required for normal physiological function that cannot be synthesized by the body, and thus must be obtained from a dietary source. Apart from water, which is universally required for the maintenance of homeostasis, essential nutrients are indispensable for the metabolic processes of cells, as well as the proper physiological functions of tissues and organs. In the case of humans, there are nine amino acids, two fatty acids, thirteen vitamins and fifteen minerals that are considered essential nutrients. In addition, there are several molecules that are considered conditionally essential nutrients since they are indispensable in certain developmental and pathological states.

Amino Acids

An essential amino acid is an amino acid that cannot be synthesized *de novo* (from scratch) by an organism, and therefore must be supplied in its diet. Out of the twenty amino acids, nine cannot be endogenously synthesized by humans: phenylalanine, valine, threonine, tryptophan, methionine, leucine, isoleucine, lysine, and histidine.

Fatty Acids

Essential fatty acids (EFAs) are fatty acids that humans and other animals must ingest because the body requires them for good health but cannot synthesize them. Only two fatty acids are known to be essential for humans: alpha-linolenic acid (an omega-3 fatty acid) and linoleic acid (an omega-6 fatty acid).

Vitamins

Vitamins are organic molecules essential for an organism that are not classified as amino acids or fatty acids. They commonly function as enzymatic cofactors, metabolic regulators or antioxidants. Humans require thirteen vitamins in their diet, most of which are actually groups of related molecules (e.g. vitamin E includes tocopherols and tocotrienols).

Minerals

Minerals are the exogenous chemical elements indispensable for an organism which are not provided by the other essential nutrients. The elements provided by essential amino acids, fatty acids and vitamins are carbon, hydrogen, oxygen, nitrogen and sulfur. For humans, the "major minerals" are calcium, phosphorus, potassium, sodium, chlorine, and magnesium. "Minor minerals" include metals such as iron, zinc, manganese and copper.

Conditionally Essential Nutrients

Conditionally essential nutrients are certain organic molecules that can normally be synthesized by an organism, but under certain conditions such biosynthesis is not enough to prevent a deficiency syndrome. In humans, such conditions include prematurity, limited nutrient intake, rapid growth, and certain disease states. Choline, inositol, taurine, arginine, glutamine and nucleotides are classified as conditionally essential and are particularly important in neonatal diet and metabolism.

Essential Amino Acid

An essential amino acid, or indispensable amino acid, is an amino acid that cannot be synthesized *de novo* (from scratch) by the organism, and thus must be supplied in its diet. The nine amino acids humans cannot synthesize are phenylalanine, valine, threonine, tryptophan, methionine, leucine, isoleucine, lysine, and histidine (i.e., F V T W M L I K H).

Six other amino acids are considered conditionally essential in the human diet, meaning their synthesis can be limited under special pathophysiological conditions, such as prematurity in the infant or individuals in severe catabolic distress. These six are arginine, cysteine, glycine, glutamine, proline, and tyrosine (i.e., R C G Q P Y). Five amino acids are dispensable in humans, meaning they can be synthesized in the body. These five are alanine, aspartic acid, asparagine, glutamic acid and serine (i.e., A D N E S).

Essentiality in Humans

Essential	Non-Essential
Histidine (H)	Alanine (A)
Isoleucine (I)	Arginine* (R)
Leucine (L)	Aspartic acid (D)
Lysine (K)	Cysteine* (C)
Methionine (M)	Glutamic acid (E)
Phenylalanine (F)	Glutamine* (Q)
Threonine (T)	Glycine* (G)
Tryptophan (W)	Proline* (P)
Valine (V)	Serine* (S)
	Tyrosine* (Y)
	Asparagine* (N)
	Selenocysteine (U)
	Pyrrolysine** (O)

(*) Essential only in certain cases.

(**) Pyrrolysine, sometimes considered "the 22nd amino acid", is not used by humans.

Eukaryotes can synthesize some of the amino acids from other substrates. Consequently, only a subset of the amino acids used in protein synthesis are essential nutrients.

Minimum Daily Intake

Estimating the daily requirement for the indispensable amino acids has proven to be difficult; these numbers have undergone considerable revision over the last 20 years. The following table lists the WHO recommended daily amounts currently in use for essential amino acids in adult humans, together with their standard one-letter abbreviations. Food sources are identified based on the USDA National Nutrient Database Release.

Amino acid(s)	mg per kg body weight	mg per 70 kg	mg per 100 kg
H Histidine	10	700	1000
I Isoleucine	20	1400	2000
L Leucine	39	2730	3900
K Lysine	30	2100	3000
M Methionine + **C** Cysteine	10.4 + 4.1 (15 total)	1050	1500

F Phenylalanine + **Y** Tyrosine	25 (total)	1750	2500
T Threonine	15	1050	1500
W Tryptophan	4	280	400
V Valine	26	1820	2600

The recommended daily intakes for children aged three years and older is 10% to 20% higher than adult levels and those for infants can be as much as 150% higher in the first year of life. Cysteine (or sulphur-containing amino acids), tyrosine (or aromatic amino acids), and arginine are always required by infants and growing children.

Relative Amino Acid Composition of Protein Sources

Various attempts have been made to express the "quality" or "value" of various kinds of protein. Measures include the biological value, net protein utilization, protein efficiency ratio, protein digestibility-corrected amino acid score and complete proteins concept. These concepts are important in the livestock industry, because the relative lack of one or more of the essential amino acids in animal feeds would have a limiting effect on growth and thus on feed conversion ratio. Thus, various feedstuffs may be fed in combination to increase net protein utilization, or a supplement of an individual amino acid (methionine, lysine, threonine, or tryptophan) can be added to the feed.

Although proteins from plant sources tend to have a relatively lower concentrations of protein by mass in comparison to protein from eggs or milk, they are nevertheless "complete" in that they contain at least trace amounts of all of the amino acids that are essential in human nutrition. Eating various plant foods in combination can provide a protein of higher biological value. Certain native combinations of foods, such as corn and beans, soybeans and rice, or red beans and rice, contain the essential amino acids necessary for humans in adequate amounts.

Additionally, certain types of algae and marine phytoplankton predate the division between animal and plant life on the planet; they have both chlorophyll as do plants, and also all the essential amino acids, as do animal proteins.

Protein Per Calorie

It can be shown that common vegetable sources contain adequate protein, often more protein per Calorie than the standard reference, whole raw egg, while other plant sources, particularly fruits contain less. For example, while 100 g of raw broccoli only provides 28 kcal and 3 g of protein, it has over 100 mg of protein per kcal. An egg contains five times as many calories (143 kcal) but only four times as much protein, roughly 90 mg of protein per kcal. However, a carrot has only 23 mg protein per kcal or twice the minimum recommendation, a banana meets the minimum, and an apple is below recommendation. It is recommended that adult humans obtain 10–35% of their calories as protein, or roughly 11–39 mg of protein per kcal per day (22–78 g for 2000 kcal). The US FDA daily reference value of 50 g protein per 2000 kcal is 25 mg/kcal per day.

Source	protein (g)	Calories (kcal)	protein/ Calorie (mg / kcal)	L (mg)	T (mg)	W (mg)	M+C (mg)
Apples, raw (100 g)	0.26	52	5	12	6	1	2
Minimum daily reference	22	2000	11				
Bananas, raw (100 g)	1	89	11	500	28	9	17
Carrot, raw (100 g)	1	41	24	101	191	12	103
US FDA daily / WHO (70 kg)	50	2000	25	2730	1050	280	1050
Upper daily reference	78	2000	39				
Peanut, valencia, raw (100 g)	48	570	84	1,627	859	244	630
Soybeans, mature seeds, dry roasted (100 g)	43	449	96	3223	1719	575	1172
Egg, whole, raw (100 g)	13	143	91	912	556	167	652
Broccoli, raw (100 g)	3	28	107	141	91	29	54
Soy Sauce, typical (100 g)	11	60	183	729	403	182	576
Beef, Australian, imported, grass-fed, ground, 85% lean / 15% fat, raw (100 g)	18	234	77	1430	780	200	690

Complete Proteins in Non-human Animals

Scientists had known since the early 20th century that rats could not survive on a diet whose only protein source was zein, which comes from maize (corn), but recovered if they were fed casein from cow's milk. This led William Cumming Rose to the discovery of the essential amino acid threonine. Through manipulation of rodent diets, Rose was able to show that ten amino acids are essential for rats: lysine, tryptophan, histidine, phenylalanine, leucine, isoleucine, methionine, valine, and arginine, in addition to threonine. Rose's later work showed that eight amino acids are essential for adult human beings, with histidine also being essential for infants. Longer term studies established histidine as also essential for adult humans.

Interchangeability

The distinction between essential and non-essential amino acids is somewhat unclear, as some amino acids can be produced from others. The sulfur-containing amino acids, methionine and homocysteine, can be converted into each other but neither can be synthesized *de novo* in humans. Likewise, cysteine can be made from homocysteine but cannot be synthesized on its own. So, for convenience, sulfur-containing amino acids are sometimes considered a single pool of nutritionally equivalent amino acids as are the aromatic amino acid pair, phenylalanine and tyrosine. Likewise arginine, ornithine, and citrulline, which are interconvertible by the urea cycle, are considered a single group.

Effects of Deficiency

If one of the essential amino acids is less than needed for an individual the utilization of other amino acids will be hindered and thus protein synthesis will be less than what it usually is, even in the presence of adequate total nitrogen intake.

Protein deficiency has been shown to affect all of the body's organs and many of its systems, including the brain and brain function of infants and young children; the immune system, thus elevating risk of infection; gut mucosal function and permeability, which affects absorption and vulnerability to systemic disease; and kidney function. The physical signs of protein deficiency include edema, failure to thrive in infants and children, poor musculature, dull skin, and thin and fragile hair. Biochemical changes reflecting protein deficiency include low serum albumin and low serum transferrin.

The amino acids that are essential in the human diet were established in a series of experiments led by William Cumming Rose. The experiments involved elemental diets to healthy male graduate students. These diets consisted of cornstarch, sucrose, butterfat without protein, corn oil, inorganic salts, the known vitamins, a large brown "candy" made of liver extract flavored with peppermint oil (to supply any unknown vitamins), and mixtures of highly purified individual amino acids. The main outcome measure was nitrogen balance. Rose noted that the symptoms of nervousness, exhaustion, and dizziness were encountered to a greater or lesser extent whenever human subjects were deprived of an essential amino acid.

Essential amino acid deficiency should be distinguished from protein-energy malnutrition, which can manifest as marasmus or kwashiorkor. Kwashiorkor was once attributed to pure protein deficiency in individuals who were consuming enough calories ("sugar baby syndrome"). However, this theory has been challenged by the finding that there is no difference in the diets of children developing marasmus as opposed to kwashiorkor. Still, for instance in Dietary Reference Intakes (DRI) maintained by the USDA, lack of one or more of the essential amino acids is described as protein-energy malnutrition.

Essential Fatty Acid

Essential fatty acids, or EFAs, are fatty acids that humans and other animals must ingest because the body requires them for good health but cannot synthesize them. Those not essential are non-essential fatty acids.

The term "essential fatty acid" refers to fatty acids required for biological processes but does not include the fats that only act as fuel. Essential fatty acids should not be confused with essential oils, which are "essential" in the sense of being a concentrated *essence*.

Only two fatty acids are known to be essential for humans: alpha-linolenic acid (an omega-3 fatty acid) and linoleic acid (an omega-6 fatty acid). Some other fatty acids are sometimes classified as "conditionally essential," meaning that they can become essential under some developmental or disease conditions; examples include docosahexaenoic acid (an omega-3 fatty acid) and gamma-linolenic acid (an omega-6 fatty acid).

When the two EFAs were discovered in 1923, they were designated "vitamin F", but in 1929, research on rats showed that the two EFAs are better classified as fats rather than vitamins.

Functions

In the body, essential fatty acids serve multiple functions. In each of these, the balance between dietary ω-3 and ω-6 strongly affects function.

- They are modified to make
    - the classic eicosanoids (affecting inflammation and many other cellular functions)
    - the endocannabinoids (affecting mood, behavior and inflammation)
    - the lipoxins which are a group of eicosanoid derivatives formed via the lipoxygenase pathway from ω-6 EFAs and resolvins from ω-3 (in the presence of acetylsalicylic acid, downregulating inflammation)
    - the isofurans, neurofurans, isoprostanes, hepoxilins, epoxyeicosatrienoic acids (EETs) and Neuroprotectin D
- They form lipid rafts (affecting cellular signaling)
- They act on DNA (activating or inhibiting transcription factors such as NF-κB, which is linked to pro-inflammatory cytokine production)

Nomenclature and Terminology

Fatty acids are straight chain hydrocarbons possessing a carboxyl (COOH) group at one end. The carbon next to the carboxylate is known as α, the next carbon β, and so forth. Since biological fatty acids can be of different lengths, the last position is labelled as a "ω", the last letter in the Greek alphabet. The physiological properties of unsaturated fatty acids largely depend on the position of the first unsaturation relative to the end position and not the carboxylate. For example, the term ω-3 signifies that the first double bond exists as the third carbon-carbon bond from the terminal CH_3 end (ω) of the carbon chain. The number of carbons and the number of double bonds are also listed.

ω-3 18:4 (stearidonic acid) or 18:4 ω-3 or 18:4 n−3 indicates an 18-carbon chain with 4 double bonds, and with the first double bond in the third position from the CH_3 end. Double bonds are *cis* and separated by a single methylene (CH_2) group unless otherwise noted. So in free fatty acid form, the chemical structure of stearidonic acid is:

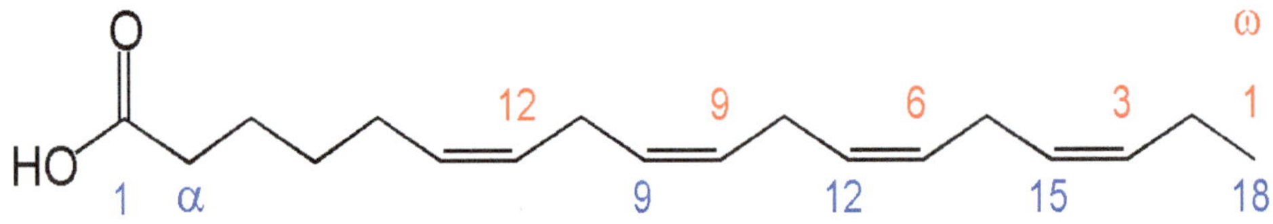

Examples

The essential fatty acids start with the short chain polyunsaturated fatty acids (SC-PUFA):

- ω-3 fatty acids:
  - α-Linolenic acid or ALA (18:3n-3)
- ω-6 fatty acids:
  - Linoleic acid or LA (18:2n-6)

These two fatty acids cannot be synthesized by humans because humans lack the desaturase enzymes required for their production.

They form the starting point for the creation of longer and more desaturated fatty acids, which are also referred to as long-chain polyunsaturated fatty acids (LC-PUFA):

- ω-3 fatty acids:
  - eicosapentaenoic acid or EPA (20:5n-3)
  - docosahexaenoic acid or DHA (22:6n-3)
- ω-6 fatty acids:
  - gamma-linolenic acid or GLA (18:3n-6)
  - dihomo-gamma-linolenic acid or DGLA (20:3n-6)
  - arachidonic acid or AA (20:4n-6)

ω-9 fatty acids are not essential in humans because they can be synthesized from carbohydrates or other fatty acids.

Essential Fatty Acids

Mammals lack the ability to introduce double bonds in fatty acids beyond carbon 9 and 10, hence ω-6 linoleic acid (18:2,9,12), abbreviated LA (18:2n-6), and the ω-3 linolenic acid (18:3,9,12,15), abbreviated ALA (18:3n-3), are essential for humans in the diet. In humans, arachidonic acid (20:4,5,8,11,14, abbreviated 20:4n-6) can be synthesized from LA by alternative desaturation and chain elongation.

Humans can convert both LA and ALA to docosapentaenoic acid (22:5n-6) and docosahexaenoic acid (22:6n-3; DHA) respectively, although the conversion to DHA is limited, resulting in lower blood levels of DHA than through direct ingestion. This is illustrated by studies in vegans and vegetarians. If there is relatively more LA than ALA in the diet it favors the formation of docosapentaenoic acid (22:5n-6) from LA rather than docosahexaenoic acid (22:6n-3) from ALA. This effect can be altered by changing the relative ratio of LA:ALA, but is more effective when total intake of polyunsaturated fatty acids is low. However, the capacity to convert LA to AA and ALA to DHA in the preterm infant is limited, and preformed AA and DHA may be required to meet the needs of the developing brain. Both AA and DHA are present in breastmilk and contribute along with the parent fatty acids LA and ALA to meeting the requirements of the newborn infant. Many infant formulas have AA and DHA added to them with an aim to make them more equivalent to human milk.

Essential nutrients are defined as those that cannot be synthesized de novo in sufficient quantities for normal physiological function. This definition is met for LA and ALA but not the longer chain derivatives in adults. The longer chain derivatives particularly, however, have pharmacological properties that can modulate disease processes, but this should not be confused with dietary essentiality.

Between 1930 and 1950, arachidonic acid and linolenic acid were termed 'essential' because each was more or less able to meet the growth requirements of rats given fat-free diets. However, they were yet to be recognized as essential nutrients for humans. In the 1950s Arild Hansen showed that infants fed skimmed milk developed essential fatty acid deficiency. It was characterized by an increased food intake, poor growth, and a scaly dermatitis, and was cured by the administration of corn oil.

Later work by Hansen randomized 426 children, mainly black, to four treatments: modified cow's milk formula, skimmed milk formula, skimmed milk formula with coconut oil, or cow's milk formula with corn oil. The infants who received the skimmed milk formula or the formula with coconut oil developed essential fatty acid deficiency signs and symptoms. This could be cured by administration of ethyl linoleate (the ethyl ester of linoleic acid) with about 1% of the energy intake.

Collins et al. 1970 were the first to demonstrate linoleic acid deficiency in adults. They found that patients undergoing intravenous nutrition with glucose became isolated from their fat supplies and rapidly developed biochemical signs of essential fatty acid deficiency (an increase in 20:3n-9/20:4n-6 ratio in plasma) and skin symptoms. This could be treated by infusing lipids, and later studies showed that topical application of sunflower oil would also resolve the dermal symptoms. Linoleic acid has a specific role in maintaining the skin water-permeability barrier, probably as constituents of acylglycosylceramides. This role cannot be met by any ω-3 fatty acids or by arachidonic acid.

The main physiological requirement for ω-6 fatty acids is attributed to arachidonic acid. Arachidonic acid is the major precursor of prostaglandins, leukotrienes, and anandamides that play a vital role in cell signaling. Metabolites from the ω-3 pathway, mainly from eicosapentaenoic acid, are mostly inactive, and this explains why ω-3 fatty acids do not correct the reproductive failure in rats where arachidonic is needed to make active prostaglandins that cause uterine contraction. To some extent, any ω-3 or ω-6 can contribute to the growth-promoting effects of EFA deficiency, but only ω-6 fatty acids can restore reproductive performance and correct the dermatitis in rats. Particular fatty acids are still needed at critical life stages (e.g. lactation) and in some disease states.

In nonscientific writing, common usage is that the term *essential fatty acid* comprises all the ω-3 or -6 fatty acids. Conjugated fatty acids like calendic acid are not considered essential. Authoritative sources include the whole families, but generally only make dietary recommendations for LA and ALA with the exception of DHA for infants under the age of 6 months. Recent reviews by WHO/FAO in 2009 and the European Food Safety Authority have reviewed the evidence and made recommendations for minimal intakes of LA and ALA and have also recommended intakes of longer chain ω-3 fatty acids based on the association of oily fish consumption with a lower risk of cardiovascular disease. Some earlier review lumped all polyunsaturated fatty acids together without qualification whether they were short or long-chain PUFA or whether they were ω-3 and ω-6 PUFA.

Conditionally Essential

Traditionally speaking, the LC-PUFAs are not essential. Because the LC-PUFA are sometimes required, they may be considered conditionally essential fatty acids, or not essential to healthy adults.

Food Sources

Some of the food sources of ω-3 and ω-6 fatty acids are fish and shellfish, flaxseed (linseed) and flaxseed oil, hemp seed, olive oil, soya oil, canola (rapeseed) oil, chia seeds, pumpkin seeds, sunflower seeds, leafy vegetables, and walnuts; but most of these food sources are poor sources of EFA's. Flaxseeds are the best source of ω-3 EFA, next is chiaseed, lastly hempseed; sunflower and starflower seeds are the best sources of ω-6 EFA.

Essential fatty acids play a part in many metabolic processes, and there is evidence to suggest that low levels of essential fatty acids, or the wrong balance of types among the essential fatty acids, may be a factor in a number of illnesses, including osteoporosis.

Fish is the main source of the longer omega-3 fats; eicosapentaenoic acid (EPA) and docosahexaenoic acid (DHA). Some plant-based foods contain omega-3 in the form of alpha-linolenic acid (ALA), which appears to have a modest benefit for cardiovascular health. The human body can (and in case of a purely vegetarian diet often must unless certain algae or supplements derived from them are consumed) convert ALA to EPA and subsequently DHA. This elongation of ALA is inefficient. Interestingly, conversion to DHA is higher in women than in men; this is thought to reflect the need to provide DHA to the fetus and infant during pregnancy and breast feeding.

The *IUPAC Lipid Handbook* provides a very large and detailed listing of fat contents of animal and vegetable fats, including ω-3 and -6 oils. The National Institutes of Health's EFA Education group publishes *Essential Fats in Food Oils.* This lists 40 common oils, more tightly focused on EFAs and sorted by n-6:3 ratio. *Vegetable Lipids as Components of Functional Food* lists notable vegetable sources of EFAs as well as commentary and an overview of the biosynthetic pathways involved. Careful readers will note that these sources are not in excellent agreement. EFA content of vegetable sources varies with cultivation conditions. Animal sources vary widely, both with the animal's feed and that the EFA makeup varies markedly with fats from different body parts.

Human Health

Almost all the polyunsaturated fats in the human diet are EFAs. Essential fatty acids play an important role in the life and death of cardiac cells.

Reference Intake Values

Reference intake values for as published by the Panel on Dietetic Products, Nutrition and Allergies of the European Food Safety Authority (EFSA).

Common name	Type	Reference intake values
alpha-Linolenic acid (ALA)	Omega-3	2g Gram
Linoleic acid (LA)	Omega-6	10g Gram

In the United States, the recommendations for omega-3 fatty acids covers ALA, EPA and DHA, and for adults the values are 1.6 g/day for men and 1.1. g/day for women. The recommendation for omega-6 fatty acids is for linoleic acid: 17 g/day for younger men, dropping to 14 g/day for older men; for women 12 and 11 g/day.

Essential Fatty Acid Deficiency

Essential fatty acid deficiency results in a dermatitis similar to that seen in zinc or biotin deficiency.

Nutrition

Nutrition is the science that interprets the interaction of nutrients and other substances in food in relation to maintenance, growth, reproduction, health and disease of an organism. It includes food intake, absorption, assimilation, biosynthesis, catabolism and excretion.

The diet of an organism is what it eats, which is largely determined by the availability, the processing and palatability of foods. A healthy diet includes preparation of food and storage methods that preserve nutrients from oxidation, heat or leaching, and that reduce risk of foodborne illness.

Registered dietitian nutritionists (RDs or RDNs) are health professionals qualified to provide safe, evidence-based dietary advice which includes a review of what is eaten, a thorough review of nutritional health, and a personalized nutritional treatment plan. They also provide preventive and therapeutic programs at work places, schools and similar institutions. Certified Clinical Nutritionists or CCNs, are trained health professionals who also offer dietary advice on the role of nutrition in chronic disease, including possible prevention or remediation by addressing nutritional deficiencies before resorting to drugs. Government regulation especially in terms of licensing, is currently less universal for the CCN than that of RD or RDN. Another advanced Nutrition Professional is a Certified Nutrition Specialist or CNS. These Board Certified Nutritionists typically specialize in obesity and chronic disease. In order to become board certified, potential CNS candidate must pass an examination, much like Registered Dieticians. This exam covers specific domains within the health sphere including; Clinical Intervention and Human Health.

A poor diet may cause health problems, causing deficiency diseases such as blindness, anemia, scurvy, preterm birth, stillbirth and cretinism; health-threatening conditions like obesity and metabolic syndrome; and such common chronic systemic diseases as cardiovascular disease, diabetes, and osteoporosis. A poor diet can cause the wasting of kwashiorkor in acute cases, and the stunting of marasmus in chronic cases of malnutrition.

History

Antiquity

The first recorded dietary advice, carved into a Babylonian stone tablet in about 2500 BC, cautioned those with pain inside to avoid eating onions for three days. Scurvy, later found to be a vitamin C deficiency, was first described in 1500 BC in the Ebers Papyrus.

According to Walter Gratzer, the study of nutrition probably began during the 6th century BC. In China, the concept of *Qi* developed, a spirit or "wind" similar to what Western Europeans later called *pneuma*. Food was classified into "hot" (for example, meats, blood, ginger, and hot spices) and "cold" (green vegetables) in China, India, Malaya, and Persia. *Humours* developed perhaps first in China alongside *qi*. Ho the Physician concluded that diseases are caused by deficiencies of elements (Wu Xing: fire, water, earth, wood, and metal), and he classified diseases as well as prescribed diets. About the same time in Italy, Alcmaeon of Croton (a Greek) wrote of the importance of equilibrium between what goes in and what goes out, and warned that imbalance would result in disease marked by obesity or emaciation.

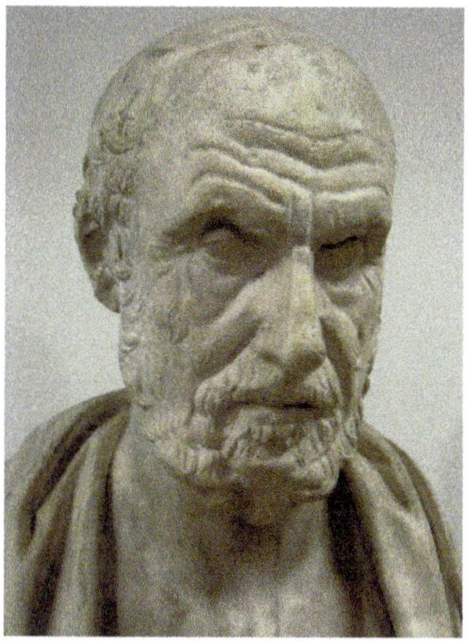

Hippocrates lived about 400 BC, and Galen and the understanding of nutrition followed him for centuries.

The first recorded nutritional experiment with human subjects is found in the Bible's Book of Daniel. Daniel and his friends were captured by the king of Babylon during an invasion of Israel. Selected as court servants, they were to share in the king's fine foods and wine. But they objected, preferring vegetables (pulses) and water in accordance with their Jewish dietary restrictions. The king's chief steward reluctantly agreed to a trial. Daniel and his friends received their diet for ten days and were then compared to the king's men. Appearing healthier, they were allowed to continue with their diet.

Around 475 BC, Anaxagoras stated that food is absorbed by the human body and, therefore, contains "homeomerics" (generative components), suggesting the existence of nutrients. Around 400 BC, Hippocrates, who recognized and was concerned with obesity, which may have been common in southern Europe at the time, said, "Let food be your medicine and medicine be your food." The works that are still attributed to him, *Corpus Hippocraticum*, called for moderation and emphasized exercise.

Salt, pepper and other spices were prescribed for various ailments in various preparations for example mixed with vinegar. In the 2nd century BC, Cato the Elder believed that cabbage (or the urine of cabbage-eaters) could cure digestive diseases, ulcers, warts, and intoxication. Living about the turn of the millennium, Aulus Celsus, an ancient Roman doctor, believed in "strong" and "weak" foods (bread for example was strong, as were older animals and vegetables).

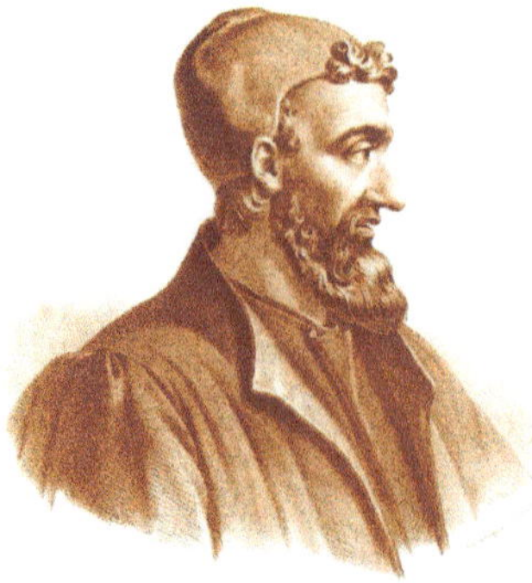

Followed for a millennium and a half, Galen (1st century) created the first coherent (although mistaken) theory of nutrition.

Galen to Lind

One mustn't overlook the doctrines of Galen: In use from his life in the 1st century AD until the 17th century, it was heresy to disagree with him for 1500 years. Galen was physician to gladiators in Pergamon, and in Rome, physician to Marcus Aurelius and the three emperors who succeeded him. Most of Galen's teachings were gathered and enhanced in the late 11th century by Benedictine monks at the School of Salerno in *Regimen sanitatis Salernitanum*, which still had users in the 17th century. Galen believed in the bodily *humours* of Hippocrates, and he taught that *pneuma* is the source of life. Four elements (earth, air, fire and water) combine into "complexion", which combines into states (the four temperaments: sanguine, phlegmatic, choleric, and melancholic). The states are made up of pairs of attributes (hot and moist, cold and moist, hot and dry, and cold and dry), which are made of four humours: blood, phlegm, green (or yellow) bile, and black bile (the bodily form of the elements). Galen thought that for a person to have gout, kidney stones, or arthritis was scandalous, which Gratzer likens to Samuel Butler's *Erehwon* (1872) where sickness is a crime.

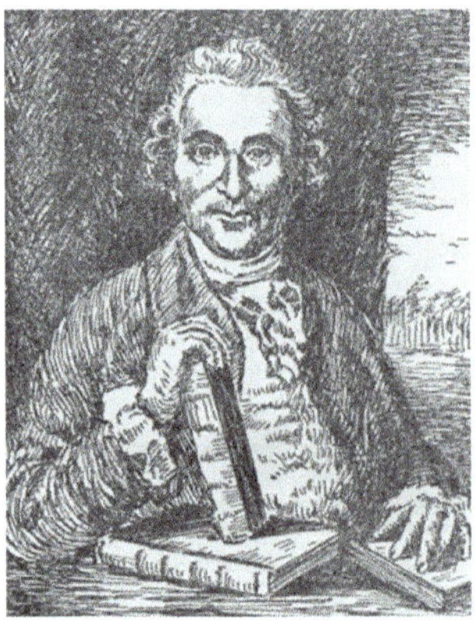

James Lind conducted in 1747 the first controlled clinical trial in modern times, and in 1753 published *Treatise on Scurvy*.

In the 1500s, Paracelsus was probably the first to criticize Galen publicly. Also in the

16th century, scientist and artist Leonardo da Vinci compared metabolism to a burning candle. Leonardo did not publish his works on this subject, but he was not afraid of thinking for himself and he definitely disagreed with Galen. Ultimately, 16th century works of Andreas Vesalius, sometimes called the father of modern medicine, overturned Galen's ideas. He was followed by piercing thought amalgamated with the era's mysticism and religion sometimes fueled by the mechanics of Newton and Galileo. Jan Baptist van Helmont, who discovered several gases such as carbon dioxide, performed the first quantitative experiment. Robert Boyle advanced chemistry. Sanctorius measured body weight. Physician Herman Boerhaave modeled the digestive process. Physiologist Albrecht von Haller worked out the difference between nerves and muscles.

Sometimes overlooked during his life, James Lind, a physician in the British navy, performed the first scientific nutrition experiment in 1747. Lind discovered that lime juice saved sailors that had been at sea for years from scurvy, a deadly and painful bleeding disorder. Between 1500 and 1800, an estimated two million sailors had died of scurvy. The discovery was ignored for forty years, after which British sailors became known as "limeys." The essential vitamin C within citrus fruits would not be identified by scientists until 1932.

Lavoisier and Modern Science

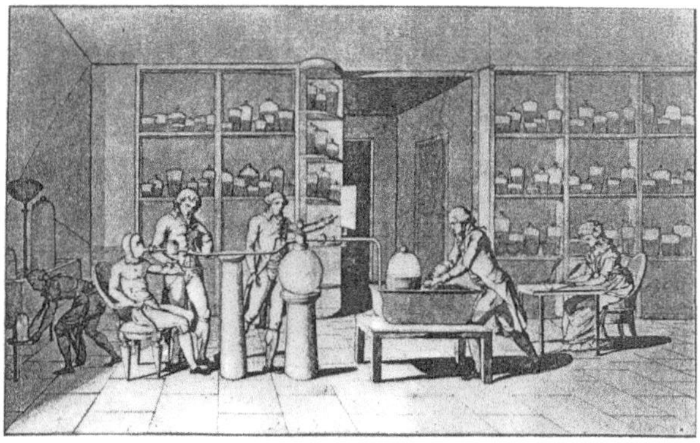

By containing his assistant, Armand Seguin, inside a rubber suit fitted with a tube sealed to his mouth with putty, Antoine Lavoisier first measured basal metabolic rate. Drawing by Madame Lavoisier (seated at right).

Around 1770, Antoine Lavoisier discovered the details of metabolism, demonstrating that the oxidation of food is the source of body heat. Called the most fundamental chemical discovery of the 18th century, Lavoisier discovered the principle of conservation of mass. His ideas made the phlogiston theory of combustion obsolete.

In 1790, George Fordyce recognized calcium as necessary for the survival of fowl. In the early 19th century, the elements carbon, nitrogen, hydrogen, and oxygen were recognized as the primary components of food, and methods to measure their proportions were developed.

In 1816, François Magendie discovered that dogs fed only carbohydrates (sugar), fat (olive oil), and water died evidently of starvation, but dogs also fed protein survived, identifying protein as an essential dietary component. William Prout in 1827 was the first person to divide foods into carbohydrates, fat, and protein. During the 19th century, Jean-Baptiste Dumas and Justus von Liebig quarrelled over their shared belief that animals get their protein directly from plants (animal and plant protein are the same and that humans do not create organic compounds). With a reputation as the leading organic chemist of his day but with no credentials in animal physiology, Liebig grew rich making food extracts like beef bouillon and infant formula that were later found to be of questionable nutritious value. In the 1860s, Claude Bernard discovered that body fat can be synthesized from carbohydrate and protein, showing that the energy in blood glucose can be stored as fat or as glycogen.

In the early 1880s, Kanehiro Takaki observed that Japanese sailors (whose diets consisted almost entirely of white rice) developed beriberi (or endemic neuritis, a disease causing heart problems and paralysis), but British sailors and Japanese naval officers did not. Adding various types of vegetables and meats to the diets of Japanese sailors prevented the disease, (not because of the increased protein as Takaki supposed but because it introduced a few parts per million of thiamine to the diet, later understood as a cure).

In 1896, Eugen Baumann observed iodine in thyroid glands. In 1897, Christiaan Eijkman worked with natives of Java, who also suffered from beriberi. Eijkman observed that chickens fed the native diet of white rice developed the symptoms of beriberi but remained healthy when fed unprocessed brown rice with the outer bran intact. Eijkman cured the natives by feeding them brown rice, discovering that food can cure disease. Over two decades later, nutritionists learned that the outer rice bran contains vitamin B1, also known as thiamine.

From 1900 to the Present

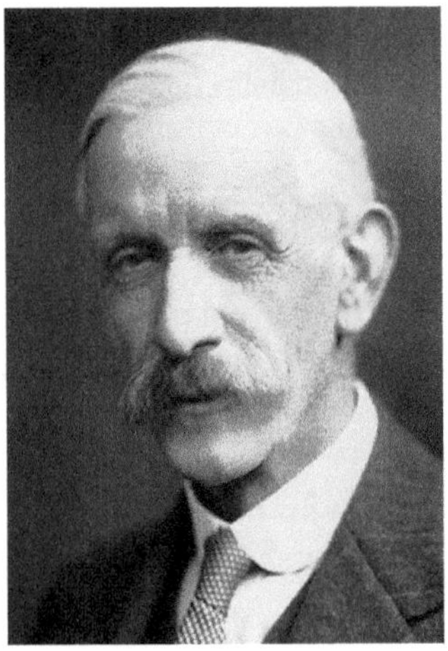

Frederick Hopkins discovered vitamins, for which he shared a Nobel prize with Eijkman.

In the early 20th century, Carl von Voit and Max Rubner independently measured caloric energy expenditure in different species of animals, applying principles of physics in nutrition. In 1906, Edith G. Willcock and Frederick Hopkins showed that the amino acid tryptophan aids the well-being of mice but it did not assure their growth. In the middle of twelve years of attempts to isolate them, Hopkins said in a 1906 lecture that "unsuspected dietetic factors," other than calories, protein, and minerals, are needed to prevent deficiency diseases. In 1907, Stephen M. Babcock and Edwin B. Hart conducted the single-grain experiment, which took nearly four years to complete.

Vitamin	Year Isolated
Thiamin	1926
Vitamin C	1926
Vitamin A	1939
Vitamin D	1931
Vitamin E	1936
Niacin	1937
Biotin	1939
Vitamin K	1939
Pantothenic acid	1939
Folate	1939
Riboflavin	1933
Vitamin B6	1936

Oxford University closed down its nutrition department after World War II because the subject seemed to have been completed between 1912 and 1944.

In 1912, Casimir Funk coined the term vitamin, a vital factor in the diet, from the words "vital" and "amine," because these unknown substances preventing scurvy, beriberi, and pellagra, were thought then to be derived from ammonia. The vitamins were studied in the first half of the 20th century.

In 1913, Elmer McCollum and Marguerite Davis discovered the first vitamin, fat-soluble vitamin A, then water-soluble vitamin B (in 1915; now known to be a complex of several water-soluble vitamins) and named vitamin C as the then-unknown substance preventing scurvy. Lafayette Mendel and Thomas Osborne also performed pioneering work on vitamins A and B. In 1919, Sir Edward Mellanby incorrectly identified rickets as a vitamin A deficiency because he could cure it in dogs with cod liver oil. In 1922, McCollum destroyed the vitamin A in cod liver oil, but found that it still cured rickets. Also in 1922, H.M. Evans and L.S. Bishop discover vitamin E as essential for rat pregnancy, originally calling it "food factor X" until 1925.

In 1925, Hart discovered that trace amounts of copper are necessary for iron absorption. In 1927, Adolf Otto Reinhold Windaus synthesized vitamin D, and was awarded the Nobel Prize in Chemistry in 1928. In 1928, Albert Szent-Györgyi isolated ascorbic acid, and in 1932 proved that it is vitamin C by preventing scurvy. In 1935, he synthesized it, and in 1937, he won a Nobel Prize for his efforts. Szent-Györgyi concurrently elucidated much of the citric acid cycle.

In the 1930s, William Cumming Rose identified essential amino acids, necessary protein components that the body cannot synthesize. In 1935, Underwood and Marston independently discovered the necessity of cobalt. In 1936, Eugene Floyd DuBois showed that work and school performance are related to caloric intake. In 1938, Erhard Fernholz discovered the chemical structure of vitamin E and then he tragically disappeared. It was synthesised the same year by Paul Karrer.

In 1940, rationing in the United Kingdom during and after World War II took place according to nutritional principles drawn up by Elsie Widdowson and others. In 1941, the first Recommended Dietary Allowances (RDAs) were established by the National Research Council.

In 1992, The U.S. Department of Agriculture introduced the Food Guide Pyramid. In 2002, a Natural Justice study showed a relation between nutrition and violent behavior. In 2005, one inconclusive study found that obesity could be caused by adenovirus in addition to bad nutrition.

World leaders are looking at alternatives like genetically modified foods to tackle the problem of world hunger and food shortages.

Nutrients

The list of nutrients that people are known to require is, in the words of Marion Nestle, "almost certainly incomplete". As of 2014, nutrients are thought to be of two types: macro-nutrients which are needed in relatively large amounts, and micronutrients which are needed in smaller quantities. A type of carbohydrate, dietary fiber, i.e. non-digestible material such as cellulose, is required, for both mechanical and biochemical reasons, although the exact reasons remain unclear. Other micronutrients include antioxidants and phytochemicals, which are said to influence (or protect) some body systems. Their necessity is not as well established as in the case of, for instance, vitamins.

Most foods contain a mix of some or all of the nutrient types, together with other substances, such as toxins of various sorts. Some nutrients can be stored internally (e.g., the fat-soluble vitamins), while others are required more or less continuously. Poor health can be caused by a lack of required nutrients or, in extreme cases, too much of a required nutrient. For example, both salt and water (both absolutely required) will cause illness or even death in excessive amounts.

Macronutrients

The macronutrients are carbohydrates, fiber, fats, protein, and water. The macronutrients (excluding fiber and water) provide structural material (amino acids from which proteins are built, and lipids from which cell membranes and some signaling molecules are built) and energy. Some of the structural material can be used to generate energy internally, and in either case it is measured in Joules or kilocalories (often called "Calories" and written with a capital *C* to distinguish them from little 'c' calories). Carbohydrates and proteins provide 17 kJ approximately (4 kcal) of energy per gram, while fats provide 37 kJ (9 kcal) per gram, though the net energy from either depends on such factors as absorption and digestive effort, which vary substantially from instance to instance. Vitamins, minerals, fiber, and water do not provide energy, but are required for other reasons.

Molecules of carbohydrates and fats consist of carbon, hydrogen, and oxygen atoms. Carbohydrates range from simple monosaccharides (glucose, fructose, galactose) to complex polysaccharides (starch). Fats are triglycerides, made of assorted fatty acid monomers bound to a glycerol backbone. Some fatty acids, but not all, are essential in the diet: they cannot be synthesized in the body. Protein molecules contain nitrogen atoms in addition to carbon, oxygen, and hydrogen. The fundamental components of protein are nitrogen-containing amino acids, some of which are essential in the sense that humans cannot make them internally. Some of the amino acids are convertible (with the expenditure of energy) to glucose and can be used for energy production, just as ordinary glucose, in a process known as gluconeogenesis. By breaking down existing protein, the carbon skeleton of the various amino acids can be metabolized to intermediates in cellular respiration; the remaining ammonia is discarded primarily as urea in urine. This occurs normally only during prolonged starvation.

Carbohydrates

Carbohydrates may be classified as monosaccharides, disaccharides, or polysaccharides depending on the number of monomer (sugar) units they contain. They constitute a large part of foods such as rice, noodles, bread, and other grain-based products. Monosaccharides, disaccharides, and polysaccharides contain one, two, and three or more sugar units, respectively. Polysaccharides are often referred to as *complex* carbohydrates because they are typically long, multiple branched chains of sugar units.

Traditionally, simple carbohydrates are believed to be absorbed quickly, and therefore to raise blood-glucose levels more rapidly than complex carbohydrates. This, however, is not accurate. Some simple carbohydrates (e.g., fructose) follow different metabolic pathways (e.g., fructolysis) that result in only a partial catabolism to glucose, while, in essence, many complex carbohydrates may be digested at the same rate as simple carbohydrates. Glucose stimulates the production of insulin through food entering the bloodstream, which is grasped by the beta cells in the pancreas.

Fiber

Dietary fiber is a carbohydrate that is incompletely absorbed in humans and in some animals. Like all carbohydrates, when it is metabolized it can produce four Calories (kilocalories) of energy per gram. However, in most circumstances it accounts for less than that because of its limited absorption and digestibility. Dietary fiber consists mainly of cellulose, a large carbohydrate polymer which is indigestible as humans do not have the required enzymes to disassemble it. There are two subcategories: soluble and insoluble fiber. Whole grains, fruits (especially plums, prunes, and figs), and vegetables are good sources of dietary fiber. There are many health benefits of a high-fiber diet. Dietary fiber helps reduce the chance of gastrointestinal problems such as constipation and diarrhea by increasing the weight and size of stool and softening it. Insoluble fiber, found in whole wheat flour, nuts and vegetables, especially stimulates peristalsis – the rhythmic muscular contractions of the intestines, which move digesta along the digestive tract. Soluble fiber, found in oats, peas, beans, and many fruits, dissolves in water in the intestinal tract to produce a gel that slows the movement of food through the intestines. This may help lower blood glucose levels because it can slow the absorption of sugar. Additionally, fiber, perhaps especially that from whole grains, is thought to possibly help lessen insulin spikes, and therefore reduce the risk of type 2 diabetes. The link between increased fiber consumption and a decreased risk of colorectal cancer is still uncertain.

Fat

A molecule of dietary fat typically consists of several fatty acids (containing long chains of carbon and hydrogen atoms), bonded to a glycerol. They are typically found as triglycerides (three fatty acids attached to one glycerol backbone). Fats may be classified as saturated or unsaturated depending on the detailed structure of the fatty acids involved. Saturated fats have all of the carbon atoms in their fatty acid chains bonded to hydrogen atoms, whereas unsaturated fats have some of these carbon atoms double-bonded, so their molecules have relatively fewer hydrogen atoms than a saturated fatty acid of the same length. Unsaturated fats may be further classified as monounsaturated (one double-bond) or polyunsaturated (many double-bonds). Furthermore, depending on the location of the double-bond in the fatty acid chain, unsaturated fatty acids are classified as omega-3 or omega-6 fatty acids. Trans fats are a type of unsaturated fat with *trans*-isomer bonds; these are rare in nature and in foods from natural sources; they are typically created in an industrial process called (partial) hydrogenation. There are nine kilocalories in each gram of fat. Fatty acids such as conjugated linoleic acid, catalpic acid, eleostearic acid and punicic acid, in addition to providing energy, represent potent immune modulatory molecules.

Saturated fats (typically from animal sources) have been a staple in many world cultures for millennia. Unsaturated fats (e. g., vegetable oil) are considered healthier, while trans fats are to be avoided. Saturated and some trans fats are typically solid at room temperature (such as butter or lard), while unsaturated fats are typically liquids (such as olive oil or flaxseed oil). Trans fats are very rare in nature, and have been shown to be highly detrimental to human health, but have properties useful in the food processing industry, such as rancidity resistance.

Essential Fatty Acids

Most fatty acids are non-essential, meaning the body can produce them as needed, generally from other fatty acids and always by expending energy to do so. However, in humans, at least two fatty acids are essential and must be included in the diet. An appropriate balance of essential fatty acids—omega-3 and omega-6 fatty acids—seems also important for health, although definitive experimental demonstration has been elusive. Both of these "omega" long-chain polyunsaturated fatty acids are substrates for a class of eicosanoids known as prostaglandins, which have roles throughout the human body. They are hormones, in some respects. The omega-3 eicosapentaenoic acid (EPA), which can be made in the human body from the omega-3 essential fatty acid alpha-linolenic acid (ALA), or taken in through marine food sources, serves as a building block for series 3 prostaglandins (e.g., weakly inflammatory PGE3). The omega-6 dihomo-gamma-linolenic acid (DGLA) serves as a building block for series 1 prostaglandins (e.g. anti-inflammatory PGE1), whereas arachidonic acid (AA) serves as a building block for series 2 prostaglandins (e.g. pro-inflammatory PGE 2). Both DGLA and AA can be made from the omega-6 linoleic acid (LA) in the human body, or can be taken in directly through food. An appropriately balanced intake of omega-3 and omega-6 partly determines the relative production of different prostaglandins, which is one reason why a balance between omega-3 and omega-6 is believed important for cardiovascular health. In industrialized societies, people typically consume large amounts of processed vegetable oils, which have reduced amounts of the essential fatty acids along with too much of omega-6 fatty acids relative to omega-3 fatty acids.

The conversion rate of omega-6 DGLA to AA largely determines the production of the prostaglandins PGE1 and PGE2. Omega-3 EPA prevents AA from being released from membranes, thereby skewing prostaglandin balance away from pro-inflammatory PGE2 (made from AA) toward anti-inflammatory PGE1 (made from DGLA). Moreover, the conversion (desaturation) of DGLA to AA is controlled by the enzyme delta-5-desaturase, which in turn is controlled by hormones such as insulin (up-regulation) and glucagon (down-regulation). The amount and type of carbohydrates consumed, along with some types of amino acid, can influence processes involving insulin, glucagon, and other hormones; therefore, the ratio of omega-3 versus omega-6 has wide effects on general health, and specific effects on immune function and inflammation, and mitosis (i.e., cell division).

Protein

Proteins are structural materials in much of the animal body (e.g. muscles, skin, and hair). They also form the enzymes that control chemical reactions throughout the body.

Each protein molecule is composed of amino acids, which are characterized by inclusion of nitrogen and sometimes sulphur (these components are responsible for the distinctive smell of burning protein, such as the keratin in hair). The body requires amino acids to produce new proteins (protein retention) and to replace damaged proteins (maintenance). As there is no protein or amino acid storage provision, amino acids must be present in the diet. Excess amino acids are discarded, typically in the urine. For all animals, some amino acids are *essential* (an animal cannot produce them internally) and some are *non-essential* (the animal can produce them from other nitrogen-containing compounds). About twenty amino acids are found in the human body, and about ten of these are essential and, therefore, must be included in the diet. A diet that contains adequate amounts of amino acids (especially those that are essential) is particularly important in some situations: during early development and maturation, pregnancy, lactation, or injury (a burn, for instance). A *complete* protein source contains all the essential amino acids; an *incomplete* protein source lacks one or more of the essential amino acids.

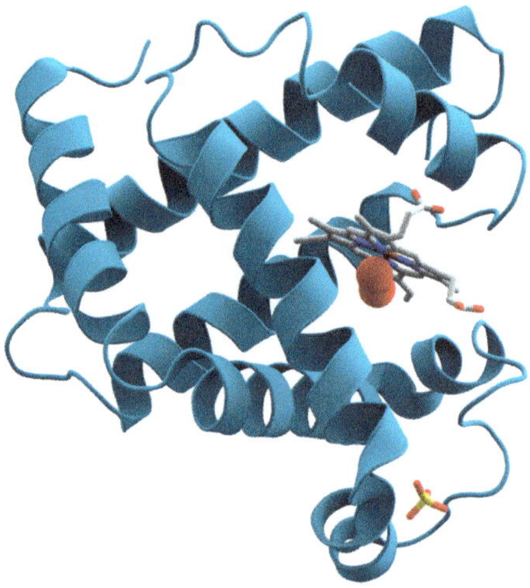

Proteins are chains of amino acids found in most nutritional foods.

It is possible with protein combinations of two incomplete protein sources (e.g., rice and beans) to make a complete protein source, and characteristic combinations are the basis of distinct cultural cooking traditions. However, complementary sources of protein do not need to be eaten at the same meal to be used together by the body. Excess amino acids from protein can be converted into glucose and used for fuel through a process called gluconeogenesis. The amino acids remaining after such conversion are discarded.

Water

Water is excreted from the body in multiple forms; including urine and feces, sweating, and by water vapour in the exhaled breath. Therefore, it is necessary to adequately rehydrate to replace lost fluids.

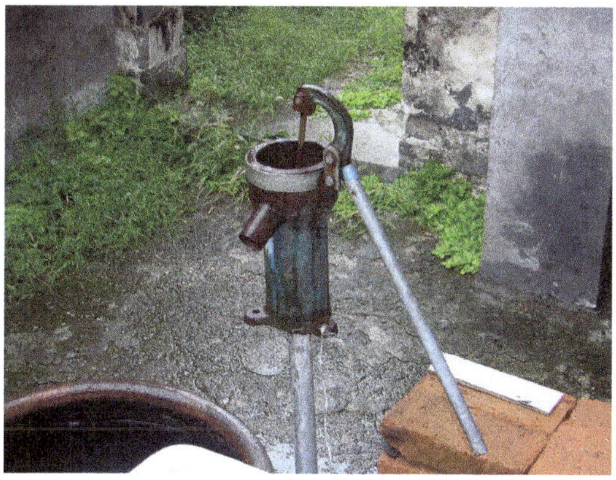

A manual water pump in China

Early recommendations for the quantity of water required for maintenance of good health suggested that 6–8 glasses of water daily is the minimum to maintain proper hydration. However the notion that a person should consume eight glasses of water per day cannot be traced to a credible scientific source. The original water intake recommendation in 1945 by the Food and Nutrition Board of the National Research Council read: "An ordinary standard for diverse persons is 1 milliliter for each calorie of food. Most of this quantity is contained in prepared foods." More recent comparisons of well-known recommendations on fluid intake have revealed large discrepancies in the volumes of water we need to consume for good health. Therefore, to help standardize guidelines, recommendations for water consumption are included in two recent European Food Safety Authority (EFSA) documents (2010): (i) Food-based dietary guidelines and (ii) Dietary reference values for water or adequate daily intakes (ADI). These specifications were provided by calculating adequate intakes from measured intakes in populations of individuals with "desirable osmolarity values of urine and desirable water volumes per energy unit consumed." For healthful hydration, the current EFSA guidelines recommend total water intakes of 2.0 L/day for adult females and 2.5 L/day for adult males. These reference values include water from drinking water, other beverages, and from food. About 80% of our daily water requirement comes from the beverages we drink, with the remaining 20% coming from food. Water content varies depending on the type of food consumed, with fruit and vegetables containing more than cereals, for example. These values are estimated using country-specific food balance sheets published by the Food and Agriculture Organisation of the United Nations. Other guidelines for nutrition also have implications for the beverages we consume for healthy hydration- for example, the World Health Organization (WHO) recommend that added sugars should represent no more than 10% of total energy intake.

The EFSA panel also determined intakes for different populations. Recommended intake volumes in the elderly are the same as for adults as despite lower energy consumption, the water requirement of this group is increased due to a reduction in renal concentrating capacity. Pregnant and breastfeeding women require additional fluids to stay hydrated. The EFSA panel proposes that pregnant women should consume the same volume of water as non-pregnant women, plus an increase in proportion to the higher energy requirement, equal to 300 mL/day. To compensate for additional fluid output, breastfeeding women require an additional 700 mL/day above the recommended intake values for non-lactating women.

For those who have healthy kidneys, it is somewhat difficult to drink too much water, but (especially in warm humid weather and while exercising) it is dangerous to drink too little. While overhydration is much less common than dehydration, it is also possible to drink far more water than necessary, which can result in water intoxication, a serious and potentially fatal condition. In particular, large amounts of de-ionized water are dangerous.

Micronutrients

The micronutrients are minerals, vitamins, and others.

Minerals

Dietary minerals are inorganic chemical elements required by living organisms, other than the four elements carbon, hydrogen, nitrogen, and oxygen that are present in nearly all organic molecules. The term "mineral" is archaic, since the intent is to describe simply the less common elements in the diet. Some are heavier than the four just mentioned, including several metals, which often occur as ions in the body. Some dietitians recommend that these be supplied from foods in which they occur naturally, or at least as complex compounds, or sometimes even from natural inorganic sources (such as calcium carbonate from ground oyster shells). Some minerals are absorbed much more readily in the ionic forms found in such sources. On the other hand, minerals are often artificially added to the diet as supplements; the most famous is likely iodine in iodized salt which prevents goiter.

Macrominerals

Many elements are essential in relative quantity; they are usually called "bulk minerals". Some are structural, but many play a role as electrolytes. Elements with recommended dietary allowance (RDA) greater than 150 mg/day are, in alphabetical order (with informal or folk-medicine perspectives in parentheses):

- Calcium, a common electrolyte, but also needed structurally (for muscle and digestive system health, bone strength, some forms neutralize acidity, may help clear toxins, provides signaling ions for nerve and membrane functions)
- Chlorine as chloride ions; very common electrolyte
- Magnesium, required for processing ATP and related reactions (builds bone, causes strong peristalsis, increases flexibility, increases alkalinity)

- Phosphorus, required component of bones; essential for energy processing
- Potassium, a very common electrolyte (heart and nerve health)
- Sodium, a very common electrolyte; in general not found in dietary supplements, despite being needed in large quantities, because the ion is very common in food: typically as sodium chloride, or common salt. Excessive sodium consumption can deplete calcium and magnesium, leading to high blood pressure and osteoporosis
- Sulfur, for three essential amino acids and therefore many proteins (skin, hair, nails, liver, and pancreas). Sulfur is not consumed alone, but in the form of sulfur-containing amino acids

Trace Minerals

Many elements are required in trace amounts, usually because they play a catalytic role in enzymes. Some trace mineral elements (RDA < 200 mg/day) are, in alphabetical order:

- Cobalt required for biosynthesis of vitamin B12 family of coenzymes. Animals cannot biosynthesize B12, and must obtain this cobalt-containing vitamin in their diet
- Copper required component of many redox enzymes, including cytochrome c oxidase
- Chromium required for sugar metabolism
- Iodine required not only for the biosynthesis of thyroxine but also — it is presumed — for other important organs as breast, stomach, salivary glands, thymus, etc.; for this reason iodine is needed in larger quantities than others in this list, and sometimes classified with the macrominerals
- Iron required for many enzymes, and for hemoglobin and some other proteins
- Manganese (processing of oxygen)
- Molybdenum required for xanthine oxidase and related oxidases
- Selenium required for peroxidase (antioxidant proteins)
- Zinc required for several enzymes such as carboxypeptidase, liver alcohol dehydrogenase, and carbonic anhydrase

Vitamins

As with the minerals discussed above, some vitamins are recognized as organic essential nutrients, necessary in the diet for good health. (Vitamin D is the exception: it can be synthesized in the skin, in the presence of UVB radiation.) Certain vitamin-like compounds that are recommended in the diet, such as carnitine, are thought useful for survival and health, but these are not "essential" dietary nutrients because the human body has some capacity to produce them from other compounds. Moreover, thousands of different phytochemicals have recently been discovered in food (particularly in fresh vegetables), which may have desirable properties including antioxidant activity; however, experimental demonstration has been suggestive but inconclusive. Other essential nutrients that are not classified as vitamins include essential amino acids, choline, essential fatty acids, and the minerals.

Vitamin deficiencies may result in disease conditions, including goitre, scurvy, osteoporosis, impaired immune system, disorders of cell metabolism, certain forms of cancer, symptoms of premature aging, and poor psychological health (including eating disorders), among many others. Excess levels of some vitamins are also dangerous to health (notably vitamin A). Deficient or excess levels of minerals can also have serious health consequences.

Healthy Diets

Whole Plant Food Diet

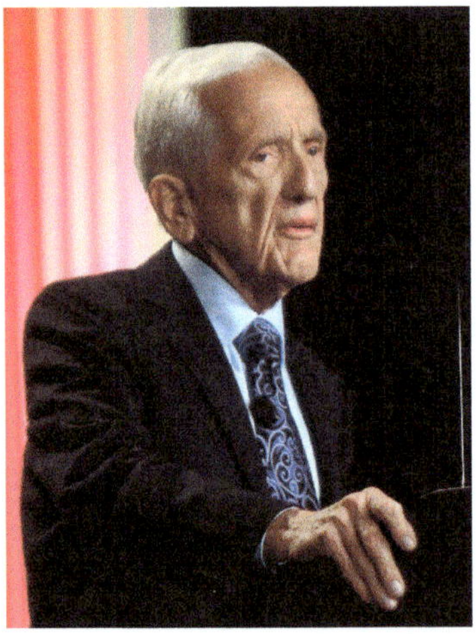

T. Colin Campbell is among the scientists who advocate a plant-based diet.

Heart disease, cancer, obesity, and diabetes are commonly called "Western" diseases because these maladies were once rarely seen in developing countries. An international study in China found some regions had virtually no cancer or heart disease, while in other areas they reflected "up to a 100-fold increase" coincident with shifts from diets that were found to be entirely plant-based to heavily animal-based, respectively. In contrast, diseases of affluence like cancer and heart disease are common throughout the developed world, including the United States. Adjusted for age and exercise, large regional clusters of people in China rarely suffered from these "Western" diseases possibly because their diets are rich in vegetables, fruits, and whole grains, and have little dairy and meat products. There are arguments for and against this controversial issue.

In particular, the consumption of whole-plant foods slows digestion and allows better absorption, and a more favorable balance of essential nutrients per Calorie.

The United Healthcare/Pacificare nutrition guideline recommends a whole plant food diet, and recommends using protein only as a condiment with meals. A *National Geographic* cover article from November 2005, entitled *The Secrets of Living Longer*, also recommends a whole plant food diet. The article is a lifestyle survey of three populations, Sardinians, Okinawans, and Adventists, who generally display longevity and "suffer a fraction of the diseases that commonly kill people in other parts of the developed world, and enjoy more healthy years of life." In common with all three groups is to "Eat fruits, vegetables, and whole grains."

The French "Paradox"

The French paradox is the observation that the French suffer a relatively low incidence of coronary heart disease, despite having a diet relatively rich in saturated fats. A number of explanations have been suggested:

- Saturated fat consumption does not cause heart disease.
- Reduced consumption of processed carbohydrate and other junk foods.
- Regular consumption of red wine.
- Higher consumption of artificially produced trans-fats by Americans, which has been shown to have greater lipoprotein effects per gram than saturated fat.

However, statistics collected by the World Health Organization from 1990–2000 show that the incidence of heart disease in France may have been underestimated and, in fact, may be similar to that of neighboring countries.

Phytochemicals

Phytochemicals such as polyphenols are compounds produced naturally in plants (phyto means "plant" in Greek). In general, the term is used to refer to those chemicals under research to assess whether they have biological significance. To date, there is no evidence in humans that polyphenols or other non-nutrient compounds from plants have health effects. Further, dietary supplements containing phytochemicals also have no proven health benefit.

While initial studies sought to reveal if antioxidant or phytochemical supplements might promote health, later large clinical trials did not detect any benefit and showed instead that excess supplementation could be harmful.

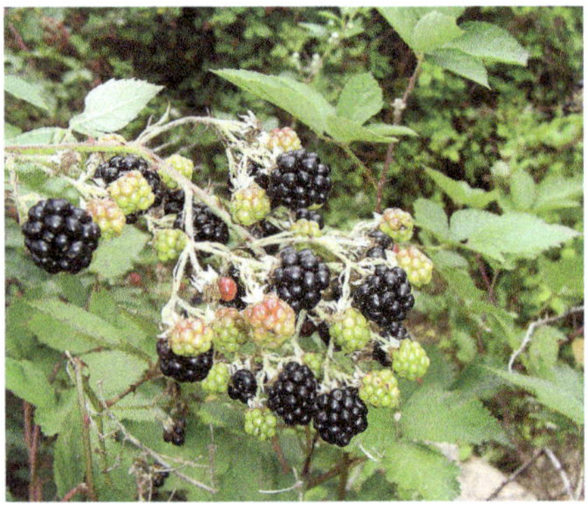

Blackberries are a source of polyphenols.

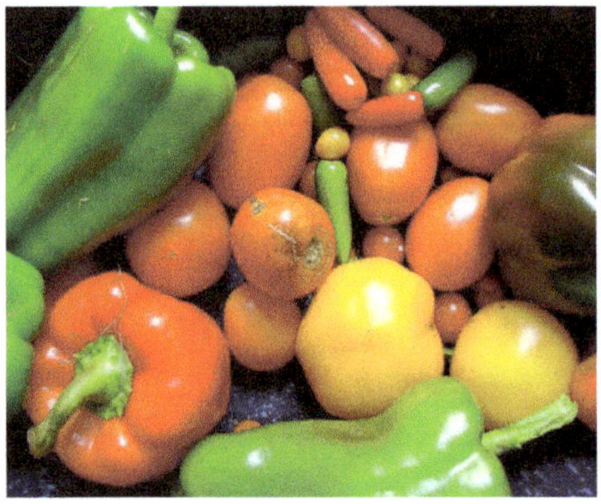

Colorful fruits and vegetables can be components of a healthy diet.

Intestinal Bacterial Flora

Animal intestines contain a large population of gut flora. In humans, the four dominant phyla are Firmicutes, Bacteroidetes, Actinobacteria, and Proteobacteria. They are essential to digestion and are also affected by food that is consumed. Bacteria in the gut perform many important functions for humans, including breaking down and aiding in the absorption of otherwise indigestible food; stimulating cell growth; repressing the growth of harmful bacteria, training the immune system to respond only to pathogens; producing vitamin B_{12}; and defending against some infectious diseases.

Animal Nutrition

Carnivore and herbivore diets are contrasting, with basic nitrogen and carbon proportions vary for their particular foods. Many herbivores rely on bacterial fermentation to create digestible nutrients from indigestible plant cellulose, while obligate carnivores must eat animal meats to obtain certain vitamins or nutrients their bodies cannot otherwise synthesize.

Plant Nutrition

Plant nutrition is the study of the chemical elements that are necessary for plant growth. There are several principles that apply to plant nutrition. Some elements are directly involved in plant metabolism. However, this principle does not account for the so-called beneficial elements, whose presence, while not required, has clear positive effects on plant growth.

A nutrient that is able to limit plant growth according to Liebig's law of the minimum is considered an essential plant nutrient if the plant cannot complete its full life cycle without it. There are 16 essential plant soil nutrients, besides the three major elemental nutrients carbon and oxygen that are obtained by photosynthetic plants from carbon dioxide in air, and hydrogen, which is obtained from water.

Plants uptake essential elements from the soil through their roots and from the air (consisting of mainly nitrogen and oxygen) through their leaves. Green plants obtain their carbohydrate supply from the carbon dioxide in the air by the process of photosynthesis. Carbon and oxygen are absorbed from the air, while other nutrients are absorbed from the soil. Nutrient uptake in the soil is achieved by cation exchange, wherein root hairs pump hydrogen ions (H^+) into the soil through proton pumps. These hydrogen ions displace cations attached to negatively charged soil particles so that the cations are available for uptake by the root. In the leaves, stomata open to take in carbon dioxide and expel oxygen. The carbon dioxide molecules are used as the carbon source in photosynthesis.

Although nitrogen is plentiful in the Earth's atmosphere, very few plants can use this directly. Most plants, therefore, require nitrogen compounds to be present in the soil in which they grow. This is made possible by the fact that largely inert atmospheric nitrogen is changed in a nitrogen fixation process to biologically usable forms in the soil by bacteria.

Plant nutrition is a difficult subject to understand completely, partially because of the variation between different plants and even between different species or individuals of a given clone. Elements present at low levels may cause deficiency symptoms, and toxicity is possible at levels that are too high. Furthermore, deficiency of one element may present as symptoms of toxicity from another element, and vice versa.

Environmental Nutrition

Research in the field of nutrition has greatly contributed in finding out the essential facts about how environmental depletion can lead to crucial nutrition-related health problems like contamination, spread of contagious diseases, malnutrition, etc. Moreover, environmental contamination due to discharge of agricultural as well as industrial chemicals like organocholrines, heavy metal, and radionucleotides may adversely affect the human and the ecosystem as a whole. As far as safety of the human health is concerned, then these environmental contaminants can reduce people's nutritional status and health. This could directly or indirectly cause drastic changes in their diet habits. Hence, food-based remedial as well as preventive strategies are essential to address global issues like hunger and malnutrition and to enable the susceptible people to adapt themselves to all these environmental as well as socio-economic alterations.

Advice and Guidance

Government Policies

Canada's Food Guide is another example government-run nutrition program. Produced by Health Canada, the guide advises food quantities, provides education on balanced nutrition, and promotes physical activity in accordance with government-mandated nutrient needs. Like other nutrition programs around the world, Canada's Food Guide divides nutrition into four main food groups: vegetables and fruit, grain products, milk and alternatives, and meat and alternatives. It is interesting to note that, unlike its American counterpart, the Canadian guide references and provides alternative to meat and dairy, which can be attributed to the growing vegan and vegetarian movements.

In the US, dietitians are registered (RD) or licensed (LD) with the Commission for Dietetic Registration and the American Dietetic Association, and are only able to use the title "dietitian," as described by the business and professions codes of each respective state, when they have met specific educational and experiential prerequisites and passed a national registration or licensure examination, respectively. In California, registered dietitians must abide by the *"Business and Professions Code of Section 2585-2586.8"*.Anyone may call themselves a nutritionist, including unqualified dietitians, as this term is unregulated. Some states, such as the State of Florida, have begun to include the title "nutritionist" in state licensure requirements. Most governments provide guidance on nutrition, and some also impose mandatory disclosure/labeling requirements for processed food manufacturers and restaurants to assist consumers in complying with such guidance.

In the US, nutritional standards and recommendations are established jointly by the US Department of Agriculture and US Department of Health and Human Services. Dietary and physical activity guidelines from the USDA are presented in the concept of MyPlate, which superseded the food pyramid, which replaced the Four Food Groups. The Senate committee currently responsible for oversight of the USDA is the *Agriculture, Nutrition and Forestry Committee*. Committee hearings are often televised on C-SPAN. The U.S. Department of Health and Human Services provides a sample week-long menu that fulfills the nutritional recommendations of the government.

Government Programs

Governmental organisations have been working on nutrition literacy interventions in non-primary health care settings to address the nutrition information problem in the U.S. Some programs include:

The Family Nutrition Program (FNP) is a free nutrition education program serving low-income adults around the U.S. This program is funded by the Food Nutrition Service's (FNS) branch of the United States Department of Agriculture (USDA) usually through a local state academic institution that runs the program. The FNP has developed a series of tools to help families participating in the Food Stamp Program stretch their food dollar and form healthful eating habits including nutrition education.

Expanded Food and Nutrition Education Program (ENFEP) is a unique program that currently operates in all 50 states and in American Samoa, Guam, Micronesia, Northern Marianas, Puerto Rico, and the Virgin Islands. It is designed to assist limited-resource audiences in acquiring the knowledge, skills, attitudes, and changed behavior necessary for nutritionally sound diets, and to contribute to their personal development and the improvement of the total family diet and nutritional well-being.

An example of a state initiative to promote nutrition literacy is Smart Bodies, a public-private partnership between the state's largest university system and largest health insurer, Louisiana State Agricultural Center and Blue Cross and Blue Shield of Louisiana Foundation. Launched in 2005, this program promotes lifelong healthful eating patterns and physically active lifestyles for children and their families. It is an interactive educational program designed to help prevent childhood obesity through classroom activities that teach children healthful eating habits and physical exercise.

Education

Nutrition is taught in schools in many countries. In England and Wales, the Personal and Social Education and Food Technology curricula include nutrition, stressing the importance of a balanced diet and teaching how to read nutrition labels on packaging. In many schools, a Nutrition class will fall within the Family and Consumer Science or Health departments. In some American schools, students are required to take a certain number of FCS or Health related classes. Nutrition is offered at many schools, and, if it is not a class of its own, nutrition is included in other FCS or Health classes such as: Life Skills, Independent Living, Single Survival, Freshmen Connection, Health etc. In many Nutrition classes, students learn about the food groups, the food pyramid, Daily Recommended Allowances, calories, vitamins, minerals, malnutrition, physical activity, healthful food choices, portion sizes, and how to live a healthy life.

A 1985, US National Research Council report entitled *Nutrition Education in US Medical Schools* concluded that nutrition education in medical schools was inadequate. Only 20% of the schools surveyed taught nutrition as a separate, required course. A 2006 survey found that this number had risen to 30%. Membership by physicians in leading professional nutrition societies such as the American Society for Nutrition has generally declined from the 1990s.

Nutrition Literacy

At the time of this entry, we were not able to identify any specific nutrition literacy studies in the U.S. at a national level. However, the findings of the 2003 National Assessment of Adult Literacy (NAAL) provide a basis upon which to frame the nutrition literacy problem in the U.S. NAAL introduced the first ever measure of "the degree to which individuals have the capacity to obtain, process and understand basic health information and services needed to make appropriate health decisions" – an objective of Healthy People 2010 and of which nutrition literacy might be considered an important subset. On a scale of below basic, basic, intermediate and proficient, NAAL found 13 percent of adult Americans have proficient health literacy, 44% have intermediate literacy, 29 percent have basic literacy and 14 percent have below basic health literacy. The study found that health literacy increases with education and people living below the level of poverty have lower health literacy than those above it.

Another study examining the health and nutrition literacy status of residents of the lower Mississippi Delta found that 52 percent of participants had a high likelihood of limited literacy skills. While a precise comparison between the NAAL and Delta studies is difficult, primarily because of methodological differences, Zoellner et al. suggest that health literacy rates in the Mississippi Delta region are different from the U.S. general population and that they help establish the scope of the problem of health literacy among adults in the Delta region. For example, only 12 percent of study participants identified the My Pyramid graphic two years after it had been launched by the USDA. The study also found significant relationships between nutrition literacy and income level and nutrition literacy and educational attainment further delineating priorities for the region.

These statistics point to the complexities surrounding the lack of health/nutrition literacy and reveal the degree to which they are embedded in the social structure and interconnected with other problems. Among these problems are the lack of information about food choices, a lack of understanding of nutritional information and its application to individual circumstances, limited or difficult access to healthful foods, and a range of cultural influences and socioeconomic constraints such as low levels of education and high levels of poverty that decrease opportunities for healthful eating and living.

The links between low health literacy and poor health outcomes has been widely documented and there is evidence that some interventions to improve health literacy have produced successful results in the primary care setting. More must be done to further our understanding of nutrition literacy specific interventions in non-primary care settings in order to achieve better health outcomes.

Malnutrition

Malnutrition refers to insufficient, excessive, or imbalanced consumption of nutrients by an organism. In developed countries, the diseases of malnutrition are most often associated with nutritional imbalances or excessive consumption. In developing countries, malnutrition is more likely to be caused by poor access to a range of nutritious foods or inadequate knowledge. In Mali the International Crops Research Institute for the Semi-Arid Tropics (ICRISAT) and the Aga Khan Foundation, trained women's groups to make *equinut*, a healthy and nutritional version of the traditional recipe *di-dègué* (comprising peanut paste, honey and millet or rice flour). The aim was to boost nutrition and livelihoods by producing a product that women could make and sell, and which would be accepted by the local community because of its local heritage.

Although there are more organisms in the world who are malnourished due to insufficient consumption, increasingly more organisms suffer from excessive over-nutrition; a problem caused by an over abundance of sustenance coupled with the instinctual desire (by animals in particular) to consume all that it can.

Nutritionism is the view that excessive reliance on food science and the study of nutrition can lead to poor nutrition and to ill health. It was originally credited to Gyorgy Scrinis, and was popularized by Michael Pollan. Since nutrients are invisible, policy makers rely on nutrition experts to advise on food choices. Because science has an incomplete understanding of how food affects the human body, Pollan argues, nutritionism can be blamed for many of the health problems relating to diet in the Western World today.

Insufficient

In general, *under-consumption* refers to the long-term consumption of insufficient sustenance in relation to the energy that an organism expends or expels, leading to poor health.

Excessive

In general, *over-consumption* refers to the long-term consumption of excess sustenance in relation to the energy that an organism expends or expels, leading to poor health and, in animals, obesity. It can cause excessive hair loss, brittle nails, and irregular premenstrual cycles for females.

Unbalanced

When too much of one or more nutrients is present in the diet to the exclusion of the proper amount of other nutrients, the diet is said to be unbalanced.

Illnesses Caused by Improper Nutrient Consumption

Nutrients	Deficiency	Excess
Macronutrients		
Calories	Starvation, marasmus	Obesity, diabetes mellitus, cardiovascular disease
Simple carbohydrates	Low energy levels.	Obesity, diabetes mellitus, cardiovascular disease
Complex carbohydrates	Micronutrient deficiency	Obesity, cardiovascular disease (high glycemic index foods)
Protein	Kwashiorkor	Rabbit starvation
Saturated fat	Low testosterone levels, vitamin deficiencies.	Obesity, cardiovascular disease

Trans fat	None	Obesity, cardiovascular disease
Unsaturated fat	Fat-soluble vitamin deficiency	Obesity, cardiovascular disease
Micronutrients		
Vitamin A	Xerophthalmia and night blindness	Hypervitaminosis A (cirrhosis, hair loss)
Vitamin B_1	Beri-Beri	?
Vitamin B_2	Skin and corneal lesions	?
Niacin	Pellagra	Dyspepsia, cardiac arrhythmias, birth defects
Vitamin B_{12}	Pernicious anemia	?
Vitamin C	Scurvy	Diarrhea causing dehydration
Vitamin D	Rickets	Hypervitaminosis D (dehydration, vomiting, constipation)
Vitamin E	Neurological disease	Hypervitaminosis E (anticoagulant: excessive bleeding)
Vitamin K	Hemorrhage	Liver damage
Omega-3 fats	Cardiovascular Disease	Bleeding, Hemorrhages, Hemorrhagic stroke, reduced glycemic control among diabetics
Omega-6 fats	None	Cardiovascular Disease, Cancer
Cholesterol	None	Cardiovascular Disease
Macrominerals		
Calcium	Osteoporosis, tetany, carpopedal spasm, laryngospasm, cardiac arrhythmias	Fatigue, depression, confusion, nausea, vomiting, constipation, pancreatitis, increased urination, kidney stones
Magnesium	Hypertension	Weakness, nausea, vomiting, impaired breathing, and hypotension
Potassium	Hypokalemia, cardiac arrhythmias	Hyperkalemia, palpitations
Sodium	Hyponatremia	Hypernatremia, hypertension
Trace minerals		
Iron	Anemia	Cirrhosis, Hereditary hemochromatosis, heart disease
Iodine	Goiter, hypothyroidism	Iodine toxicity (goiter, hypothyroidism)

Mental Agility

Research indicates that improving the awareness of nutritious meal choices and establishing long-term habits of healthy eating have a positive effect on cognitive and spatial memory capacity, with potential to increase a student's ability to process and retain academic information.

Some organizations have begun working with teachers, policymakers, and managed foodservice contractors to mandate improved nutritional content and increased nutritional resources in school cafeterias from primary to university level institutions. Health and nutrition have been proven to have close links with overall educational success. Currently, less than 10% of American college students report that they eat the recommended five servings of fruit and vegetables daily. Better nutrition has been shown to affect both cognitive and spatial memory performance; a study showed those with higher blood sugar levels performed better on certain memory tests. In another study, those who consumed yogurt performed better on thinking tasks when compared to those that consumed caffeine-free diet soda or confections. Nutritional deficiencies have been shown to have a negative effect on learning behavior in mice as far back as 1951.

> "Better learning performance is associated with diet-induced effects on learning and memory ability".
>
> The "nutrition-learning nexus" demonstrates the correlation between diet and learning and has application in a higher education setting.
>
> "We find that better-nourished children perform significantly better in school, partly because they enter school earlier and thus have more time to learn but mostly because of greater learning productivity per year of schooling."
>
> 91% of college students feel that they are in good health, whereas only 7% eat their recommended daily allowance of fruits and vegetables.
>
> Nutritional education is an effective and workable model in a higher education setting.
>
> More "engaged" learning models that encompass nutrition is an idea that is picking up steam at all levels of the learning cycle.

There is limited research available that directly links a student's Grade Point Average (G.P.A.) to their overall nutritional health. Additional substantive data is needed to prove that overall intellectual health is closely linked to a person's diet, rather than just another correlation fallacy.

Mental Disorders

Nutritional supplement treatment may be appropriate for major depression, bipolar disorder, schizophrenia, and obsessive compulsive disorder, the four most common mental disorders in developed countries. Supplements that have been studied most for mood elevation and stabilization include eicosapentaenoic acid and docosahexaenoic acid (each of which an omega-3 fatty acid contained in fish oil but not in flaxseed oil), vitamin B12, folic acid, and inositol.

Cancer

Cancer is now common in developing countries. According to a study by the International Agency for Research on Cancer, "In the developing world, cancers of the liver, stomach and esophagus were more common, often linked to consumption of carcinogenic preserved foods, such as smoked or salted food, and parasitic infections that attack organs." Lung cancer rates are rising rapidly in poorer nations because of increased use of tobacco. Developed countries "tended to have cancers linked to affluence or a 'Western lifestyle' — cancers of the colon, rectum, breast and prostate — that can be caused by obesity, lack of exercise, diet and age."

Metabolic Syndrome

Several lines of evidence indicate lifestyle-induced hyperinsulinemia and reduced insulin function (i.e., insulin resistance) as a decisive factor in many disease states. For example, hyperinsulinemia and insulin resistance are strongly linked to chronic inflammation, which in turn is strongly linked to a variety of adverse developments such as arterial microinjuries and clot formation (i.e., heart disease) and exaggerated cell division (i.e., cancer). Hyperinsulinemia and insulin resistance (the so-called metabolic syndrome) are characterized by a combination of abdominal obesity, elevated blood sugar, elevated blood pressure, elevated blood triglycerides, and reduced HDL cholesterol. The negative effect of hyperinsulinemia on prostaglandin PGE1/PGE2 balance may be significant.

The state of obesity clearly contributes to insulin resistance, which in turn can cause type 2 diabetes. Virtually all obese and most type 2 diabetic individuals have marked insulin resistance. Although the association between overweight and insulin resistance is clear, the exact (likely multifarious) causes of insulin resistance remain less clear. It is important to note that it has been demonstrated that appropriate exercise, more regular food intake, and reducing glycemic load all can reverse insulin resistance in overweight individuals (and thereby lower blood sugar levels in those with type 2 diabetes).

Obesity can unfavourably alter hormonal and metabolic status via resistance to the hormone leptin, and a vicious cycle may occur in which insulin/leptin resistance and obesity aggravate one another. The vicious cycle is putatively fuelled by continuously high insulin/leptin stimulation and fat storage, as a result of high intake of strongly insulin/leptin stimulating foods and energy. Both insulin and leptin normally function as satiety signals to the hypothalamus in the brain; however, insulin/leptin resistance may reduce this signal and therefore allow continued overfeeding despite large body fat stores. In addition, reduced leptin signalling to the brain may reduce leptin's normal effect to maintain an appropriately high metabolic rate.

There is a debate about how and to what extent different dietary factors— such as intake of processed carbohydrates, total protein, fat, and carbohydrate intake, intake of saturated and trans fatty acids, and low intake of vitamins/minerals—contribute to the development of insulin and leptin resistance. In any case, analogous to the way modern man-made pollution may possess the potential to overwhelm the environment's ability to maintain homeostasis, the recent explosive introduction of high glycemic index and processed foods into the human diet may possess the potential to overwhelm the body's ability to maintain homeostasis and health (as evidenced by the metabolic syndrome epidemic).

Hyponatremia

Excess water intake, without replenishment of sodium and potassium salts, leads to hyponatremia, which can further lead to water intoxication at more dangerous levels. A well-publicized case occurred in 2007, when Jennifer Strange died while participating in a water-drinking contest. More usually, the condition occurs in long-distance endurance events (such as marathon or triathlon competition and training) and causes gradual mental dulling, headache, drowsiness, weakness, and confusion; extreme cases may result in coma, convulsions, and death. The primary damage comes from swelling of the brain, caused by increased osmosis as blood salinity decreases. Effective fluid replacement techniques include water aid stations during running/cycling races, trainers providing water during team games, such as soccer, and devices such as Camel Baks, which can provide water for a person without making it too hard to drink the water.

Antinutrient

Antinutrients are natural or synthetic compounds that interfere with the absorption of nutrients. Nutrition studies focus on antinutrients commonly found in food sources and beverages.

Sugar Consumption in The United States

The relatively recent increased consumption of sugar has been linked to the rise of some afflictions such as diabetes, obesity, and more recently heart disease. Increased consumption of sugar has been tied to these three, among others. Obesity levels have more than doubled in the last 30 years among adults, going from 15% to 35% in the United States. Obesity and diet also happen to be high risk factors for diabetes. In the same time span that obesity doubled, diabetes numbers quadrupled in America. Increased weight, especially in the form of belly fat, and high sugar intake are also high risk factors for heart disease. Both sugar intake and fatty tissue increase the probability of elevated LDL cholesterol in the bloodstream. Elevated amounts of Low-density lipoprotein (LDL) cholesterol, is the primary factor in heart disease. In order to avoid all the dangers of sugar, moderate consumption is paramount.

Processed Foods

Since the Industrial Revolution some two hundred years ago, the food processing industry has invented many technologies that both help keep foods fresh longer and alter the fresh state of food as they appear in nature. Cooling is the primary technology used to maintain freshness, whereas many more technologies have been invented to allow foods to last longer without becoming spoiled. These latter technologies include pasteurisation, autoclavation, drying, salting, and separation of various components, all of which appearing to alter the original nutritional contents of food. Pasteurisation and autoclavation (heating techniques) have no doubt improved the safety of many common foods, preventing epidemics of bacterial infection. But some of the (new) food processing technologies have downfalls as well.

Modern separation techniques such as milling, centrifugation, and pressing have enabled concentration of particular components of food, yielding flour, oils, juices, and so on, and even separate fatty acids, amino acids, vitamins, and minerals. Inevitably, such large-scale concentration changes the nutritional content of food, saving certain nutrients while removing others. Heating techniques may also reduce food's content of many heat-labile nutrients such as certain vitamins and phytochemicals, and possibly other yet-to-be-discovered substances. Because of reduced nutritional value, processed foods are often 'enriched' or 'fortified' with some of the most critical nutrients (usually certain vitamins) that were lost during processing. Nonetheless, processed foods tend to have an inferior nutritional profile compared to whole, fresh foods, regarding content of both sugar and high GI starches, potassium/sodium, vitamins, fiber, and of intact, unoxidized (essential) fatty acids. In addition, processed foods often contain potentially harmful substances such as oxidized fats and trans fatty acids.

A dramatic example of the effect of food processing on a population's health is the history of epidemics of beri-beri in people subsisting on polished rice. Removing the outer layer of rice by polishing it removes with it the essential vitamin thiamine, causing beri-beri. Another example is the development of scurvy among infants in the late 19th century in the United States. It turned out that the vast majority of sufferers were being fed milk that had been heat-treated (as suggested by Pasteur) to control bacterial disease. Pasteurisation was effective against bacteria, but it destroyed the vitamin C.

As mentioned, lifestyle- and obesity-related diseases are becoming increasingly prevalent all around the world. There is little doubt that the increasingly widespread application of some modern food processing technologies has contributed to this development. The food processing industry is a major part of modern economy, and as such it is influential in political decisions (e.g., nutritional recommendations, agricultural subsidising). In any known profit-driven economy, health considerations are hardly a priority; effective production of cheap foods with a long shelf-life is more the trend. In general, whole, fresh foods have a relatively short shelf-life and are less profitable to produce and sell than are more processed foods. Thus, the consumer is left with the choice between more expensive, but nutritionally superior, whole, fresh foods, and cheap, usually nutritionally inferior, processed foods. Because processed foods are often cheaper, more convenient (in both purchasing, storage, and preparation), and more available, the consumption of nutritionally inferior foods has been increasing throughout the world along with many nutrition-related health complications.

Healthy Diet

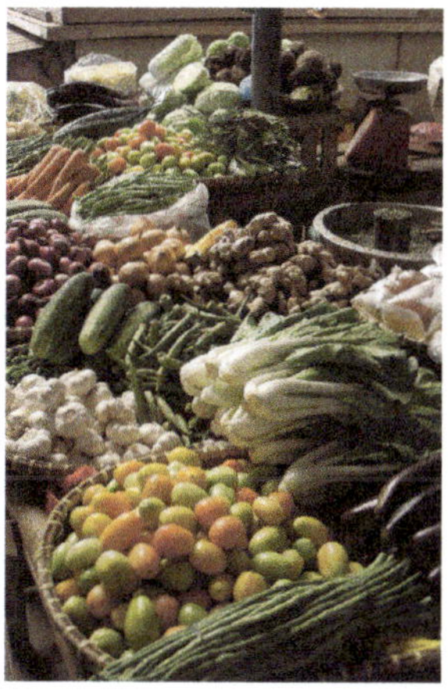

Leafy green, allium, and cruciferous vegetables are key components of a healthy diet.

A healthy diet is one that helps to maintain or improve overall health.

A healthy diet provides the body with essential nutrition: fluid, adequate essential amino acids from protein, essential fatty acids, vitamins, minerals, and adequate calories. The requirements for a healthy diet can be met from a variety of plant-based and animal-based foods. A healthy diet supports energy needs and provides for human nutrition without exposure to toxicity or excessive weight gain from consuming excessive amounts. Where lack of calories is not an issue, a properly balanced diet (in addition to exercise) is also thought to be important for lowering health risks, such as obesity, heart disease, type 2 diabetes, hypertension and cancer.

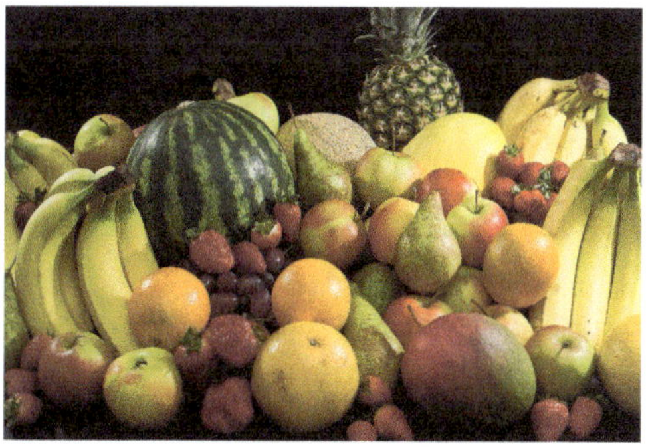

Common colorful culinary fruits. Apples, pears, strawberries, oranges, bananas, grapes, canary melons, watermelon, cantaloupe, pineapple and mango.

Various nutrition guides are published by medical and governmental institutions to educate the public on what they should be eating to promote health. Nutrition facts labels are also mandatory in some countries to allow consumers to choose between foods based on the components relevant to health.

The idea of dietary therapy (using dietary choices to maintain health and improve poor health) is quite old and thus has both modern scientific forms (medical nutrition therapy) and prescientific forms (such as dietary therapy in traditional Chinese medicine).

Mainstream Science

Healthy eating is simple, according to Marion Nestle, who expresses the mainstream view among scientists who study nutrition:

The basic principles of good diets are so simple that I can summarize them in just ten words: eat less, move more, eat lots of fruits and vegetables. For additional clarification, a five-word modifier helps: go easy on junk foods. Follow these precepts and you will go a long way toward preventing the major diseases of our overfed society—coronary heart disease, certain cancers, diabetes, stroke, osteoporosis, and a host of others. These precepts constitute the bottom line of what seem to be the far more complicated dietary recommendations of many health organizations and national and international governments—the forty-one "key recommendations" of the 2005 Dietary Guidelines, for example. Although you may feel as though advice about nutrition is constantly changing, the basic ideas behind my four precepts have not changed in half a century. And they leave plenty of room for enjoying the pleasures of food.

David L. Katz, who reviewed the most prevalent popular diets in 2014, noted:

The weight of evidence strongly supports a theme of healthful eating while allowing for variations on that theme. A diet of minimally processed foods close to nature, predominantly plants, is decisively associated with health promotion and disease prevention and is consistent with the salient components of seemingly distinct dietary approaches. Efforts to improve public health through diet are forestalled not for want of knowledge about the optimal feeding of Homo sapiens but for distractions associated with exaggerated claims, and our failure to convert what we reliably know into what we routinely do. Knowledge in this case is not, as of yet, power; would that it were so.

Recommendations

World Health Organization

The World Health Organization (WHO) makes the following 5 recommendations with respect to both populations and individuals:

- Eat roughly the same amount of calories that your body is using and maintain a healthy weight.
- Limit intake of fats, and prefer unsaturated fats to saturated fats and trans fats.
- Increase consumption of plant foods, particularly fruits, vegetables, legumes, whole grains and nuts.

- Limit the intake of sugar. A 2003 report recommends less than 10% of calorie intake from simple sugars.
- Limit salt / sodium consumption from all sources and ensure that salt is iodized.

Other recommendations include:

- Essential micronutrients such as vitamins and certain minerals.
- Avoiding directly poisonous (e.g. heavy metals) and carcinogenic (e.g. benzene) substances.
- Avoiding foods contaminated by human pathogens (e.g. *E. coli*, tapeworm eggs).

WHO recommends an intake of less than 5 grams of salt per day for the prevention of cardiovascular disease.

United States Department of Agriculture

The Dietary Guidelines for Americans by the United States Department of Agriculture (USDA) recommends three healthy patterns of diet, summarized in table below, for a 2000 kcal diet.

It emphasizes both health and environmental sustainability and a flexible approach: the committee that drafted it wrote: "The major findings regarding sustainable diets were that a diet higher in plant-based foods, such as vegetables, fruits, whole grains, legumes, nuts, and seeds, and lower in calories and animal-based foods is more health promoting and is associated with less environmental impact than is the current U.S. diet. This pattern of eating can be achieved through a variety of dietary patterns, including the "Healthy U.S.-style Pattern," the "Healthy Mediterranean-style Pattern," and the "Healthy Vegetarian Pattern". Food group amounts per day, unless noted per week.

Food group/subgroup (units)	Healthy US patterns	Healthy Vegetarian patterns	Healthy Med-style patterns
Fruits (cup eq)	2	2	2.5
Vegetables (cup eq)	2.5	2.5	2.5
Dark green	1.5/wk	1.5/wk	1.5/wk
Red/orange	5.5/wk	5.5/wk	5.5/wk
Starchy	5/wk	5/wk	5/wk
Legumes	1.5/wk	3/wk	1.5/wk
Others	4/wk	4/wk	4/wk
Grains (oz eq)	6	6.5	6
Whole	3	3.5	3
Refined	3	3	3

Dairy (cup eq)	3	3	2
Protein Foods (oz eq)	5.5	3.5	6.5
Meat (red and processed)	12.5/wk	--	12.5/wk
Poultry	10.5/wk	--	10.5/wk
Seafood	8/wk	--	15/wk
Eggs	3/wk	3/wk	3/wk
Nuts/seeds	4/wk	7/wk	4/wk
Processed Soy (including tofu)	0.5/wk	8/wk	0.5/wk
Oils (grams)	27	27	27
Solid fats limit (grams)	18	21	17
Added sugars limit (grams)	30	36	29

American Heart Association / World Cancer Research Fund / American Institute for Cancer Research

The American Heart Association, World Cancer Research Fund, and American Institute for Cancer Research recommends a diet that consists mostly of unprocessed plant foods, with emphasis a wide range of whole grains, legumes, and non-starchy vegetables and fruits. This healthy diet is full of a wide range of various non-starchy vegetables and fruits, that provide different colors including red, green, yellow, white, purple, and orange. They note that tomato cooked with oil, allium vegetables like garlic, and cruciferous vegetables like cauliflower, provide some protection against cancer. This healthy diet is low in energy density, which may protect against weight gain and associated diseases. Finally, limiting consumption of sugary drinks, limiting energy rich foods, including "fast foods" and red meat, and avoiding processed meats improves health and longevity. Overall, researchers and medical policy conclude that this healthy diet can reduce the risk of chronic disease and cancer.

In children less than 25 gms of added sugar (100 calories) is recommended per day. Other recommendations include no extra sugars in those under 2 years old and less than one soft drink per week.

Harvard School of Public Health

The Nutrition Source of Harvard School of Public Health makes the following 10 recommendations for a healthy diet:

- Choose good carbohydrates: whole grains (the less processed the better), vegetables, fruits and beans. Avoid white bread, white rice, and the like as well as pastries, sugared sodas, and other highly processed food.

- Pay attention to the protein package: good choices include fish, poultry, nuts, and beans. Try to avoid red meat.
- Choose foods containing healthy fats. Plant oils, nuts, and fish are the best choices. Limit consumption of saturated fats, and avoid foods with trans fat.
- Choose a fiber-filled diet which includes whole grains, vegetables, and fruits.
- Eat more vegetables and fruits—the more colorful and varied, the better.
- Calcium is important, but milk is not its best or only source. Good sources of calcium are collards, bok choy, fortified soy milk, baked beans, and supplements which contain calcium and vitamin D.
- Water is the best source of liquid. Avoid sugary drinks, and limit intake of juices and milk. Coffee, tea, artificially-sweetened drinks, 100-percent fruit juices, low-fat milk and alcohol can fit into a healthy diet but are best consumed in moderation. Sports drinks are recommended only for people who exercise more than an hour at a stretch to replace substances lost in sweat.
- Limit salt intake. Choose more fresh foods, instead of processed ones.
- Moderate alcohol drinking has health benefits, but is not recommended for everyone.
- Daily multivitamin and extra vitamin D intake has potential health benefits.

Other than nutrition, the guide recommends frequent physical exercise and maintaining a healthy body weight.

For Specific Conditions

In addition to dietary recommendations for the general population, there are many specific diets that have primarily been developed to promote better health in specific population groups, such as people with high blood pressure (as in low sodium diets or the more specific DASH diet), or people who are overweight or obese (in weight control diets). However, some of them may have more or less evidence for beneficial effects in normal people as well.

Hypertension

A low sodium diet is beneficial for people with high blood pressure. A Cochrane review published in 2008 concluded that a long term (more than 4 weeks) low sodium diet has a useful effect to reduce blood pressure, both in people with hypertension and in people with normal blood pressure.

The DASH diet (Dietary Approaches to Stop Hypertension) is a diet promoted by the National Heart, Lung, and Blood Institute (part of the NIH, a United States government organization) to control hypertension. A major feature of the plan is limiting intake of sodium, and it also generally encourages the consumption of nuts, whole grains, fish, poultry, fruits and vegetables while lowering the consumption of red meats, sweets, and sugar. It is also "rich in potassium, magnesium, and calcium, as well as protein".

The Mediterranean diet has also been shown to improve cardiovascular outcomes.

Obesity

Weight control diets aim to maintain a controlled weight. In most cases dieting is used in combination with physical exercise to lose weight in those who are overweight or obese.

Diets to promote weight loss are divided into four categories: low-fat, low-carbohydrate, low-calorie, and very low calorie. A meta-analysis of six randomized controlled trials found no difference between the main diet types (low calorie, low carbohydrate, and low fat), with a 2–4 kilogram weight loss in all studies. At two years, all calorie-reduced diet types cause equal weight loss irrespective of the macronutrients emphasized.

Reduced Disease Risk

There may be a relationship between lifestyle including food consumption and potentially lowering the risk of cancer or other chronic diseases. A diet high in fruits and vegetables appears to decrease the risk of cardiovascular disease and death but not cancer.

A healthy diet may consist mostly of whole plant foods, with limited consumption of energy dense foods, red meat, alcoholic drinks and salt while reducing consumption of sugary drinks, and processed meat. A healthy diet may contain non-starchy vegetables and fruits, including those with red, green, yellow, white, purple or orange pigments. Tomato cooked with oil, allium vegetables like garlic, and cruciferous vegetables like cauliflower "probably" contain compounds which are under research for their possible anti-cancer activity.

A healthy diet is low in energy density, lowering caloric content, thereby possibly inhibiting weight gain and lowering risk against chronic diseases. Chronic Western diseases are associated with pathologically increased IGF-1 levels. Findings in molecular biology and epidemiologic data suggest that milk consumption is a promoter of chronic diseases of Western nations, including atherosclerosis, carcinogenesis and neurodegenerative diseases.

Unhealthy Diets

The Western pattern diet which is typically eaten by Americans and increasingly adapted by people in the developing world as they leave poverty is unhealthy: it is "rich in red meat, dairy products, processed and artificially sweetened foods, and salt, with minimal intake of fruits, vegetables, fish, legumes, and whole grains."

An unhealthy diet is a major risk factor for a number of chronic diseases including: high blood pressure, diabetes, abnormal blood lipids, overweight/obesity, cardiovascular diseases, and cancer.

The WHO estimates that 2.7 million deaths are attributable to a diet low in fruits and vegetables every year. Globally it is estimated to cause about 19% of gastrointestinal cancer, 31% of ischaemic heart disease, and 11% of strokes, thus making it one of the leading preventable causes of death worldwide.

Popular Diets

Popular diets, often referred to as fad diets, make promises of weight loss or other health advantages such as longer life without backing by solid science, and in many cases are characterized by highly restrictive or unusual food choices. Celebrity endorsements (including celebrity doctors) are frequently associated with popular diets, and the individuals who develop and promote these programs often profit handsomely.

Public Health

Fears of high cholesterol were frequently voiced up until the mid-1990s. However, more recent research has shown that the distinction between high- and low-density lipoprotein ('good' and 'bad' cholesterol, respectively) must be addressed when speaking of the potential ill effects of cholesterol. Different types of dietary fat have different effects on blood levels of cholesterol. For example, polyunsaturated fats tend to decrease both types of cholesterol; monounsaturated fats tend to lower LDL and raise HDL; saturated fats tend to either raise HDL, or raise both HDL and LDL; and trans fat tend to raise LDL and lower HDL.

While dietary cholesterol is only found in animal products such as meat, eggs, and dairy, studies have not found a link between eating cholesterol and blood levels of cholesterol.

Vending machines in particular have come under fire as being avenues of entry into schools for junk food promoters. However, there is little in the way of regulation and it is difficult for most people to properly analyze the real merits of a company referring to itself as "healthy." Recently, the Committee of Advertising Practice in the United Kingdom launched a proposal to limit media advertising for food and soft drink products high in fat, salt or sugar. The British Heart Foundation released its own government-funded advertisements, labeled "Food4Thought", which were targeted at children and adults to discourage unhealthy habits of consuming junk food.

Cultural and Psychological Factors

From a psychological and cultural perspective, a healthier diet may be difficult to achieve for people with poor eating habits. This may be due to tastes acquired in childhood and preferences for sugary, salty and/or fatty foods.

Sports Nutrition

Sports nutrition is the study and practice of nutrition and diet with regards to improving one's athletic performance. Nutrition is an important part of many sports training regimens, being popular in strength sports (such as weightlifting and bodybuilding) and endurance sports (e.g. cycling, running, swimming, rowing). Sports Nutrition focuses its studies on the type, as well as the quantity of fluids and food taken by an athlete. In addition, it deals with the consumption of nutrients such as vitamins, minerals, supplements and organic substances that include carbohydrates, proteins and fats.

Supplements

Dietary supplements contain one or more dietary ingredients (including vitamins; minerals; amino acids; herbs or other botanicals; and other substances) or their constituents is intended to be taken by mouth as a pill, capsule, tablet, or liquid. Athletes may choose to consider taking dietary supplements to assist in improving their athletic performance. There are many other supplements out there that include performance enhancing supplements (steroids, blood doping, creatine, human growth hormone), energy supplements (caffeine), and supplements that aid in recovery (protein, BCAAs).

Performance Enhancing Supplements

In the extreme case of performance-enhancing supplements, athletes, particularly bodybuilders may choose to use illegal substances such as anabolic steroids. These compounds which are related to the hormone testosterone, can quickly build mass and strength, but have many adverse effects such as high blood pressure and negative gender specific effects. Blood doping, another illegal ergogenic, was discovered in the 1940's when it was used by World War II pilots. Blood doping also known as blood transfusions, increases oxygen delivery to exercising tissues and has been demonstrated to improve performance in endurance sports, such as long-distance cycling.

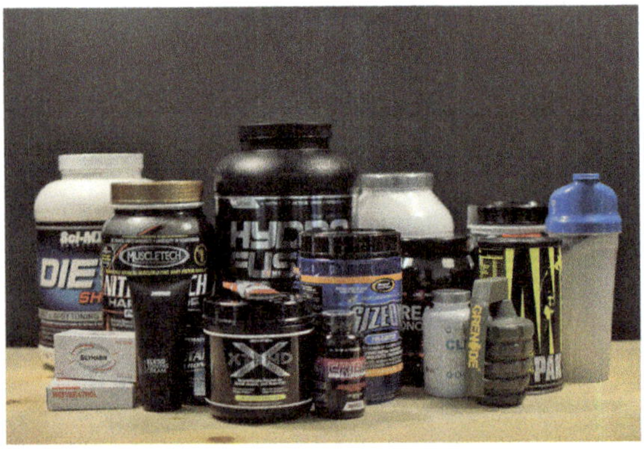

An assortment of supplements.

The supplement, Creatine, may be helpful for well-trained athletes to increase exercise performance and strength in relation with their dietary regimen. The substance glutamine, found in whey fiber supplements, is the most abundant free amino acid found in the human body. It is considered that glutamine may have a possible role in stimulated anabolic processes such as muscle glycogen and protein synthesis, for well-trained and well-nourished athletes. Other popular studies done on supplements include androstenedione, chromium, and ephedra. The findings show that there are no substantial benefits from the extra intake of these supplements, yet higher health risks and costs.

Energy Supplements

Athletes sometimes turn to energy supplements to increase their ability to exercise more often. Common supplements to increase an athlete's energy include: Caffeine, Guarana, Vitamin B12, and Asian ginseng. Caffeine, a common energy supplement, can be found in many different forms such as pills, tablets or capsules, and can also be found in common foods, such as coffee and tea. Caffeine is used to improve energy and increases metabolism. Guarana is another supplement that athletes take to enhance their athletic ability, it is frequently used for weight loss and as an energy supplement.

A 2009 study from the University of Texas reports that caffeinated energy drinks decrease sporting performance. They found that after drinking an energy drink, 83% of participants improved their physical activity parameters by an average of 4.7%. This was attributed to the effects of caffeine, sucrose and Vitamin B in the drink - however scientific consensus does not support the efficacy of using Vitamin B as a performance enhancer. To explain the performance improvement the writers report an increase in blood levels of epinephrine, norepinephrine and beta-Endorphin. The adenosine receptor antagonism of caffeine accounts for the first two, while the latter is accounted for by the Neurobiological effects of physical exercise.

Caffeine has been around since the 1900's and became popularly used in the 1970's when its power of masking fatigue became highly recognized. Similarly, the caffeine found in energy drinks and coffee shows an increased reaction performance and feelings of energy, focus and alertness in quickness and reaction anaerobic power tests. In other words, consuming an energy drink or any drink with caffeine increases short time/rapid exercise performance (like short full-speed sprints and heavy power weight lifting). Caffeine is chemically similar to adenosine, a type of sugar that helps in the regulation of important body processes, including the firing of neurotransmitters. Caffeine takes the place of adenosine in your brain, attaching itself to the same neural receptors affected by adenosine, and causing your neurons to fire more rapidly, hence caffeine's stimulating effects.

Recovery Supplements

Common supplements to help athletes recover from exercising, include protein and amino acid supplements. The main use for athletes to take dietary proteins are for hormones, oxygen transport, cellular repair, enzymes and conversion to fuel. The intake of protein is a part of the nutrient requirements for the normal athlete and is an important component of exercise training. In addition, it aids in performance and recovery. Dietary protein intake for well-trained athletes should occur before, during and after physical activity as it is advantageous in gaining muscle mass and strength. However, if too much protein and amino acid supplements is consumed it can be more harmful to the body than it is beneficial; health risks include: dehydration, gout, calcium loss, liver, renal damage, diarrhea, bloating, and water loss. A bountiful protein diet must be paired with a healthy, well-rounded meal plan and regular resistance exercise. Characteristics of this particular diet include the type of exercise, intensity, duration and carbohydrate values of diet. The most effective way to secure the natural nutrients required by your body for optimum health and physiological performance is by eating your vitamins, minerals, proteins, fats, sugars and carbohydrates, which can be procured from fresh fruits and vegetables.

Post-exercise nutrition is an important factor in a nutrition plan for athletes as it pertains to the recovery of the body. Traditionally, sports drinks such as Gatorade and Powerade, are consumed during and after exercise because they effectively rehydrate the body by refueling the body with minerals and electrolytes. Electrolytes regulate the bodies nerve and muscle function, blood pH, blood pressure, and the rebuilding of damaged tissue. These types of drink are commonly made of glucose and sucrose in water and has been seen to improve the football players' performance.

A substitute for sports drinks is milk, which contains many electrolytes, nutrients and other elements that help to make it an effective post-exercise beverage. It is true that milk helps replace fluids and electrolytes lost after the athlete has worked out. A recovery drink is supposed to replenish the sugar lost, and help recover the muscles to be able to workout at full intensity by the next time they workout. When compared to plain water or sports drinks, research suggests that chocolate milk is more effective at replacing fluids lost through sweat and maintaining normal body fluid levels. Athletes drinking chocolate milk following exercise-induced dehydration had fluid levels about 2 percent higher (on initial body mass) than those using other post-exercise recovery beverages. These results allowed for prolonged performance, especially in repeated bouts of exercise or training.

Factors Influencing Nutritional Requirements

Differing conditions and objectives suggest the need for athletes to ensure that their sports nutritional approach is appropriate for their situation. Factors that may affect an athlete's nutritional needs include type of activity (aerobic vs. anaerobic), gender, weight, height, body mass index, workout or activity stage (pre-workout, intro-workout, recovery), and time of day (e.g. some nutrients are utilized by the body more effectively during sleep than while awake).Most culprits that get in the way of performance are fatigue, injury and soreness. A proper diet will reduce these disturbances in performance. The key to a proper diet is to get a variety of food, and to consume all the macro-nutrients, vitamins, and minerals needed. According to Eblere's article (2008), it is ideal to choose raw foods, for example unprocessed foods such as oranges instead of orange juice. Eating foods that are natural means the athlete is getting the most nutritional value out of the food. When foods are processed, the nutritional value is normally reduced.

Anaerobic Exercise

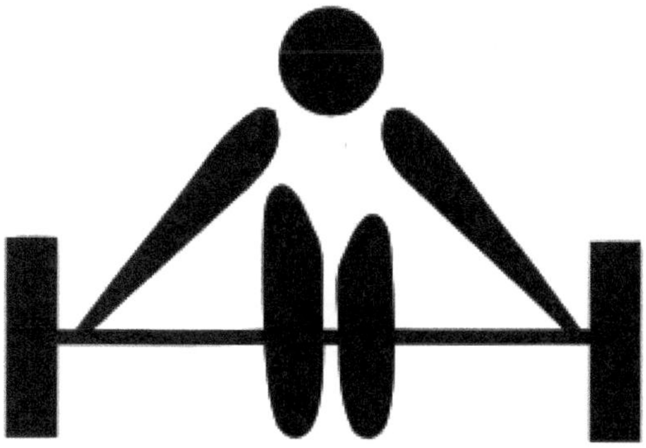

Weightlifting is an anaerobic exercise

During anaerobic exercise, the process of glycolysis breaks down the sugars from carbohydrates for energy without the use of oxygen. This type of exercise occurs in physical activity such as power sprints, strength resistances and quick explosive movement where the muscles are being used for power and speed, with short-time energy use. After this type of exercise, there is a need to refill glycogen storage sites in the body (the long simple sugar chains in the body that store energy), although they are not likely fully depleted.

To compensate for this glycogen reduction, athletes will often take in large amounts of carbohydrates, immediately following their exercise. Typically, high-glycemic-index carbohydrates are preferred for their ability to rapidly raise blood glucose levels.For the purpose of protein synthesis, protein or individual amino acids are ingested as well. Branched-chain amino acids are important since they are most responsible for the synthesis of protein. According to Lemon et al. (1995) female endurance runners have the hardest time getting enough protein in their diet. Endurance athletes in general need more protein in their diet than the sedentary person.Research has shown that endurance athletes are recommended to have 1.2 to 1.4 g of protein per kg of body weight in order to repair damaged tissue. If the athlete consumes too few calories for the body's needs, lean tissue will be broken down for energy and repair. Protein deficiency can cause many problems such as early and extreme fatigue, particularly long recovery, and poor wound healing. Complete proteins such as meat, eggs, and soy provide the athlete with all essential amino acids for synthesizing new tissues. However, vegetarian and vegan athletes frequently combine legumes with a whole grain to provide the body with a complete protein across the day's food intake. A popular combination being rice and beans.

Spada's research on endurance sports nutrition (2000) and where the types of carbohydrates come from will be explained. He advises for carbohydrates to be unprocessed and/or whole grains for optimal performance while training. These carbohydrates offer the most fuel, nutritional value, and satiety. Fruits and vegetables contribute important carbohydrate foundation for an athlete's diet. They provide vitamins and minerals that are lost through exercise and later needed to be replenished. Both fruits and vegetables improve healing, aid in recovery, and reduce risks of cancer, high blood pressure, and constipation. Vegetables offer a little more nutritional value than fruits for the amount of calories, therefore an athlete should strive to eat more vegetables than fruits. Dark-colored vegetables usually have more nutritional value than pale colored ones.(add info) A general rule is the darker the color the more nutrient dense it is. Like all foods, it is very important to have a variety. To get the most nutritional value out of fruits and vegetables it is important to eat them in their natural, unprocessed form with no other nutrient (sugar) added.

Often in the continuation of this anaerobic exercise, the product from this metabolic mechanism builds up in what is called lactic acid fermentation. Lactate is produced more quickly than it is being removed and it serves to regenerate NAD^+ cells on where it's needed. During intense exercise when oxygen is not being used, a high amount of ATP is produced and pH levels fall causing acidosis or more specifically lactic acidosis. Lactic acid build up can be treated by staying well-hydrated throughout and especially after the workout, having an efficient cool down routine and good post-workout stretching.

Intense activity can cause significant and permanent damage to bodily tissues. In order to repair, vitamin E and other antioxidants are needed to protect muscle damage. Oxidation damage and muscle tissue breakdown happens during endurance running so athletes need to eat foods high in protein in order to repair these muscle tissues. It is important for female endurance runners to consume proper nutrients in their diet that will repair, fuel, and minimize fatigue and injury. To keep a female runner's body performing at its best, the ten nutrients need to be included in their diets.

Prenatal Nutrition

Nutrition and weight management before and during pregnancy has a profound effect on the development of infants. This is a rather critical time for healthy fetal development as infants rely heavily on maternal stores and nutrient for optimal growth and health outcome later in life. Prenatal nutrition addresses nutrient recommendations before and during pregnancy. Prenatal nutrition has a strong influence on birth weight and further development of the infant.There was a study at the National Institution of Health were they found out that babies born from an obese mother, have a higher probability to fail tests of fine motor skills which is the movement of small muscles such as the hands and fingers.

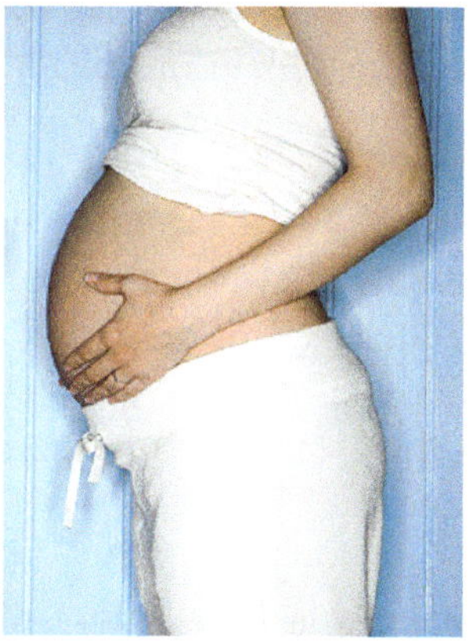

Pregnancy

A common saying that 'a woman is eating for two while pregnant' implies that a mother should consume twice as much during pregnancy. However, in reality this is not true. Although maternal consumption will directly affect both herself and the growing fetus, over eating excessively will compromise the baby's health as the infant will have to work extra hard to become healthy in the future. Compared with the infant, the mother possesses the least biological risk. Therefore, excessive calories, rather than going to the infant, often get stored as fat in the mother. On the other hand, insufficient consumption will result in lower birth weight.

Maintaining a healthy weight during gestation lowers adverse risks on infants such as birth defects, as well as chronic conditions in adulthood such as obesity, diabetes, and cardiovascular disease (CVD). Ideally, the rate of weight gain should be monitored during pregnancy to support the most ideal infant development.

Background

Barker's Hypothesis – Influences of Birth Weight on Health in Later Life

The "Barker Hypothesis", or Thrifty phenotype, states that conditions during pregnancy will have long-term effects on adult health. Associated risk of lifelong diseases includes cardiovascular disease, type-2 diabetes, obesity, and hypertension. Babies born lighter in weight appear to have an increased rate of mortality than babies born at a heavier weight. This does not mean that heavy babies are less of a concern. Death rate would rise as birth weight increases beyond normal birth weight range. Therefore, it is important to maintain a healthy gestational weight gain throughout pregnancy for achieving the optimal infant birth weight.

When this theory was first proposed, it was not well accepted and was met with much skepticism. The main criticism was that confounding variables such as environmental factors could attribute to many of the chronic diseases such that low birth weight alone should not be dictated as an independent risk factor. Subsequent research studies supporting the theory attempted to adjust these environmental factors and in turn, provided more convincing results with minimal confounding variables.

"Barker's Hypothesis" is also known as "Fetal Programming Hypothesis". The word "programming" illustrates the idea that during critical periods in early fetal development, there are persisting changes in the body structure and function that are caused by environmental stimuli. This relates to the concept of developmental plasticity where our genes can express different ranges of physiological or morphological states in response to the environmental conditions during fetal development.

If the mother has an inadequate diet then it signals the baby that the living condition in the long term will be impoverished. Consequently, the baby adapts by changing its body size and metabolism to prepare for harsh conditions of food shortages after birth. Physiological and metabolic processes in the body undergo long-term changes as a result of restricted growth. When the living environment switches from the condition of malnutrition to a society of abundant supply of nutrients, this exposes the baby to a bountiful environment that goes against what its body is designed for and this places the baby at a higher risk of adult diseases later in adulthood. By the same token, if the fetus growing in the womb of a healthy mother is exposed to prolonged famine after birth, the infant would be less adaptive to the harsh environment than low-birth-weight babies.

Pedersen's hypothesis – Influences of Maternal Glucose Concentration on Fetal Growth

In 1952 the Danish physician Jørgen Pedersen of the University of Copenhagen, formulated the hypothesis that maternal hyperglycemia during pregnancy might cause fetal hyperglycemia, thus exposing the fetus to elevated insulin levels. This would result in an increased risk of fetal macrosomia and neonatal hypoglycemia.

The blood glucose concentration in humans is mainly dependent on diet, especially energy-ingestion and the percentage of carbohydrates in the diet. High glucose concentrations in the blood of pregnant women cause an intensified transfer of nutrient to the fetus, increasing fetal growth. Studies could link higher maternal glucose to an increase in infant birth weight as well as different extents of morbidity, among other things the incidence of congenital malformations, supporting the Hypothesis, that even moderately increased blood glucose in the absence of diabetes positively influences growth in the fetus.

Subsequently alterations of Pedersen's Hypothesis took place: Nutrients other than sugar and their linkage to fetal overgrowth in diabetic pregnancy were taken into account too; but the crucial role of the fetal hyperinsulinism and monitoring of motherly glucose was nevertheless stressed. Recent studies pointed out that diabetes in the mother could foster even more lasting effects on the child's health than previously thought, even raising the risk of obesity and type 2 diabetes.

Historical Cases

Various nutritional conditions, both times of scarcity and of abundance occurred time and again in different societies at different times, and thus in some cases epidemiological studies have exposed a correlation between the nutritional status of pregnant women and the health of their children or even grandchildren.

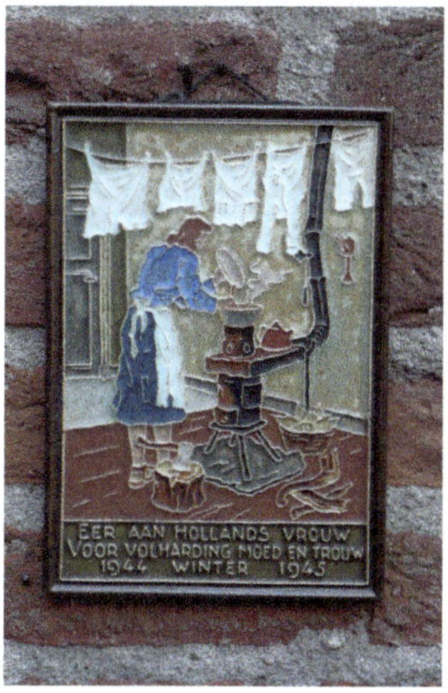
EER AAN HOLLANDS VROUW
VOOR VOLHARDING MOED EN TROUW
1944 WINTER 1945

A tile tribute to the Dutch Famine

The Dutch Famine

Since small birth weight is associated with an increased risk of chronic diseases in later life, and poor maternal nutrition during gestation contributes to restricted fetal development, maternal malnutrition may be a cause of increased disease susceptibility in adulthood.

The Dutch famine of 1944 or the "Hunger Winter" during World War II serves as an epidemiological study that is used to examine the effects of maternal under-nutrition during different gestational stages. The famine was a period (roughly five to six months) of extreme food shortage in the west of Netherlands. The famine was imposed on a previously well-nourished population and the official daily ration for the general adult population gradually decreased from 1800 calories in December 1943 to 1400 calories in October 1944 to below 1000 calories in the late November 1944. December 1944 to April 1945 was the peak of the famine where the official daily ration fell abruptly to about 400~800 calories. Even though pregnant and lactating women had extra food during the famine, these extra supplies could no longer be provided at the height of the famine. In the early May 1945, the liberation of the Netherlands restored the food supply. The daily ration had increased to more than 2000 calories in June 1945. What is unique about Dutch Famine as an experimental study on the effects of maternal malnutrition is that the population was strictly circumscribed in time and place and the sudden onset and relief of the famine was imposed on a previously well-nourished population.

The Dutch Famine during World War II had a profound effect on the health condition of the general public, especially women who conceived during the period of time. The period of maternal starvation is shown to have limited intrauterine growth and has been identified as one of the most important contributor to coronary heart disease as well as other chronic diseases later in life. These findings agree well with Barker's hypothesis; it supports the theory that maternal under-nutrition leads to a lower birth weight due to restricted intrauterine development and ultimately leads to higher risks of chronic conditions in adult life.

The French Paradox

The French paradox regards the seemingly paradoxical fact that people living in France since many generations suffer from a relatively little incidence of heart disease, although the traditional French cuisine is high in saturated fatty acids.

One explanation suggested for the paradox is the potential impact of nutritional enhancements during pregnancy and the first months and years of life that would positively influence the health of following generations: After the defeat in the Franco-German War, a nutrition program for pregnant women and small children with the aim of strengthening future generations of soldiers was introduced by the French Government. This might be one explanation for positive health-outcomes in following generations.

Recommendations for Pregnant Women

Gestation Stages

Gestation is the period of embryo development from conception to birth. Gestation is about 40 weeks in humans and is divided into three trimesters, each spanning 3 months. Gestational stages, on the other hand, are based on physiological fetal development, which include blastogenesis, embryonic stage and fetal stage.

Blastogenesis is the stage from fertilization to about 2 weeks. The fertilized egg or the zygote becomes a blastocyst where the outer layer and the inner cell mass differentiate to form placenta and the fetus respectively. Implantation occurs at this stage where the blastocyst becomes buried in the endometrium.

Embryonic stage is approximately from 2 weeks to 8 weeks. It is also in this stage where the blastocyst develops into an embryo, where all major features of human are present and operational by the end of this stage.

Fetal stage is from 9 weeks to term. During this period of time, the embryo develops rapidly and becomes a fetus. Pregnancy becomes visible at this stage.

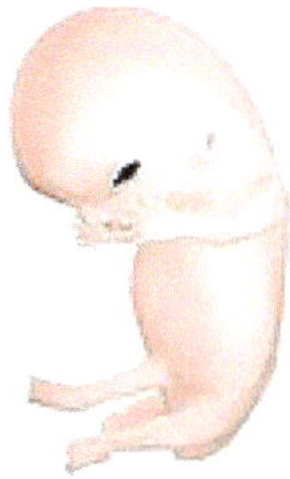

Embryo at 8 weeks after fertilization

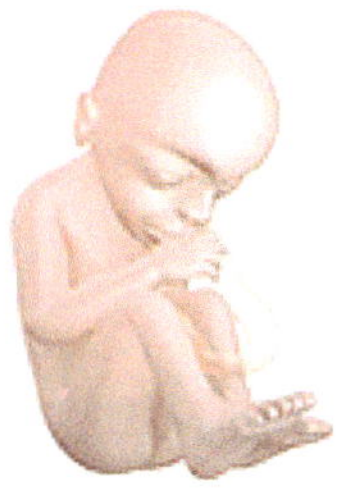

Fetus at 18 weeks after fertilization

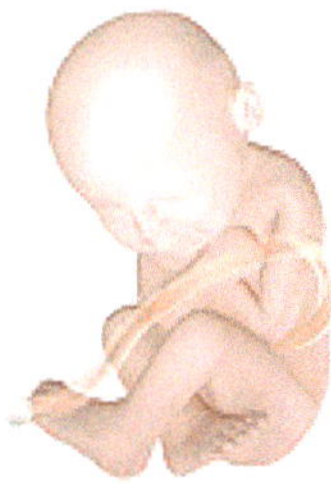

Fetus at 38 weeks after fertilization

Pre-pregnancy Weight and Gestational Weight Gain

The pattern and amount of weight gain is closely associated with gestational stages. Additional energy is required during pregnancy due to the expansion of maternal tissues and stores in order to support fetal development.

In the first trimester (blastogenesis and early embryonic stages), the mother experiences a minimal weight gain (approximately 0.5-2 kilograms), while the embryo weighs only 6 grams, which is approximately the weight of 6 raisins.

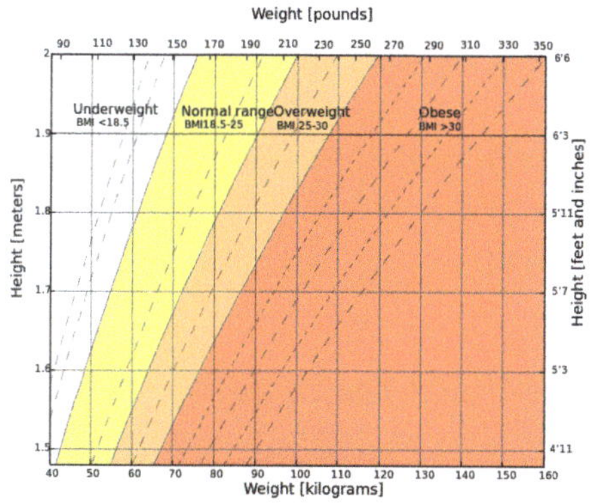

BMI chart

In the second trimester and third trimester (late embryonic and fetal stages), the fetus undergoes rapid weight growth and the weight increases to about 3000~4000 grams. It is also in this period that the mother experiences the bulk of her gestational weight gain but the amount of weight gain varies greatly. The amount of weight gain depends strongly on their pre-pregnant weight.

Generally, a normal weight is strongly recommended for mothers when entering gestation, as it promotes overall health of infants. Maternal body weight is determined by the Body Mass Index (BMI) which is defined as the weight in kilograms divided by the square of the height in meters. While pregnant, body weight should be managed within the recommended gestational weight gain range as it is shown to have a positive effect on pregnancy outcomes. Gestational weight gain should also be progressive and the recommended weight depends on pre-pregnant body weight.

Since the total weight gain depends on pre-pregnant body weight, it is recommended that underweight women should undergo a larger weight gain for healthy pregnancy outcomes, and overweight or obese women should undergo a smaller weight gain.

Normal Weight Women

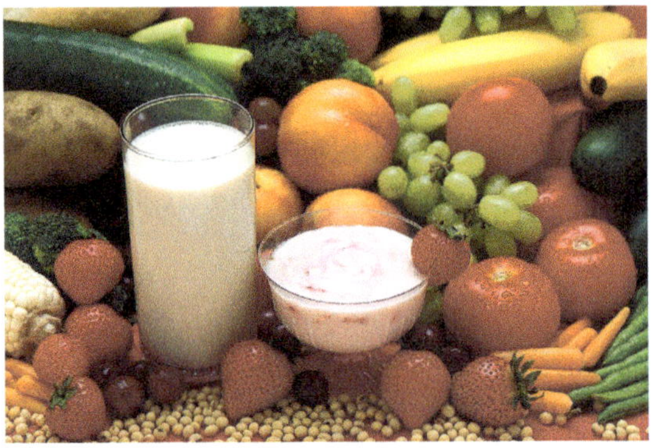

Health choices such as low-fat milk and alternatives, fruits, and vegetables should be emphasized for pregnant women.

Women having a BMI of 18.5~24.9 are classified as having a *normal or healthy* body weight. This group have the lowest risk of adverse birth outcomes. Their babies are least likely to either be low-birth weight or high-birth weight. It is advised that women with a normal weight before pregnancy should gain a total of 11.5 kilograms to 16.0 kilograms throughout gestation, which is approximately 0.4 kilogram per week in the second and third trimesters.

In order to maintain a steady weight gain, the mother should engage in mild physical activities. Participating in aerobic activities such as walking and swimming 3 to 4 times a week is usually adequate. Vigorous physical activity is not recommended since an excessive loss of calories is induced which is not sufficient to support fetal development.

A proper diet is also essential to healthy weight gain. The common saying "a woman is eating for two" often leads to mothers thinking that they should eat twice as much. In reality, only a small increase in caloric intake is needed to provide for the fetus; approximately 350 calories more in the second trimester and 450 calories more in the third trimester. Also, healthy choices should be emphasized for these extra calories such as whole grain products, fruits and vegetables as well as low-fat dairy alternatives.

Underweight Women

Women are classified as *underweight* if they have a pre-pregnant BMI of 18.5 or below. Low pre-pregnancy BMI increases the risk of low birth weight infants, but the risk can be balanced by an appropriate gestational weight gain from 12.5 to 18.0 kilograms in total, or about 0.5 kilogram each week in the second and third trimesters.

Underweight women usually have inadequate nutrient stores that are not enough to provide for both herself and the fetus. While exercise and a proper diet are both needed to maintain the recommended weight gain, a balance between the two is very important. As such, underweight mothers should seek individualized advice tailored especially for themselves.

Overweight and Obese Women

Women with a high pre-pregnancy weight are classified as *overweight or obese*, defined as having a BMI of 25 or above. Women with BMI between 25 and 29.9 are in the overweight category and should gain between 7.0 and 11.5 kilograms in total, corresponding to approximately 0.28 kilogram each week during the second and third trimesters. Whereas women with BMI of 30 or above are in the obese category and should gain only between 5.0 and 9.0 kilograms overall, which equates to roughly 0.2 kilogram per week in the second and third trimesters.

Diet, exercise or a combination of both has been seen to reduce weight gain in pregnancy by 20% and reduce high blood pressure. Diet with exercise may reduce the risk of caesarean section, having a large baby and having a baby with serious breathing problems. Diet and exercise help pregnant women not gain too much weight during pregnancy when compared with giving the women no help too control weight gain or routine care (usually one session in the pregnancy).

In general, walking is encouraged for mothers classified in this category. Unfortunately, estimated energy requirements for them are not available. As such, they are encouraged to record activity and intake level. This can be done with the help of tools such as My Food Guide Servings Tracker from Health Canada and EATracker that are available online. In extreme cases where the BMI exceeds 35, help from a registered dietitian is recommended.

Summary Table

The following table summarizes the recommended rate of weight gain and total weight gain according to pre-pregnancy BMI for singleton pregnancies. The first column categorizes the type of body weight based on the Body Mass Index. The second column summarizes the total recommended weight gain for each type of body weight, and the third column presents the corresponding weekly weight gain during the period when the fetus undergoes rapid growth (during second and third trimesters). In extreme cases, the amount of total and weekly weight gain can vary by a factor of two depending on a woman's pre-pregnant weight. For example, a woman in the obese category is recommended to gain a total of 5~9 kilograms, whereas an underweight woman needs to gain up to 18 kilograms in weight.

Pre-pregnancy BMI Category	**Recommendated Total Weight Gain**	**Weekly Weight Gain** (after 12 weeks)
Underweight BMI <18.5	12.5~18 kg (28~40 lb)	0.5 kg (1.0 lb)
Healthy weight BMI 18.5~ 24.9	11.5~16 kg (25~35 lb)	0.4 kg (1.0 lb)
Overweight BMI 25.0~ 29.9	7.0~ 11.5 kg (15~25 lb)	0.3 kg (0.6 lb)
Obese BMI > 30	5.0~9.0 kg (11~20 lb)	0.2 kg (0.5 lb)

Recommendations for Low and High Birth Weight

Diagnosis

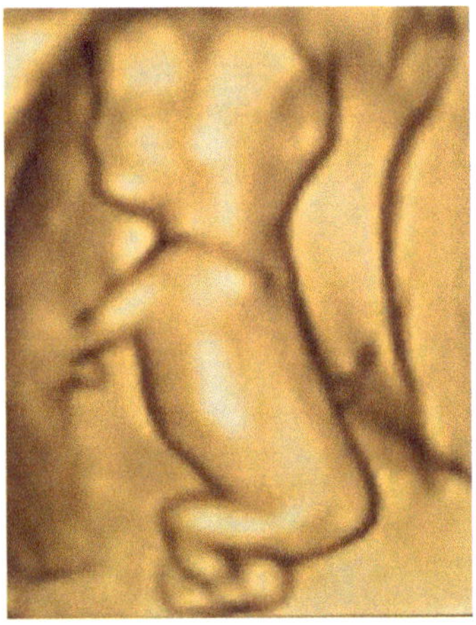

Ultrasound of fetus (~3 inches in length).

In order to have a good estimate of birth weight, ultrasonography or ultrasound during pregnancy and the date of last menstrual period are needed. Measured values from ultrasonography are compared with the growth chart to estimate fetal weight.

Crown rump length can be used as the best ultrasonographic measurement for correct diagnosis of gestational age during the first trimester. This correlation between crown rump length and gestational age would be most effectively shown when no growth defects are observed in first trimester. If growth defects were observed in the first trimester, then the measurement of the date of last menstrual period becomes quite important since the crown heel length has become less of a reliable indicator of gestational age.

After the 20th week of pregnancy, the mother would need to visit the doctor for the measurement of fundal height, which is the length from the top portion of the uterus to the pubic bone. The length measured in centimeters should correspond to the number of weeks that the mother has been pregnant. If the measured number is higher or lower than 2 centimetres, further tests using ultrasound would be needed to check the results. Another way to estimate fetal size is to look at the mother's weight gain. How much weight the mother gains can be used to indicate fetal size.

Low Birth Weight

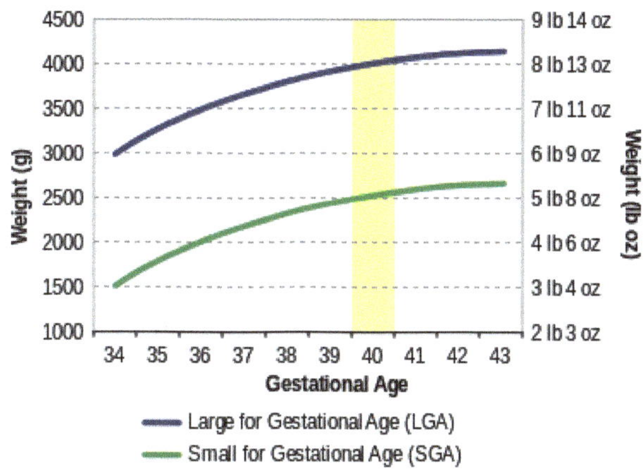

Birth weight chart

There are two ways to determine small for gestational age (SGA) infants. Many research studies agree that SGA babies are those with birth weight or crown heel length measured at two standard deviations or more below the mean of the infant's gestational age, based on data consisting of a reference population. Other studies classify SGA babies as those with birth weight values below the 10th percentile of the growth chart for babies of the same gestational age. This indicates that these babies are weighing less than 90% of babies of the same gestational age.

Many factors, including maternal, placental, and fetal factors, contribute to the cause of impaired fetal growth. There are a number of maternal factors, which include age, nutritional status, alcohol abuse, smoking, and medical conditions. Insufficient utero-placental perfusion is an example of a placental factor. Chromosomal abnormalities and genetic diseases are examples of fetal factors. Identification of the causes of SGA for individual cases aids health professionals in finding ways to handle each unique case. Nutritional counseling, education, and consistent monitoring can be helpful to assist women bearing SGA infants.

Complications for the infant include limitations in body growth since the number and size of cells in tissues is smaller. The infant likely did not receive enough oxygen during pregnancy so the oxygen level is low. It is also more difficult to maintain body temperature since there is less blood flow within the small body.

As such, it is necessary to monitor oxygen level to make sure that it doesn't go too low. If the baby can't suck well, then it may be necessary for tube-feed. Since the baby cannot maintain body temperature sufficiently, a temperature-controlled bed would help to keep their bodies from losing heat. There are ways to help prevent SGA babies. Monitoring fetal growth can help identify the problem during pregnancy well before birth. It would be beneficial to seek professional help and counseling.

High Birth Weight

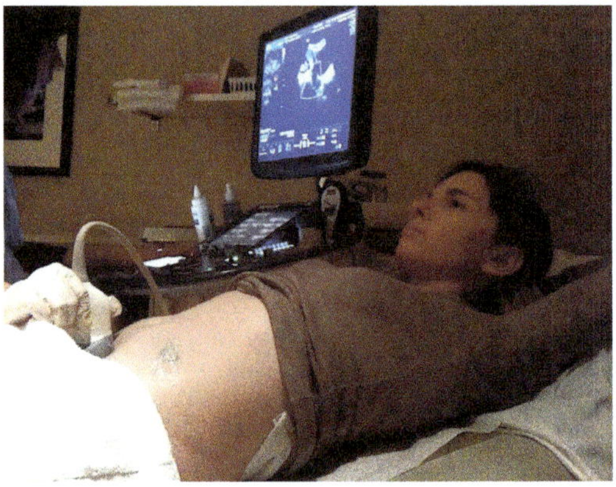

Ultrasound examination.

Research show that when birth weights of infants are greater than the 90th percentile of the growth chart for babies of the same gestational age, they are considered large for gestational age or LGA. This indicates that these babies are weighing more than 90% of babies of the same gestational age.

Many factors account for LGA babies, including genetics and excessive nutrient supply. It seems that a common factor for LGA babies is whether or not the mother has diabetes when she is pregnant. An indicator for excessive growth, regardless of gestational age, is the appearance of macrosomia. Many complications are observed for LGA babies and their mothers. A longer delivery time may be expected since it is a difficult birth. The infant would likely suffer hypoglycemia (low glucose level in the blood) after birth. The infant would also have difficulty breathing.

There might be a need for early delivery if the baby gets too big and perhaps Caesarean section would be needed. Since the baby is bigger in size, there's a higher chance of injury when coming out of the mother's body. To increase the blood glucose level in blood, a glucose/water solution can be offered to the infant.

There are ways to help prevent LGA babies. It is necessary to monitor fetal growth and perform pregnancy examinations to determine health status and detect any possibility of unrecognized diabetes. For diabetic mothers, careful management of diabetes during pregnancy period would be helpful in terms of lowering some of the risks of LGA.

Points to Consider

The goal of pregnancy is to have a healthy baby. Maintaining healthy and steady weight gain during pregnancy promotes overall health and reduces the incidence of prenatal morbidity and mortality. This, in turn, has a positive effect on the baby's health.

Since conditions during pregnancy will have long-term effects on adult health, "moderation" should be taken into account for both dietary and physical activity recommendations. Most importantly, the total recommended pregnancy weight gain depends on pre-pregnant body weight, and weight issues should be addressed before pregnancy.

Future Direction for Research

It is reasonable to expect higher weight gain for multiple gestations. Recommendations for women carrying twins are given but more research should be done to precisely determine the total weight gain, as these ranges are wide. Also, the ranges for underweight women carrying twins is unknown. There was not enough information to recommend weight gain cutoffs and guidelines for women carrying three or more babies, women of short stature (<157 centimetres), and pregnant teens. Estimated energy requirements (EER) for overweight/obese women are unavailable so more research is needed to evaluate on that. There are also important links between nutrition and mental health across pregnancy. For example, a women experiencing low mood may be more likely to smoke, use alcohol or neglect her diet.

Practical Advice for Mothers

The following general tips can be helpful to pregnant women. It would be beneficial to maintain adequate physical activity to meet energy needs from the food consumed. Eating a balanced diet would be optimal for healthy pregnancy results. To prevent problems like dehydration and constipation, it is important to drink enough fluids, especially water, to support blood volume increases during pregnancy. It is recommended to accompany regular meals with a daily prenatal vitamin supplement that has sufficient folic acid and iron content.

If the fetus is predicted to have low birth weight, in addition to the general recommendations, it would be ideal to increase caloric intake, which can be done by having extra Food Guide Servings daily. If the fetus is predicted to have high birth weight, smaller and more frequent meals should be consumed to allow better weight management. Moderate sugar intake, such as fruit juices, is also suggested. It is essential to limit food and beverages with high calories and salt content.

References

- Tina Gianoulis, "Dieting" in the St. James Encyclopedia of Popular Culture Ed. Thomas Riggs. Vol. 2. 2nd ed. Detroit: St. James Press, 2013. p106-108. ISBN 978-1-55862-847-2
- Burr, G.O., Burr, M.M. and Miller, E. (1930). "On the nature and role of the fatty acids essential in nutrition" (PDF). J. Biol. Chem. 86 (587). Retrieved 2007-01-17
- Imura K, Okada A (1998). "Amino acid metabolism in pediatric patients". Nutrition. 14 (1): 143–8. PMID 9437700. doi:10.1016/S0899-9007(97)00230-X
- Jéquier, E; Constant, F (2 September 2009). "Water as an essential nutrient: the physiological basis of hydration". European Journal of Clinical Nutrition. 64 (2): 115–123. doi:10.1038/ejcn.2009.111
- Robert S. Goodhart; Maurice E. Shils (1980). Modern Nutrition in Health and Disease (6th ed.). Philadelphia: Lea and Febinger. pp. 134–138. ISBN 0-8121-0645-8
- "App. E-3.7: Developing Vegetarian and Mediterranean-style Food Patterns - 2015 Advisory Report - health.gov". health.gov. Retrieved 2015-09-30
- Sanders TA (2009). "DHA Status of vegetarians". Prostaglandins Leukotrienes Essential Fatty Acids. 81 (2–3): 137–41. PMID 19500961. doi:10.1016/j.plefa.2009.05.013
- Rose WC, Haines WJ, Warner DT, Johnson JE (1951). "The amino acid requirements of man. II. The role of threonine and histidine". The Journal of biological chemistry. 188 (1): 49–58. PMID 14814112
- Robert S. Goodhart; Maurice E. Shils (1980). Modern Nutrition in Health and Disease (6th ed.). Philadelphia: Lea and Febinger. pp. 134–138. ISBN 0-8121-0645-8
- "British Heart Foundation launches Food4Thought campaign". British Cardiovascular Society. 22 September 2006. Retrieved 16 August 2016
- Cunnane SC (November 2003). "Problems with essential fatty acids: time for a new paradigm?". Progress in Lipid Research. 42 (6): 544–68. PMID 14559071. doi:10.1016/S0163-7827(03)00038-9
- Reiffel JA, McDonald A (August 2006). "Antiarrhythmic effects of omega-3 fatty acids". The American Journal of Cardiology. 98 (4A): 50i–60i. PMID 16919517. doi:10.1016/j.amjcard.2005.12.027
- James, William; Berger, Timothy; Elston, Dirk (2005). Andrews' Diseases of the Skin: Clinical Dermatology. (10th ed.). Saunders. ISBN 0-7216-2921-0
- "Part D. Chapter 1: Food and Nutrient Intakes, and Health: Current Status and Trends - Continued". Office of Disease Prevention and Health Promotion. 2015. Retrieved 12 May 2015
- Katz DL, Meller S (2014). "Can we say what diet is best for health?". Annu Rev Public Health. 35: 83–103. PMID 24641555. doi:10.1146/annurev-publhealth-032013-182351
- Bateson, P (2001). "Fetal experience and good adult design". International Journal of Epidemiology. 30 (5): 928–934. doi:10.1093/ije/30.5.928
- Executive Summary: Policy and Action for Cancer Prevention Food, Nutrition, and Physical Activity (PDF). World Cancer Research Fund. 2010. p. 1. ISBN 978-0-9722522-5-6
- De Leon, Victoria. "Weight Problems During Prengnacy and the Effect on Your Baby". Losing Pregnancy Weight. Retrieved 3 March 2011
- James WP (2008). "The fundamental drivers of the obesity epidemic". Obesity Research. 9 Suppl 1 (Mar;9 Suppl 1:6-13): 6–13. PMID 18307693. doi:10.1111/j.1467-789X.2007.00432.x

2

Macronutrients: An Integrated Study

Proteins are made up of one or more amino acids. They have a number of functions to perform like DNA replication, responding to stimuli, catalyzing metabolic reactions, etc. The other macronutrients explained are amino acid, fat, fatty acid, dietary fiber and carbohydrate. The major categories of macronutrients are dealt with great details in the chapter.

Protein

Proteins are large biomolecules, or macromolecules, consisting of one or more long chains of amino acid residues. Proteins perform a vast array of functions within organisms, including catalysing metabolic reactions, DNA replication, responding to stimuli, and transporting molecules from one location to another. Proteins differ from one another primarily in their sequence of amino acids, which is dictated by the nucleotide sequence of their genes, and which usually results in protein folding into a specific three-dimensional structure that determines its activity.

A linear chain of amino acid residues is called a polypeptide. A protein contains at least one long polypeptide. Short polypeptides, containing less than 20–30 residues, are rarely considered to be proteins and are commonly called peptides, or sometimes oligopeptides. The individual amino acid residues are bonded together by peptide bonds and adjacent amino acid residues. The sequence of amino acid residues in a protein is defined by the sequence of a gene, which is encoded in the genetic code. In general, the genetic code specifies 20 standard amino acids; however, in certain organisms the genetic code can include selenocysteine and—in certain archaea—pyrrolysine. Shortly after or even during synthesis, the residues in a protein are often chemically modified by post-translational modification, which alters the physical and chemical properties, folding, stability, activity, and ultimately, the function of the proteins. Sometimes proteins have non-peptide groups attached, which can be called prosthetic groups or cofactors. Proteins can also work together to achieve a particular function, and they often associate to form stable protein complexes.

Once formed, proteins only exist for a certain period of time and are then degraded and recycled by the cell's machinery through the process of protein turnover. A protein's lifespan is measured in terms of its half-life and covers a wide range. They can exist for minutes or years with an average lifespan of 1–2 days in mammalian cells. Abnormal or misfolded proteins are degraded more rapidly either due to being targeted for destruction or due to being unstable.

Like other biological macromolecules such as polysaccharides and nucleic acids, proteins are essential parts of organisms and participate in virtually every process within cells. Many proteins are enzymes that catalyse biochemical reactions and are vital to metabolism. Proteins also have structural or mechanical functions, such as actin and myosin in muscle and the proteins in the cytoskeleton, which form a system of scaffolding that maintains cell shape. Other proteins are important in cell signaling, immune responses, cell adhesion, and the cell cycle. In animals, proteins are needed in the diet to provide the essential amino acids that cannot be synthesized. Digestion breaks the proteins down for use in the metabolism.

Proteins may be purified from other cellular components using a variety of techniques such as ultracentrifugation, precipitation, electrophoresis, and chromatography; the advent of genetic engineering has made possible a number of methods to facilitate purification. Methods commonly used to study protein structure and function include immunohistochemistry, site-directed mutagenesis, X-ray crystallography, nuclear magnetic resonance and mass spectrometry.

Biochemistry

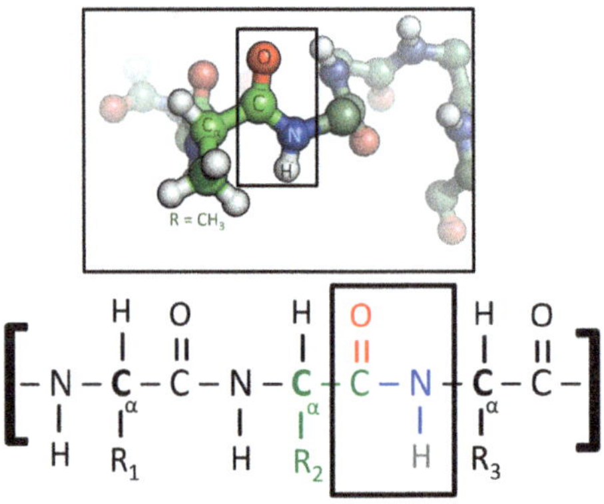

Chemical structure of the peptide bond (bottom) and the three-dimensional structure of a peptide bond between an alanine and an adjacent amino acid (top/inset).

Most proteins consist of linear polymers built from series of up to 20 different L-α-amino acids. All proteinogenic amino acids possess common structural features, including an α-carbon to which an amino group, a carboxyl group, and a variable side chain are bonded. Only proline differs from this basic structure as it contains an unusual ring to the N-end amine group, which forces the CO–NH amide moiety into a fixed conformation. The side chains of the standard amino acids, detailed in the list of standard amino acids, have a great variety of chemical structures and properties; it is the combined effect of all of the amino acid side chains in a protein that ultimately determines its three-dimensional structure and its chemical reactivity. The amino acids in a polypeptide chain are linked by peptide bonds. Once linked in the protein chain, an individual amino acid is called a *residue,* and the linked series of carbon, nitrogen, and oxygen atoms are known as the *main chain* or *protein backbone.*

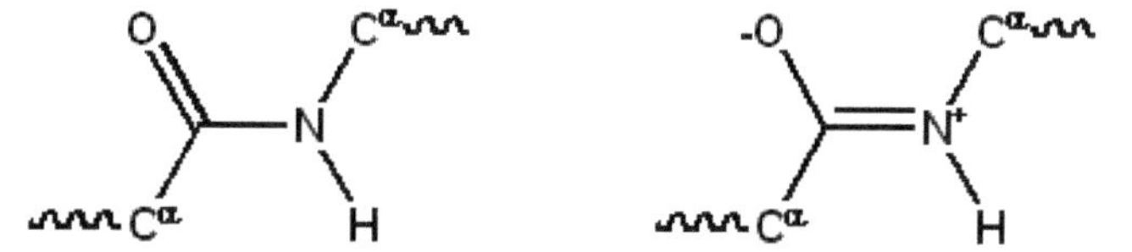

Resonance structures of the peptide bond that links individual amino acids to form a protein polymer.

The peptide bond has two resonance forms that contribute some double-bond character and inhibit rotation around its axis, so that the alpha carbons are roughly coplanar. The other two dihedral angles in the peptide bond determine the local shape assumed by the protein backbone. The end with a free amino group is known as the N-terminus or amino terminus, whereas the end of the protein with a free carboxyl group is known as the C-terminus or carboxy terminus (the sequence of the protein is written from N-terminus to C-terminus, from left to right).

The words *protein, polypeptide,* and *peptide* are a little ambiguous and can overlap in meaning. *Protein* is generally used to refer to the complete biological molecule in a stable conformation, whereas *peptide* is generally reserved for a short amino acid oligomers often lacking a stable three-dimensional structure. However, the boundary between the two is not well defined and usually lies near 20–30 residues. *Polypeptide* can refer to any single linear chain of amino acids, usually regardless of length, but often implies an absence of a defined conformation.

Abundance in Cells

It has been estimated that average-sized bacteria contain about 2 million proteins per cell (e.g. *E. coli* and *Staphylococcus aureus*). Smaller bacteria, such as *Mycoplasma* or *spirochetes* contain fewer molecules, namely on the order of 50,000 to 1 million. By contrast, eukaryotic cells are larger and thus contain much more protein. For instance, yeast cells were estimated to contain about 50 million proteins and human cells on the order of 1 to 3 billion. The concentration of individual protein copies ranges from a few molecules per cell up to 20 million. Not all genes coding proteins are expressed in most cells and their number depends on for example cell type and external stimuli. For instance, of the 20,000 or so proteins encoded by the human genome, only 6,000 are detected in lymphoblastoid cells. Moreover, the number of proteins the genome encodes correlates well with the organism complexity. Eukaryotes, bacteria, Archaea and viruses have on average 15145, 3200, 2358 and 42 proteins respectively coded in their genomes.

Synthesis

Biosynthesis

Proteins are assembled from amino acids using information encoded in genes. Each protein has its own unique amino acid sequence that is specified by the nucleotide sequence of the gene encoding this protein. The genetic code is a set of three-nucleotide sets called codons and each three-nucleotide combination designates an amino acid, for example AUG (adenine-uracil-guanine) is the code for methionine. Because DNA contains four nucleotides, the total number of possible codons is 64; hence, there is some redundancy in the genetic code, with some amino acids specified by more than one codon. Genes encoded in DNA are first transcribed into pre-messenger RNA (mRNA) by proteins such as RNA polymerase. Most organisms then process the pre-mRNA (also known as a *primary transcript*) using various forms of Post-transcriptional modification to form the mature mRNA, which is then used as a template for protein synthesis by the ribosome. In prokaryotes the mRNA may either be used as soon as it is produced, or be bound by a ribosome after having moved away from the nucleoid. In contrast, eukaryotes make mRNA in the cell nucleus and then translocate it across the nuclear membrane into the cytoplasm, where protein synthesis then takes place. The rate of protein synthesis is higher in prokaryotes than eukaryotes and can reach up to 20 amino acids per second.

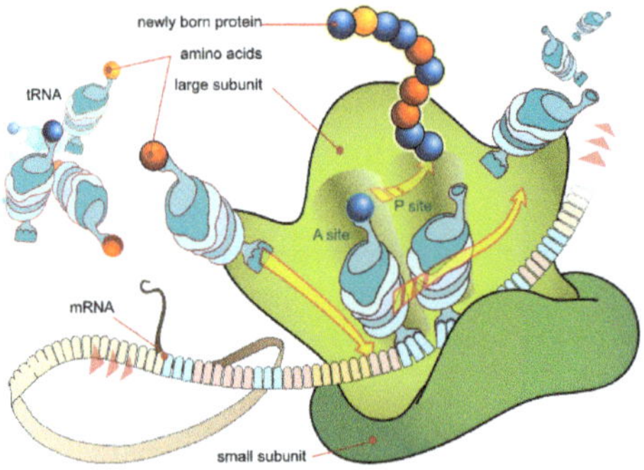

A ribosome produces a protein using mRNA as template.

The process of synthesizing a protein from an mRNA template is known as translation. The mRNA is loaded onto the ribosome and is read three nucleotides at a time by matching each codon to its base pairing anticodon located on a transfer RNA molecule, which carries the amino acid corresponding to the codon it recognizes. The enzyme aminoacyl tRNA synthetase "charges" the tRNA molecules with the correct amino acids. The growing polypeptide is often termed the *nascent chain*. Proteins are always biosynthesized from N-terminus to C-terminus.

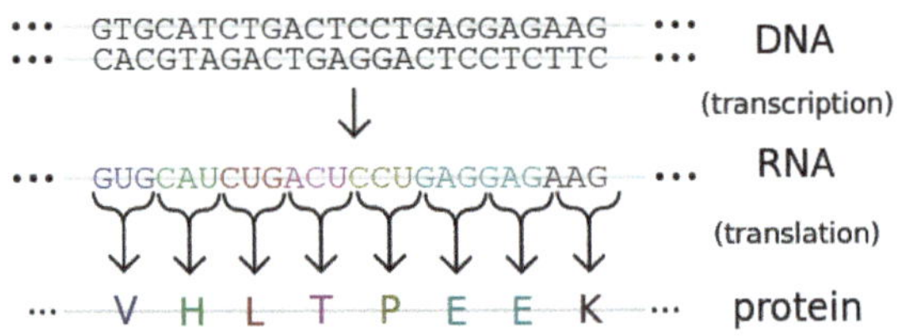

The DNA sequence of a gene encodes the amino acid sequence of a protein.

The size of a synthesized protein can be measured by the number of amino acids it contains and by its total molecular mass, which is normally reported in units of *dal-*

tons (synonymous with atomic mass units), or the derivative unit kilodalton (kDa). The average size of protein increases from Archaea, Bacteria to Eukaryote (283, 311, 438 residues and 31, 34, 49 kDa respecitvely) due bigger number of protein domains constituting proteins in higher organisms. For instance, yeast proteins are on average 466 amino acids long and 53 kDa in mass. The largest known proteins are the titins, a component of the muscle sarcomere, with a molecular mass of almost 3,000 kDa and a total length of almost 27,000 amino acids.

Chemical Synthesis

Short proteins can also be synthesized chemically by a family of methods known as peptide synthesis, which rely on organic synthesis techniques such as chemical ligation to produce peptides in high yield. Chemical synthesis allows for the introduction of non-natural amino acids into polypeptide chains, such as attachment of fluorescent probes to amino acid side chains. These methods are useful in laboratory biochemistry and cell biology, though generally not for commercial applications. Chemical synthesis is inefficient for polypeptides longer than about 300 amino acids, and the synthesized proteins may not readily assume their native tertiary structure. Most chemical synthesis methods proceed from C-terminus to N-terminus, opposite the biological reaction.

Structure

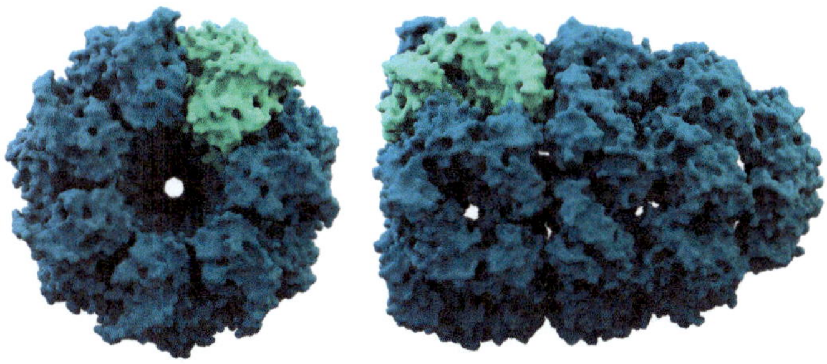

The crystal structure of the chaperonin, a huge protein complex. A single protein subunit is highlighted. Chaperonins assist protein folding.

Most proteins fold into unique 3-dimensional structures. The shape into which a protein naturally folds is known as its native conformation. Although many proteins can fold unassisted, simply through the chemical properties of their amino acids, others require the aid of molecular chaperones to fold into their native states. Biochemists often refer to four distinct aspects of a protein's structure:

- *Primary structure*: the amino acid sequence. A protein is a polyamide.
- *Secondary structure*: regularly repeating local structures stabilized by hydrogen bonds. The most common examples are the α-helix, β-sheet and turns. Because secondary structures are local, many regions of different secondary structure can be present in the same protein molecule.

- *Tertiary structure*: the overall shape of a single protein molecule; the spatial relationship of the secondary structures to one another. Tertiary structure is generally stabilized by nonlocal interactions, most commonly the formation of a hydrophobic core, but also through salt bridges, hydrogen bonds, disulfide bonds, and even posttranslational modifications. The term "tertiary structure" is often used as synonymous with the term *fold*. The tertiary structure is what controls the basic function of the protein.
- *Quaternary structure*: the structure formed by several protein molecules (polypeptide chains), usually called *protein subunits* in this context, which function as a single protein complex.

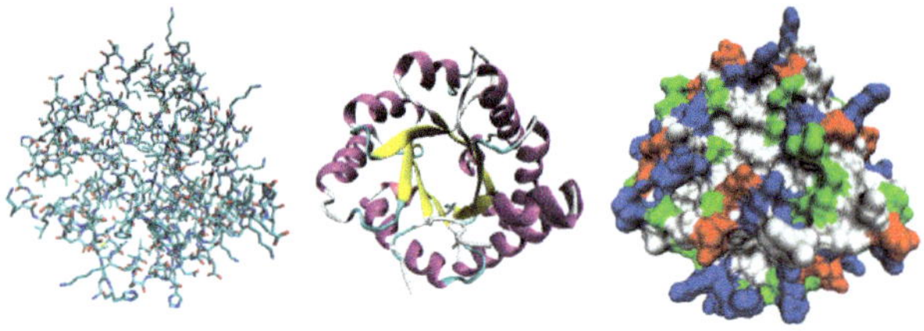

Three possible representations of the three-dimensional structure of the protein triose phosphate isomerase. Left: All-atom representation colored by atom type. Middle: Simplified representation illustrating the backbone conformation, colored by secondary structure. Right: Solvent-accessible surface representation colored by residue type (acidic residues red, basic residues blue, polar residues green, nonpolar residues white).

Proteins are not entirely rigid molecules. In addition to these levels of structure, proteins may shift between several related structures while they perform their functions. In the context of these functional rearrangements, these tertiary or quaternary structures are usually referred to as "conformations", and transitions between them are called *conformational changes*. Such changes are often induced by the binding of a substrate molecule to an enzyme's active site, or the physical region of the protein that participates in chemical catalysis. In solution proteins also undergo variation in structure through thermal vibration and the collision with other molecules.

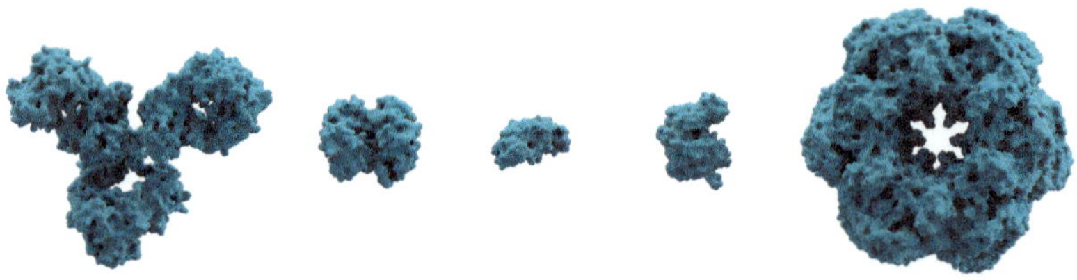

Molecular surface of several proteins showing their comparative sizes. From left to right are: immunoglobulin G (IgG, an antibody), hemoglobin, insulin (a hormone), adenylate kinase (an enzyme), and glutamine synthetase (an enzyme).

Proteins can be informally divided into three main classes, which correlate with typical tertiary structures: globular proteins, fibrous proteins, and membrane proteins. Almost all globular proteins are soluble and many are enzymes. Fibrous proteins are often structural, such as collagen, the major component of connective tissue, or keratin, the protein component of hair and nails. Membrane proteins often serve as receptors or provide channels for polar or charged molecules to pass through the cell membrane.

A special case of intramolecular hydrogen bonds within proteins, poorly shielded from water attack and hence promoting their own dehydration, are called dehydrons.

Structure Determination

Discovering the tertiary structure of a protein, or the quaternary structure of its complexes, can provide important clues about how the protein performs its function. Common experimental methods of structure determination include X-ray crystallography and NMR spectroscopy, both of which can produce information at atomic resolution. However, NMR experiments are able to provide information from which a subset of distances between pairs of atoms can be estimated, and the final possible conformations for a protein are determined by solving a distance geometry problem. Dual polarisation interferometry is a quantitative analytical method for measuring the overall protein conformation and conformational changes due to interactions or other stimulus. Circular dichroism is another laboratory technique for determining internal β-sheet / α-helical composition of proteins. Cryoelectron microscopy is used to produce lower-resolution structural information about very large protein complexes, including assembled viruses; a variant known as electron crystallography can also produce high-resolution information in some cases, especially for two-dimensional crystals of membrane proteins. Solved structures are usually deposited in the Protein Data Bank (PDB), a freely available resource from which structural data about thousands of proteins can be obtained in the form of Cartesian coordinates for each atom in the protein.

Many more gene sequences are known than protein structures. Further, the set of solved structures is biased toward proteins that can be easily subjected to the conditions required in X-ray crystallography, one of the major structure determination methods. In particular, globular proteins are comparatively easy to crystallize in preparation for X-ray crystallography. Membrane proteins, by contrast, are difficult to crystallize and are underrepresented in the PDB. Structural genomics initiatives have attempted to remedy these deficiencies by systematically solving representative structures of major fold classes. Protein structure prediction methods attempt to provide a means of generating a plausible structure for proteins whose structures have not been experimentally determined.

Cellular Functions

Proteins are the chief actors within the cell, said to be carrying out the duties specified by the information encoded in genes. With the exception of certain types of RNA, most other biological molecules are relatively inert elements upon which proteins act. Proteins make up half the dry weight of an *Escherichia coli* cell, whereas other macromolecules such as DNA and RNA make up only 3% and 20%, respectively. The set of proteins expressed in a particular cell or cell type is known as its proteome.

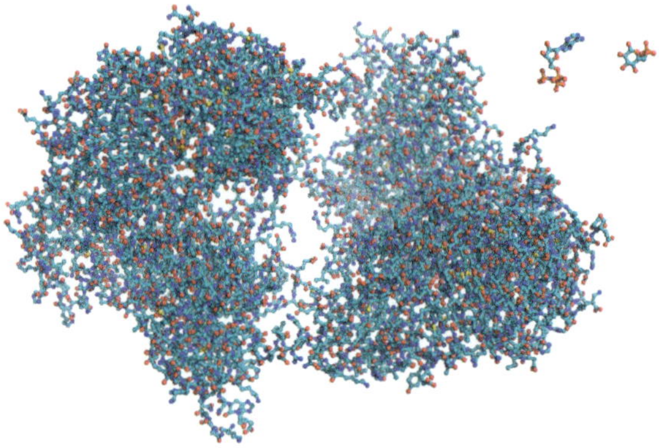

The enzyme hexokinase is shown as a conventional ball-and-stick molecular model. To scale in the top right-hand corner are two of its substrates, ATP and glucose.

The chief characteristic of proteins that also allows their diverse set of functions is their ability to bind other molecules specifically and tightly. The region of the protein responsible for binding another molecule is known as the binding site and is often a depression or "pocket" on the molecular surface. This binding ability is mediated by the tertiary structure of the protein, which defines the binding site pocket, and by the chemical properties of the surrounding amino acids' side chains. Protein binding can be extraordinarily tight and specific; for example, the ribonuclease inhibitor protein binds to human angiogenin with a sub-femtomolar dissociation constant ($<10^{-15}$ M) but does not bind at all to its amphibian homolog onconase (>1 M). Extremely minor chemical changes such as the addition of a single methyl group to a binding partner can sometimes suffice to nearly eliminate binding; for example, the aminoacyl tRNA synthetase specific to the amino acid valine discriminates against the very similar side chain of the amino acid isoleucine.

Proteins can bind to other proteins as well as to small-molecule substrates. When proteins bind specifically to other copies of the same molecule, they can oligomerize to form fibrils; this process occurs often in structural proteins that consist of globular monomers that self-associate to form rigid fibers. Protein–protein interactions also regulate enzymatic activity, control progression through the cell cycle, and allow the assembly of large protein complexes that carry out many closely related reactions with a common biological function. Proteins can also bind to, or even be integrated into, cell membranes. The ability of binding partners to induce conformational changes in proteins allows the construction of enormously complex signaling networks. As interactions between proteins are reversible, and depend heavily on the availability of different groups of partner proteins to form aggregates that are capable to carry out discrete sets of function, study of the interactions between specific proteins is a key to understand important aspects of cellular function, and ultimately the properties that distinguish particular cell types.

Enzymes

The best-known role of proteins in the cell is as enzymes, which catalyse chemical reactions. Enzymes are usually highly specific and accelerate only one or a few chemical reactions. Enzymes carry out most of the reactions involved in metabolism, as well as manipulating DNA in processes such as DNA replication, DNA repair, and transcription. Some enzymes act on other proteins to add or remove chemical groups in a process known as posttranslational modification. About 4,000 reactions are known to be catalysed by enzymes. The rate acceleration conferred by enzymatic catalysis is often enormous—as much as 10^{17}-fold increase in rate over the uncatalysed reaction in the case of orotate decarboxylase (78 million years without the enzyme, 18 milliseconds with the enzyme).

The molecules bound and acted upon by enzymes are called substrates. Although enzymes can consist of hundreds of amino acids, it is usually only a small fraction of the residues that come in contact with the substrate, and an even smaller fraction—three to four residues on average—that are directly involved in catalysis. The region of the enzyme that binds the substrate and contains the catalytic residues is known as the active site.

Dirigent proteins are members of a class of proteins that dictate the stereochemistry of a compound synthesized by other enzymes.

Cell Signaling and Ligand Binding

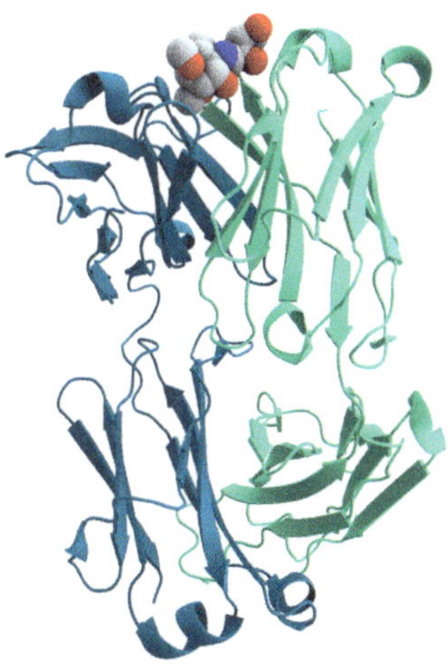

Ribbon diagram of a mouse antibody against cholera that binds a carbohydrate antigen.

Many proteins are involved in the process of cell signaling and signal transduction. Some proteins, such as insulin, are extracellular proteins that transmit a signal from the cell in which they were synthesized to other cells in distant tissues. Others are membrane proteins that act as receptors whose main function is to bind a signaling molecule and induce a biochemical response in the cell. Many receptors have a binding site exposed on the cell surface and an effector domain within the cell, which may have enzymatic activity or may undergo a conformational change detected by other proteins within the cell.

Antibodies are protein components of an adaptive immune system whose main function is to bind antigens, or foreign substances in the body, and target them for destruction. Antibodies can be secreted into the extracellular environment or anchored in the membranes of specialized B cells known as plasma cells. Whereas enzymes are limited in their binding affinity for their substrates by the necessity of conducting their reaction, antibodies have no such constraints. An antibody's binding affinity to its target is extraordinarily high.

Many ligand transport proteins bind particular small biomolecules and transport them to other locations in the body of a multicellular organism. These proteins must have a high binding affinity when their ligand is present in high concentrations, but must also release the ligand when it is present at low concentrations in the target tissues. The canonical example of a ligand-binding protein is haemoglobin, which transports oxygen from the lungs to other organs and tissues in all vertebrates and has close homologs in every biological kingdom. Lectins are sugar-binding proteins which are highly specific for their sugar moieties. Lectins typically play a role in biological recognition phenomena involving cells and proteins. Receptors and hormones are highly specific binding proteins.

Transmembrane proteins can also serve as ligand transport proteins that alter the permeability of the cell membrane to small molecules and ions. The membrane alone has a hydrophobic core through which polar or charged molecules cannot diffuse. Membrane proteins contain internal channels that allow such molecules to enter and exit the cell. Many ion channel proteins are specialized to select for only a particular ion; for example, potassium and sodium channels often discriminate for only one of the two ions.

Structural Proteins

Structural proteins confer stiffness and rigidity to otherwise-fluid biological components. Most structural proteins are fibrous proteins; for example, collagen and elastin are critical components of connective tissue such as cartilage, and keratin is found in hard or filamentous structures such as hair, nails, feathers, hooves, and some animal shells. Some globular proteins can also play structural functions, for example, actin and tubulin are globular and soluble as monomers, but polymerize to form long, stiff fibers that make up the cytoskeleton, which allows the cell to maintain its shape and size.

Other proteins that serve structural functions are motor proteins such as myosin, kinesin, and dynein, which are capable of generating mechanical forces. These proteins are crucial for cellular motility of single celled organisms and the sperm of many multicellular organisms which reproduce sexually. They also generate the forces exerted by contracting muscles and play essential roles in intracellular transport.

Methods of Study

The activities and structures of proteins may be examined *in vitro, in vivo, and in silico. In vitro* studies of purified proteins in controlled environments are useful for learning how a protein carries out its function: for example, enzyme kinetics studies explore the chemical mechanism of an enzyme's catalytic activity and its relative affinity for various possible substrate molecules. By contrast, *in vivo* experiments can provide information about the physiological role of a protein in the context of a cell or even a whole organism. *In silico* studies use computational methods to study proteins.

Protein Purification

To perform *in vitro* analysis, a protein must be purified away from other cellular components. This process usually begins with cell lysis, in which a cell's membrane is disrupted and its internal contents released into a solution known as a crude lysate. The resulting mixture can be purified using ultracentrifugation, which fractionates the various cellular components into fractions containing soluble proteins; membrane lipids and proteins; cellular organelles, and nucleic acids. Precipitation by a method known as salting out can concentrate the proteins from this lysate. Various types of chromatography are then used to isolate the protein or proteins of interest based on properties such as molecular weight, net charge and binding affinity. The level of purification can be monitored using various types of gel electrophoresis if the desired protein's molecular weight and isoelectric point are known, by spectroscopy if the protein has distinguishable spectroscopic features, or by enzyme assays if the protein has enzymatic activity. Additionally, proteins can be isolated according their charge using electrofocusing.

For natural proteins, a series of purification steps may be necessary to obtain protein sufficiently pure for laboratory applications. To simplify this process, genetic engineering is often used to add chemical features to proteins that make them easier to purify without affecting their structure or activity. Here, a "tag" consisting of a specific amino acid sequence, often a series of histidine residues (a "His-tag"), is attached to one terminus of the protein. As a result, when the lysate is passed over a chromatography column containing nickel, the histidine residues ligate the nickel and attach to the column while the untagged components of the lysate pass unimpeded. A number of different tags have been developed to help researchers purify specific proteins from complex mixtures.

Cellular Localization

The study of proteins *in vivo* is often concerned with the synthesis and localization of the protein within the cell. Although many intracellular proteins are synthesized in the cytoplasm and membrane-bound or secreted proteins in the endoplasmic reticulum, the specifics of how proteins are targeted to specific organelles or cellular structures is often unclear. A useful technique for assessing cellular localization uses genetic engineering to express in a cell a fusion protein or chimera consisting of the natural protein of interest linked to a "reporter" such as green fluorescent protein (GFP). The fused protein's position within the cell can be cleanly and efficiently visualized using microscopy, as shown in the figure opposite.

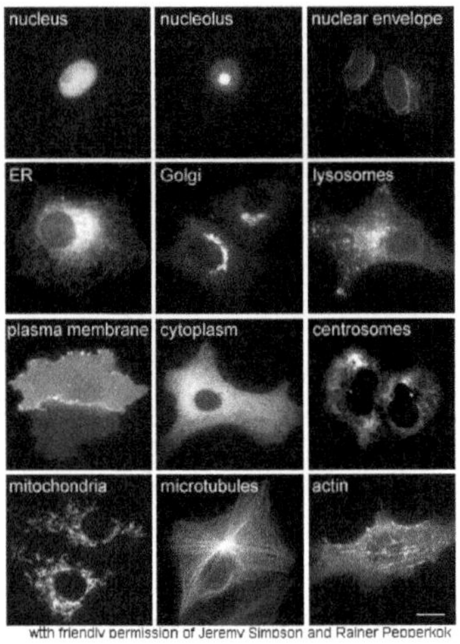

with friendly permission of Jeremy Simpson and Rainer Pepperkok

Proteins in different cellular compartments and structures tagged with green fluorescent protein (here, white).

Other methods for elucidating the cellular location of proteins requires the use of known compartmental markers for regions such as the ER, the Golgi, lysosomes or vacuoles, mitochondria, chloroplasts, plasma membrane, etc. With the use of fluorescently tagged versions of these markers or of antibodies to known markers, it becomes much simpler to identify the localization of a protein of interest. For example, indirect immunofluorescence will allow for fluorescence colocalization and demonstration of location. Fluorescent dyes are used to label cellular compartments for a similar purpose.

Other possibilities exist, as well. For example, immunohistochemistry usually utilizes an antibody to one or more proteins of interest that are conjugated to enzymes yielding either luminescent or chromogenic signals that can be compared between samples, allowing for localization information. Another applicable technique is cofractionation in sucrose (or other material) gradients using isopycnic centrifugation. While this technique does not prove colocalization of a compartment of known density and the protein of interest, it does increase the likelihood, and is more amenable to large-scale studies.

Finally, the gold-standard method of cellular localization is immunoelectron microscopy. This technique also uses an antibody to the protein of interest, along with classical electron microscopy techniques. The sample is prepared for normal electron microscopic examination, and then treated with an antibody to the protein of interest that is conjugated to an extremely electro-dense material, usually gold. This allows for the localization of both ultrastructural details as well as the protein of interest.

Through another genetic engineering application known as site-directed mutagenesis, researchers can alter the protein sequence and hence its structure, cellular localization, and susceptibility to regulation. This technique even allows the incorporation of unnatural amino acids into proteins, using modified tRNAs, and may allow the rational design of new proteins with novel properties.

Proteomics

The total complement of proteins present at a time in a cell or cell type is known as its proteome, and the study of such large-scale data sets defines the field of proteomics, named by analogy to the related field of genomics. Key experimental techniques in proteomics include 2D electrophoresis, which allows the separation of a large number of proteins, mass spectrometry, which allows rapid high-throughput identification of proteins and sequencing of peptides (most often after in-gel digestion), protein microarrays, which allow the detection of the relative levels of a large number of proteins present in a cell, and two-hybrid screening, which allows the systematic exploration of protein–protein interactions. The total complement of biologically possible such interactions is known as the interactome. A systematic attempt to determine the structures of proteins representing every possible fold is known as structural genomics.

Bioinformatics

A vast array of computational methods have been developed to analyze the structure, function, and evolution of proteins.

The development of such tools has been driven by the large amount of genomic and proteomic data available for a variety of organisms, including the human genome. It is simply impossible to study all proteins experimentally, hence only a few are subjected to laboratory experiments while computational tools are used to extrapolate to similar proteins. Such homologous proteins can be efficiently identified in distantly related organisms by sequence alignment. Genome and gene sequences can be searched by a variety of tools for certain properties. Sequence profiling tools can find restriction enzyme sites, open reading frames in nucleotide sequences, and predict secondary structures. Phylogenetic trees can be constructed and evolutionary hypotheses developed using special software like ClustalW regarding the ancestry of modern organisms and the genes they express. The field of bioinformatics is now indispensable for the analysis of genes and proteins.

Structure Prediction and Simulation

Complementary to the field of structural genomics, *protein structure prediction* develops efficient mathematical models of proteins to computationally predict their structures in theory, instead of detecting structures with laboratory observation. The most successful type of structure prediction, known as homology modeling, relies on the existence of a "template" structure with sequence similarity to the protein being modeled; structural genomics' goal is to provide sufficient representation in solved structures to model most of those that remain. Although producing accurate models remains a challenge when only distantly related template structures are available, it has been suggested that sequence alignment is the bottleneck in this process, as quite accurate models can be produced if a "perfect" sequence alignment is known. Many structure prediction methods have served to inform the emerging field of protein engineering, in which novel protein folds have already been designed. A more complex computational problem is the prediction of intermolecular interactions, such as in molecular docking and protein–protein interaction prediction.

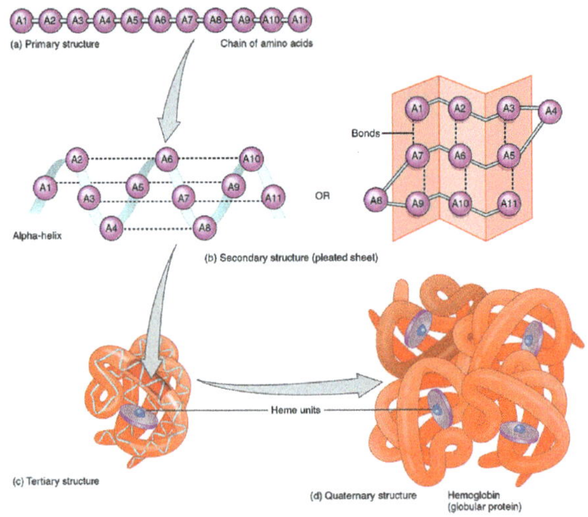

Constituent amino-acids can be analyzed to predict secondary, tertiary and quaternary protein structure, in this case hemoglobin containing heme units.

Mathematical models to simulate dynamic processes of protein folding and binding involve molecular mechanics, in particular, molecular dynamics. Monte Carlo techniques facilitate the computations, which exploit advances in parallel and distributed computing (for example, the Folding@home project which performs molecular modeling on GPUs). *In silico* simulations discovered the folding of small α-helical protein domains such as the villin headpiece and the HIV accessory protein. Hybrid methods combining standard molecular dynamics with quantum mechanical mathematics explored the electronic states of rhodopsins.

Protein Disorder and Unstructure Prediction

Many proteins (in Eucaryota ~33%) contain large unstructured but biologically functional segments and can be classified as intrinsically disordered proteins. Predicting and analysing protein disorder is, therefore, an important part of protein structure characterisation.

Nutrition

Most microorganisms and plants can biosynthesize all 20 standard amino acids, while animals (including humans) must obtain some of the amino acids from the diet. The amino acids that an organism cannot synthesize on its own are referred to as essential amino acids. Key enzymes that synthesize certain amino acids are not present in animals — such as aspartokinase, which catalyses the first step in the synthesis of lysine, methionine, and threonine from aspartate. If amino acids are present in the environment, microorganisms can conserve energy by taking up the amino acids from their surroundings and downregulating their biosynthetic pathways.

In animals, amino acids are obtained through the consumption of foods containing protein. Ingested proteins are then broken down into amino acids through digestion, which typically involves denaturation of the protein through exposure to acid and hydrolysis by enzymes called proteases. Some ingested amino acids are used for protein biosynthesis, while others are converted to glucose through gluconeogenesis, or fed into the citric acid cycle. This use of protein as a fuel is particularly important under starvation conditions as it allows the body's own proteins to be used to support life, particularly those found in muscle.

History and Etymology

Proteins were recognized as a distinct class of biological molecules in the eighteenth century by Antoine Fourcroy and others, distinguished by the molecules' ability to coagulate or flocculate under treatments with heat or acid. Noted examples at the time included albumin from egg whites, blood serum albumin, fibrin, and wheat gluten.

Proteins were first described by the Dutch chemist Gerardus Johannes Mulder and named by the Swedish chemist Jöns Jacob Berzelius in 1838. Mulder carried out elemental analysis of common proteins and found that nearly all proteins had the same empirical formula, $C_{400}H_{620}N_{100}O_{120}P_1S_1$. He came to the erroneous conclusion that they might be composed of a single type of (very large) molecule. The term "protein" to describe these molecules was proposed by Mulder's associate Berzelius; protein is derived from the Greek word (*proteios*), meaning "primary", "in the lead", or "standing in front", + *-in*. Mulder went on to identify the products of protein degradation such as the amino acid leucine for which he found a (nearly correct) molecular weight of 131 Da.

Early nutritional scientists such as the German Carl von Voit believed that protein was the most important nutrient for maintaining the structure of the body, because it was generally believed that "flesh makes flesh." Karl Heinrich Ritthausen extended known protein forms with the identification of glutamic acid. At the Connecticut Agricultural Experiment Station a detailed review of the vegetable proteins was compiled by Thomas Burr Osborne. Working with Lafayette Mendel and applying Liebig's law of the minimum in feeding laboratory rats, the nutritionally essential amino acids were established. The work was continued and communicated by William Cumming Rose. The understanding of proteins as polypeptides came through the work of Franz Hofmeister and Hermann Emil Fischer in 1902. The central role of proteins as enzymes in living organisms was not fully appreciated until 1926, when James B. Sumner showed that the enzyme urease was in fact a protein.

The difficulty in purifying proteins in large quantities made them very difficult for early protein biochemists to study. Hence, early studies focused on proteins that could be purified in large quantities, e.g., those of blood, egg white, various toxins, and digestive/metabolic enzymes obtained from slaughterhouses. In the 1950s, the Armour Hot Dog Co. purified 1 kg of pure bovine pancreatic ribonuclease A and made it freely available to scientists; this gesture helped ribonuclease A become a major target for biochemical study for the following decades.

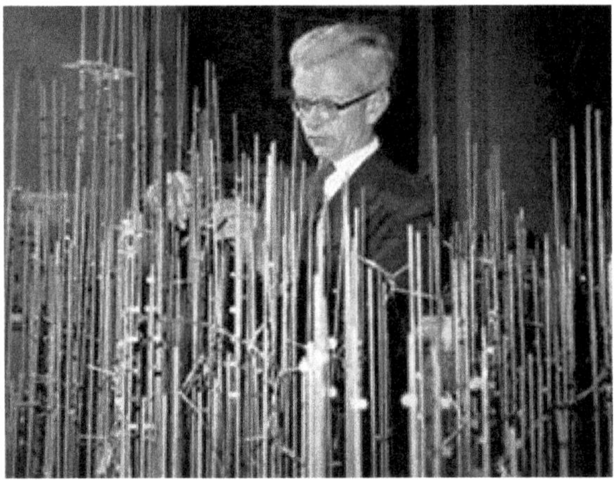

John Kendrew with model of myoglobin in progress

Linus Pauling is credited with the successful prediction of regular protein secondary structures based on hydrogen bonding, an idea first put forth by William Astbury in 1933. Later work by Walter Kauzmann on denaturation, based partly on previous studies by Kaj Linderstrøm-Lang, contributed an understanding of protein folding and structure mediated by hydrophobic interactions.

The first protein to be sequenced was insulin, by Frederick Sanger, in 1949. Sanger correctly determined the amino acid sequence of insulin, thus conclusively demonstrating that proteins consisted of linear polymers of amino acids rather than branched chains, colloids, or cyclols. He won the Nobel Prize for this achievement in 1958.

The first protein structures to be solved were hemoglobin and myoglobin, by Max Perutz and Sir John Cowdery Kendrew, respectively, in 1958. As of 2017, the Protein Data Bank has over 126,060 atomic-resolution structures of proteins. In more recent times, cryo-electron microscopy of large macromolecular assemblies and computational protein structure prediction of small protein domains are two methods approaching atomic resolution.

Amino Acid

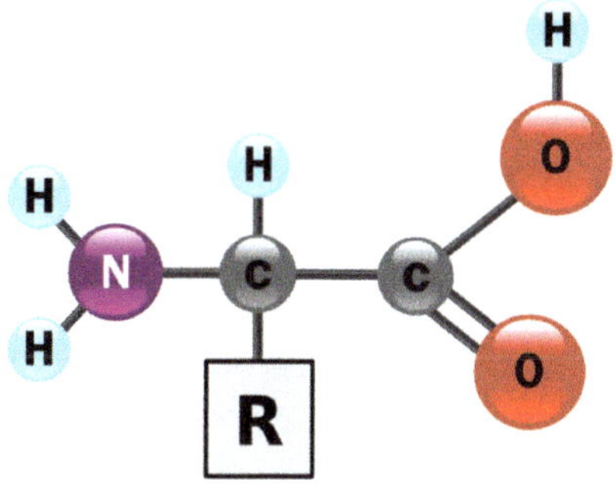

The structure of an alpha amino acid in its un-ionized form

Amino acids are organic compounds containing amine ($-NH_2$) and carboxyl (-COOH) functional groups, along with a side chain (R group) specific to each amino acid. The key elements of an amino acid are carbon, hydrogen, oxygen, and nitrogen, although other elements are found in the side chains of certain amino acids. About 500 amino acids are known (though only 20 appear in the genetic code) and can be classified in many ways. They can be classified according to the core structural functional groups' locations as alpha- (α-), beta- (β-), gamma- (γ-) or delta- (δ-) amino acids; other categories relate to polarity, pH level, and side chain group type (aliphatic, acyclic, aromatic, containing hydroxyl or sulfur, etc.). In the form of proteins, amino acid residues form the second-largest component (water is the largest) of human muscles and other tissues. Beyond their role as residues in proteins, amino acids participate in a number of processes such as neurotransmitter transport and biosynthesis.

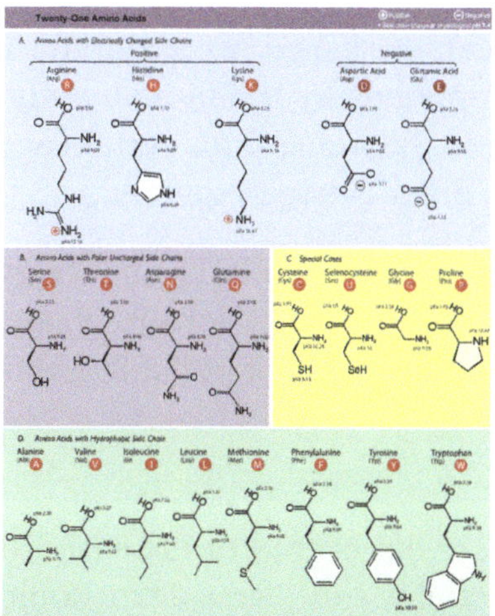

The 21 proteinogenic α-amino acids found in eukaryotes, grouped according to their side chains' pK_a values and charges carried at physiological pH 7.4

In biochemistry, amino acids having both the amine and the carboxylic acid groups attached to the first (alpha-) carbon atom have particular importance. They are known as 2-, alpha-, or α-amino acids (generic formula $H_2NCHRCOOH$ in most cases, where R is an organic substituent known as a "side chain"); often the term "amino acid" is used to refer specifically to these. They include the 22 proteinogenic ("protein-building") amino acids, which combine into peptide chains ("polypeptides") to form the building-blocks of a vast array of proteins. These are all L-stereoisomers ("left-handed" isomers), although a few D-amino acids ("right-handed") occur in bacterial envelopes, as a neuromodulator (D-serine), and in some antibiotics. Twenty of the proteinogenic amino acids are encoded directly by triplet codons in the genetic code and are known as "standard" amino acids. The other two ("non-standard" or "non-canonical") are selenocysteine (present in many prokaryotes as well as most eukaryotes, but not coded directly by DNA), and pyrrolysine (found only in some archea and one bacterium). Pyrrolysine and selenocysteine are encoded via variant codons; for example, selenocysteine is encoded by stop codon and SECIS element. *N*-formylmethionine (which is often the initial amino acid of proteins in bacteria, mitochondria, and chloroplasts) is generally considered as a form of methionine rather than as a separate proteinogenic amino acid. Codon–tRNA combinations not found in nature can also be used to "expand" the genetic code and form novel proteins known as alloproteins incorporating non-proteinogenic amino acids.

Many important proteinogenic and non-proteinogenic amino acids have biological functions. For example, in the human brain, glutamate (standard glutamic acid) and gamma-amino-butyric acid ("GABA", non-standard gamma-amino acid) are, respectively, the main excitatory and inhibitory neurotransmitters. Hydroxyproline, a major component of the connective tissue collagen), is synthesised from proline. Glycine is a biosynthetic precursor to porphyrins used in red blood cells. Carnitine is used in lipid transport.

Nine proteinogenic amino acids are called "essential" for humans because they cannot be produced from other compounds by the human body and so must be taken in as food. Others may be conditionally essential for certain ages or medical conditions. Essential amino acids may also differ between species.

Because of their biological significance, amino acids are important in nutrition and are commonly used in nutritional supplements, fertilizers, and food technology. Industrial uses include the production of drugs, biodegradable plastics, and chiral catalysts.

History

The first few amino acids were discovered in the early 19th century. In 1806, French chemists Louis-Nicolas Vauquelin and Pierre Jean Robiquet isolated a compound in asparagus that was subsequently named asparagine, the first amino acid to be discovered. Cystine was discovered in 1810, although its monomer, cysteine, remained undiscovered until 1884. Glycine and leucine were discovered in 1820. The last of the 20 common amino acids to be discovered was threonine in 1935 by William Cumming

Rose, who also determined the essential amino acids and established the minimum daily requirements of all amino acids for optimal growth.

Usage of the term *amino acid* in the English language is from 1898. Proteins were found to yield amino acids after enzymatic digestion or acid hydrolysis. In 1902, Emil Fischer and Franz Hofmeister proposed that proteins are the result of the formation of bonds between the amino group of one amino acid with the carboxyl group of another, in a linear structure that Fischer termed "peptide".

General Structure

In the structure shown at the top of the page, R represents a side chain specific to each amino acid. The carbon atom next to the carboxyl group (which is therefore numbered 2 in the carbon chain starting from that functional group) is called the α–carbon. Amino acids containing an amino group bonded directly to the alpha carbon are referred to as *alpha amino acids*. These include amino acids such as proline which contain secondary amines, which used to be often referred to as "imino acids".

Isomerism

The alpha amino acids are the most common form found in nature, but only when occurring in the L-isomer. The alpha carbon is a chiral carbon atom, with the exception of glycine which has two indistinguishable hydrogen atoms on the alpha carbon. Therefore, all alpha amino acids but glycine can exist in either of two enantiomers, called L or D amino acids, which are mirror images of each other. While L-amino acids represent all of the amino acids found in proteins during translation in the ribosome, D-amino acids are found in some proteins produced by enzyme posttranslational modifications after translation and translocation to the endoplasmic reticulum, as in exotic sea-dwelling organisms such as cone snails. They are also abundant components of the peptidoglycan cell walls of bacteria, and D-serine may act as a neurotransmitter in the brain. D-amino acids are used in racemic crystallography to create centrosymmetric crystals, which (depending on the protein) may allow for easier and more robust protein structure determination. The L and D convention for amino acid configuration refers not to the optical activity of the amino acid itself but rather to the optical activity of the isomer of glyceraldehyde from which that amino acid can, in theory, be synthesized (D-glyceraldehyde is dextrorotatory; L-glyceraldehyde is levorotatory). In alternative fashion, the *(S)* and *(R)* designators are used to indicate the absolute stereochemistry. Almost all of the amino acids in proteins are *(S)* at the α carbon, with cysteine being *(R)* and glycine non-chiral. Cysteine has its side chain in the same geometric position as the other amino acids, but the *R/S* terminology is reversed because of the higher atomic number of sulfur compared to the carboxyl oxygen gives the side chain a higher priority, whereas the atoms in most other side chains give them lower priority.

Side Chains

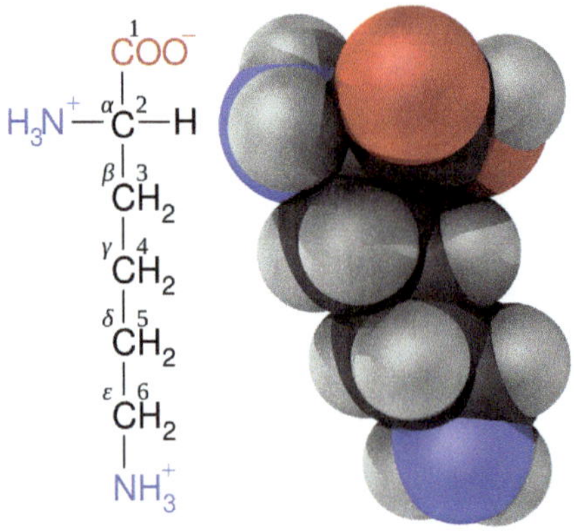

Lysine with carbon atoms labeled

In amino acids that have a carbon chain attached to the α–carbon (such as lysine) the carbons are labeled in order as α, β, γ, δ, and so on. In some amino acids, the amine group is attached to the β or γ-carbon, and these are therefore referred to as *beta* or *gamma amino acids.*

Amino acids are usually classified by the properties of their side chain into four groups. The side chain can make an amino acid a weak acid or a weak base, and a hydrophile if the side chain is polar or a hydrophobe if it is nonpolar. The chemical structures of the 22 standard amino acids, along with their chemical properties, are described.

The phrase "branched-chain amino acids" or BCAA refers to the amino acids having aliphatic side chains that are non-linear; these are leucine, isoleucine, and valine. Proline is the only proteinogenic amino acid whose side-group links to the α-amino group and, thus, is also the only proteinogenic amino acid containing a secondary amine at this position. In chemical terms, proline is, therefore, an imino acid, since it lacks a primary amino group, although it is still classed as an amino acid in the current biochemical nomenclature, and may also be called an "N-alkylated alpha-amino acid".

Zwitterions

The α-carboxylic acid group of amino acids is a weak acid, meaning that it releases a hydron (such as a proton) at moderate pH values. In other words, carboxylic acid groups ($-CO_2H$) can be deprotonated to become negative carboxylates ($-CO_2^-$). The negatively charged carboxylate ion predominates at pH values greater than the pKa of the carboxylic acid group (mean for the 20 common amino acids is about 2.2). In a complementary fashion, the α-amine of amino acids is a weak base, meaning that it accepts a proton at moderate pH values. In other words, α-amino groups (NH_2-) can be protonated to become positive α-ammonium groups ($^+NH_3-$). The positively charged α-ammonium group predominates at pH values less than the pKa of the α-ammonium group (mean for the 20 common α-amino acids is about 9.4).

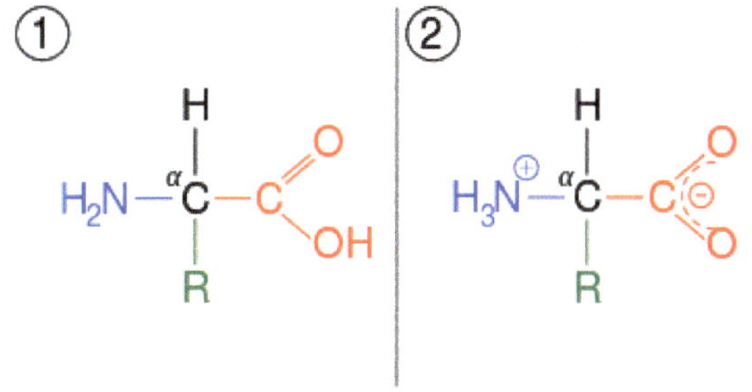

An amino acid in its (1) un-ionized and (2) zwitterionic forms

Because all amino acids contain amine and carboxylic acid functional groups, they share amphiprotic properties. Below pH 2.2, the predominant form will have a neutral carboxylic acid group and a positive α-ammonium ion (net charge +1), and above pH 9.4, a negative carboxylate and neutral α-amino group (net charge −1). But at pH between 2.2 and 9.4, an amino acid usually contains both a negative carboxylate and a positive α-ammonium group, as shown in structure (2) on the right, so has net zero charge. This molecular state is known as a zwitterion, from the German Zwitter meaning *hermaphrodite* or *hybrid.* The fully neutral form (structure (1) on the right) is a very minor species in aqueous solution throughout the pH range (less than 1 part in 10^7). Amino acids exist as zwitterions also in the solid phase, and crystallize with salt-like properties unlike typical organic acids or amines.

Isoelectric Point

The variation in titration curves when the amino acids are grouped by category can be seen here. With the exception of tyrosine, using titration to distinguish between hydrophobic amino acids is problematic.

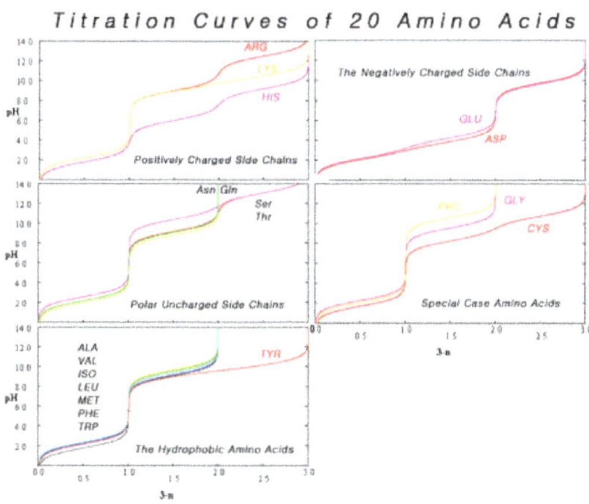

Composite of titration curves of twenty proteinogenic amino acids grouped by side chain category.

At pH values between the two pKa values, the zwitterion predominates, but coexists in dynamic equilibrium with small amounts of net negative and net positive ions. At the exact midpoint between the two pKa values, the trace amount of net negative and trace of net positive ions exactly balance, so that average net charge of all forms present is zero. This pH is known as the isoelectric point pI, so pI = ½(pKa_1 + pKa_2). The individual amino acids all have slightly different pKa values, so have different isoelectric points. For amino acids with charged side chains, the pKa of the side chain is involved. Thus for Asp, Glu with negative side chains, pI = ½(pKa_1 + pKa_R), where pKa_R is the side chain pKa. Cysteine also has potentially negative side chain with pKa_R = 8.14, so pI should be calculated as for Asp and Glu, even though the side chain is not significantly charged at neutral pH. For His, Lys, and Arg with positive side chains, pI = ½(pKa_R + pKa_2). Amino acids have zero mobility in electrophoresis at their isoelectric point, although this behaviour is more usually exploited for peptides and proteins than single amino acids. Zwitterions have minimum solubility at their isoelectric point and some amino acids (in particular, with non-polar side chains) can be isolated by precipitation from water by adjusting the pH to the required isoelectric point.

Occurrence and Functions in Biochemistry

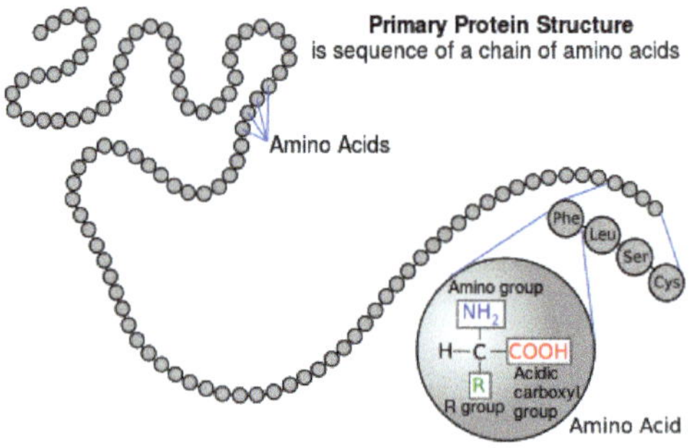

A polypeptide is an unbranched chain of amino acids.

Proteinogenic Amino Acids

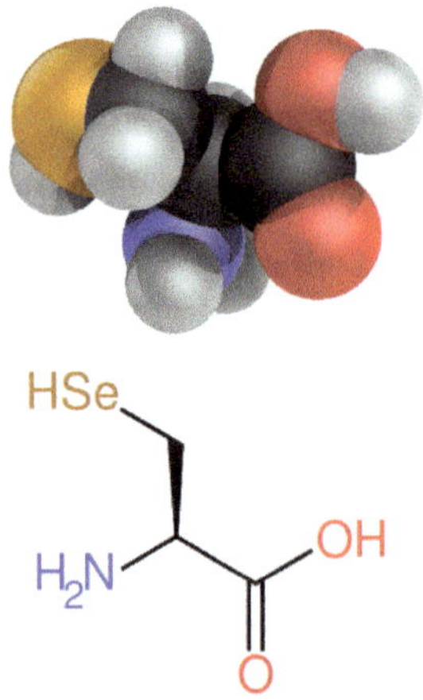

The amino acid selenocysteine

Amino acids are the structural units (monomers) that make up proteins. They join together to form short polymer chains called peptides or longer chains called either polypeptides or proteins. These polymers are linear and unbranched, with each amino acid within the chain attached to two neighboring amino acids. The process of making proteins is called *translation* and involves the step-by-step addition of amino acids to a growing protein chain by a ribozyme that is called a ribosome. The order in which the amino acids are added is read through the genetic code from an mRNA template, which is a RNA copy of one of the organism's genes.

Twenty-two amino acids are naturally incorporated into polypeptides and are called proteinogenic or natural amino acids. Of these, 20 are encoded by the universal genetic code. The remaining 2, selenocysteine and pyrrolysine, are incorporated into proteins by unique synthetic mechanisms. Selenocysteine is incorporated when the mRNA being translated includes a SECIS element, which causes the UGA codon to encode selenocysteine instead of a stop codon. Pyrrolysine is used by some methanogenic archaea in enzymes that they use to produce methane. It is coded for with the codon UAG, which is normally a stop codon in other organisms. This UAG codon is followed by a PYLIS downstream sequence.

Non-proteinogenic Amino Acids

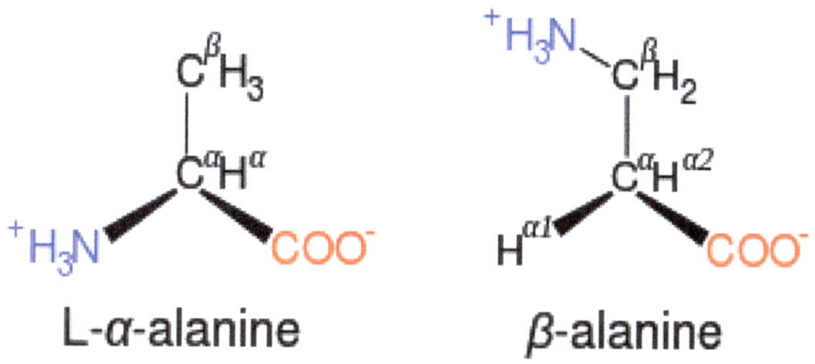

β-alanine and its α-alanine isomer

Aside from the 22 proteinogenic amino acids, many *non-proteinogenic* amino acids are known. Those either are not found in proteins (for example carnitine, GABA, Levothyroxine) or are not produced directly and in isolation by standard cellular machinery (for example, hydroxyproline and selenomethionine).

Non-proteinogenic amino acids that are found in proteins are formed by post-translational modification, which is modification after translation during protein synthesis. These modifications are often essential for the function or regulation of a protein. For example, the carboxylation of glutamate allows for better binding of calcium cations, and collagen contains hydroxyproline, generated by hydroxylation of proline. Another example is the formation of hypusine in the translation initiation factor EIF5A, through modification of a lysine residue. Such modifications can also determine the localization of the protein, e.g., the addition of long hydrophobic groups can cause a protein to bind to a phospholipid membrane.

Some non-proteinogenic amino acids are not found in proteins. Examples include 2-aminoisobutyric acid and the neurotransmitter gamma-aminobutyric acid. Non-proteinogenic amino acids often occur as intermediates in the metabolic pathways for standard amino acids – for example, ornithine and citrulline occur in the urea cycle, part of amino acid catabolism. A rare exception to the dominance of α-amino acids in biology is the β-amino acid beta alanine (3-aminopropanoic acid), which is used in plants and microorganisms in the synthesis of pantothenic acid (vitamin B_5), a component of coenzyme A.

D-amino Acid Natural Abundance

D-isomers are uncommon in live organisms. For instance, gramicidin is a polypeptide made up from mixture of D- and L-amino acids. Other compounds containing D-amino acid are tyrocidine and valinomycin. These compounds disrupt bacterial cell walls, particularly in Gram-positive bacteria. Only 837 D-amino acids were found in Swiss-Prot database (187 million amino acids analysed).

Non-standard Amino Acids

The 20 amino acids that are encoded directly by the codons of the universal genetic code are called *standard* or *canonical* amino acids. A modified form of methionine (*N*-formylmethionine) is often incorporated in place of methionine as the initial amino acid of proteins in bacteria, mitochondria and chloroplasts. Other amino acids are called *non-standard* or *non-canonical*. Most of the non-standard amino acids are also non-proteinogenic (i.e. they cannot be incorporated into proteins during translation), but two of them are proteinogenic, as they can be incorporated translationally into proteins by exploiting information not encoded in the universal genetic code.

The two non-standard proteinogenic amino acids are selenocysteine (present in many non-eukaryotes as well as most eukaryotes, but not coded directly by DNA) and pyrrolysine (found only in some archaea and one bacterium). The incorporation of these non-standard amino acids is rare. For example, 25 human proteins include selenocysteine (Sec) in their primary structure, and the structurally characterized enzymes (selenoenzymes) employ Sec as the catalytic moiety in their active sites. Pyrrolysine and selenocysteine are encoded via variant codons. For example, selenocysteine is encoded by stop codon and SECIS element.

In Human Nutrition

When taken up into the human body from the diet, the 20 standard amino acids either are used to synthesize proteins and other biomolecules or are oxidized to urea and carbon dioxide as a source of energy. The oxidation pathway starts with the removal of the amino group by a transaminase; the amino group is then fed into the urea cycle. The other product of transamidation is a keto acid that enters the citric acid cycle. Glucogenic amino acids can also be converted into glucose, through gluconeogenesis. Of the 20 standard amino acids, nine (His, Ile, Leu, Lys, Met, Phe, Thr, Trp and Val), are called essential amino acids because the human body cannot synthesize them from other compounds at the level needed for normal growth, so they must be obtained from food. In addition, cysteine, taurine, tyrosine, and arginine are considered semiessential amino-acids in children (though taurine is not technically an amino acid), because the metabolic pathways that synthesize these amino acids are not fully developed. The amounts required also depend on the age and health of the individual, so it is hard to make general statements about the dietary requirement for some amino acids. Dietary exposure to the non-standard amino acid BMAA has been linked to human neurodegenerative diseases, including ALS.

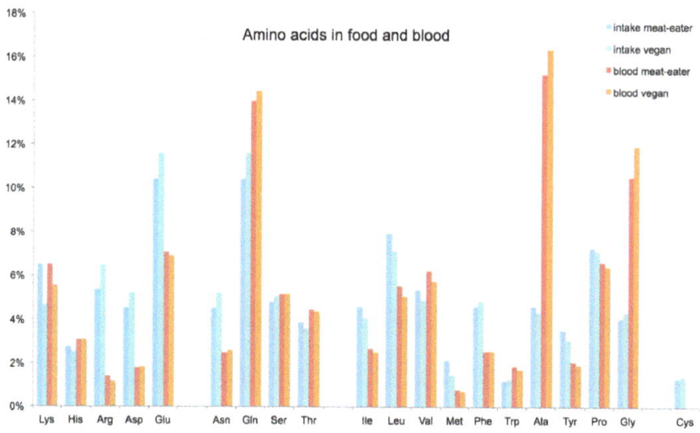

Share of amino acid in different human diets and the resulting mix of amino acids in human blood serum. Glutamate and glutamine are the most frequent in food at over 10%, while alanine, glutamine, and glycine are the most common in blood.

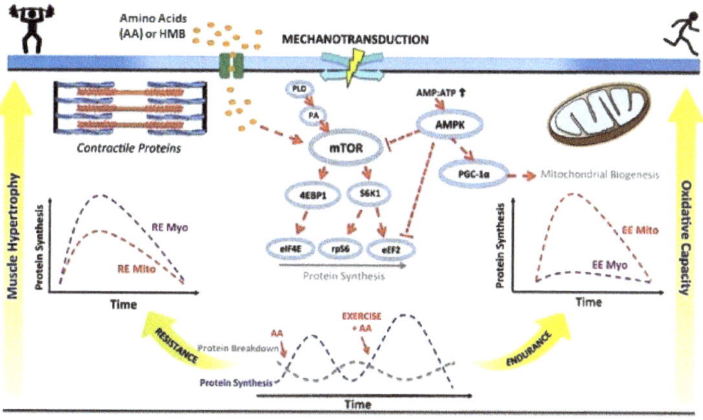

Diagram of the molecular signaling cascades that are involved in myofibrillar muscle protein synthesis and mitochondrial biogenesis in response to physical exercise and specific amino acids or their derivatives (primarily L-leucine and HMB). Many amino acids derived from food protein promote the activation of mTORC1 and increase protein synthesis by signaling through Rag GTPases.

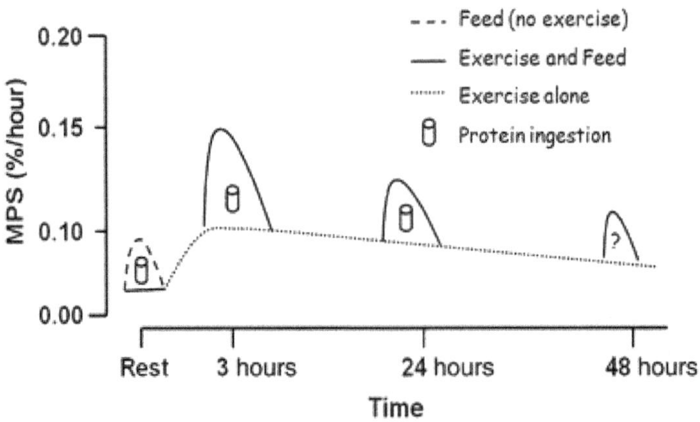

Resistance training stimulates muscle protein synthesis (MPS) for a period of up to 48 hours following exercise (shown by dotted line). Ingestion of a protein-rich meal at any point during this period will augment the exercise-induced increase in muscle protein synthesis (shown by solid lines).

Non-protein Functions

In humans, non-protein amino acids also have important roles as metabolic intermediates, such as in the biosynthesis of the neurotransmitter gamma-amino-butyric acid (GABA). Many amino acids are used to synthesize other molecules, for example:

- Tryptophan is a precursor of the neurotransmitter serotonin.
- Tyrosine (and its precursor phenylalanine) are precursors of the catecholamine neurotransmitters dopamine, epinephrine and norepinephrine and various trace amines.
- Phenylalanine is a precursor of phenethylamine and tyrosine in humans. In plants, it is a precursor of various phenylpropanoids, which are important in plant metabolism.
- Glycine is a precursor of porphyrins such as heme.
- Arginine is a precursor of nitric oxide.
- Ornithine and S-adenosylmethionine are precursors of polyamines.
- Aspartate, glycine, and glutamine are precursors of nucleotides. However, not all of the functions of other abundant non-standard amino acids are known.

Some non-standard amino acids are used as defenses against herbivores in plants. For example, canavanine is an analogue of arginine that is found in many legumes, and in particularly large amounts in *Canavalia gladiata* (sword bean). This amino acid protects the plants from predators such as insects and can cause illness in people if some types of legumes are eaten without processing. The non-protein amino acid mimosine is found in other species of legume, in particular *Leucaena leucocephala*. This compound is an analogue of tyrosine and can poison animals that graze on these plants.

Uses in Industry

Amino acids are used for a variety of applications in industry, but their main use is as additives to animal feed. This is necessary, since many of the bulk components of these feeds, such as soybeans, either have low levels or lack some of the essential amino acids: lysine, methionine, threonine, and tryptophan are most important in the production of these feeds. In this industry, amino acids are also used to chelate metal cations in order to improve the absorption of minerals from supplements, which may be required to improve the health or production of these animals.

The food industry is also a major consumer of amino acids, in particular, glutamic acid, which is used as a flavor enhancer, and aspartame (aspartyl-phenylalanine-1-methyl ester) as a low-calorie artificial sweetener. Similar technology to that used for animal nutrition is employed in the human nutrition industry to alleviate symptoms of mineral deficiencies, such as anemia, by improving mineral absorption and reducing negative side effects from inorganic mineral supplementation.

The chelating ability of amino acids has been used in fertilizers for agriculture to facilitate the delivery of minerals to plants in order to correct mineral deficiencies, such as iron chlorosis. These fertilizers are also used to prevent deficiencies from occurring and improving the overall health of the plants. The remaining production of amino acids is used in the synthesis of drugs and cosmetics.

Similarly, some amino acids derivatives are used in pharmaceutical industry. They include 5-HTP (5-hydroxytryptophan) used for experimental treatment of depression, L-DOPA (L-dihydroxyphenylalanine) for Parkinson's treatment, and eflornithine drug that inhibits ornithine decarboxylase and used in the treatment of sleeping sickness.

Expanded Genetic Code

Since 2001, 40 non-natural amino acids have been added into protein by creating a unique codon (recoding) and a corresponding transfer-RNA:aminoacyl – tRNA-synthetase pair to encode it with diverse physicochemical and biological properties in order to be used as a tool to exploring protein structure and function or to create novel or enhanced proteins.

Nullomers

Nullomers are codons that in theory code for an amino acid, however in nature there is a selective bias against using this codon in favor of another, for example bacteria prefer to use CGA instead of AGA to code for arginine. This creates some sequences that do not appear in the genome. This characteristic can be taken advantage of and used to create new selective cancer-fighting drugs and to prevent cross-contamination of DNA samples from crime-scene investigations.

Chemical Building Blocks

Amino acids are important as low-cost feedstocks. These compounds are used in chiral pool synthesis as enantiomerically pure building-blocks.

Amino acids have been investigated as precursors chiral catalysts, e.g., for asymmetric hydrogenation reactions, although no commercial applications exist.

Biodegradable Plastics

Amino acids are under development as components of a range of biodegradable polymers. These materials have applications as environmentally friendly packaging and in medicine in drug delivery and the construction of prosthetic implants. These polymers include polypeptides, polyamides, polyesters, polysulfides, and polyurethanes with amino acids either forming part of their main chains or bonded as side chains. These modifications alter the physical properties and reactivities of the polymers. An interesting example of such materials is polyaspartate, a water-soluble biodegradable polymer that may have applications in disposable diapers and agriculture. Due to its solubility and ability to chelate metal ions, polyaspartate is also being used as a biodegradeable anti-scaling agent and a corrosion inhibitor. In addition, the aromatic amino acid tyrosine is being developed as a possible replacement for toxic phenols such as bisphenol A in the manufacture of polycarbonates.

Reactions

As amino acids have both a primary amine group and a primary carboxyl group, these chemicals can undergo most of the reactions associated with these functional groups. These include nucleophilic addition, amide bond formation, and imine formation for the amine group, and esterification, amide bond formation, and decarboxylation for the carboxylic acid group. The combination of these functional groups allow amino acids to be effective polydentate ligands for metal-amino acid chelates. The multiple side chains of amino acids can also undergo chemical reactions. The types of these reactions are determined by the groups on these side chains and are, therefore, different between the various types of amino acid.

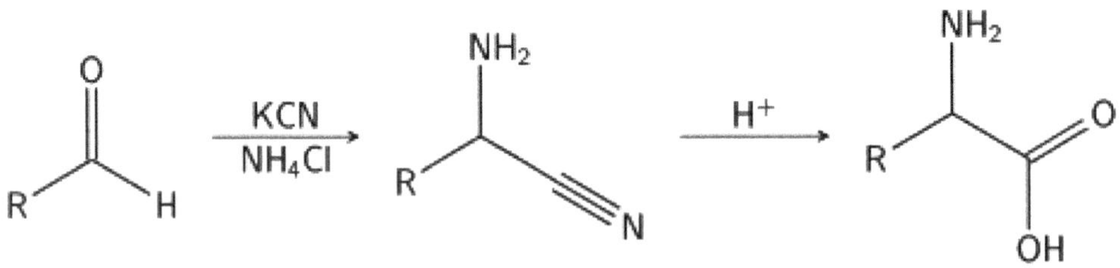

The Strecker amino acid synthesis

Chemical Synthesis

Several methods exist to synthesize amino acids. One of the oldest methods begins with the bromination at the α-carbon of a carboxylic acid. Nucleophilic substitution with ammonia then converts the alkyl bromide to the amino acid. In alternative fashion, the Strecker amino acid synthesis involves the treatment of an aldehyde with potassium cyanide and ammonia, this produces an α-amino nitrile as an intermediate. Hydrolysis of the nitrile in acid then yields a α-amino acid. Using ammonia or ammonium salts in this reaction gives unsubstituted amino acids, whereas substituting primary and secondary amines will yield substituted amino acids. Likewise, using ketones, instead of aldehydes, gives α,α-disubstituted amino acids. The classical synthesis gives racemic mixtures of α-amino acids as products, but several alternative procedures using asymmetric auxiliaries or asymmetric catalysts have been developed.

At the current time, the most-adopted method is an automated synthesis on a solid support (e.g., polystyrene beads), using protecting groups (e.g., Fmoc and t-Boc) and activating groups (e.g., DCC and DIC).

Peptide Bond Formation

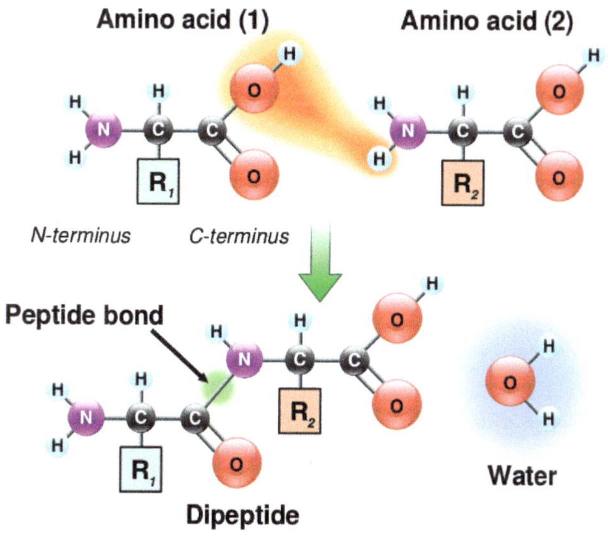

The condensation of two amino acids to form a *dipeptide* through a *peptide bond.*

As both the amine and carboxylic acid groups of amino acids can react to form amide bonds, one amino acid molecule can react with another and become joined through an amide linkage. This polymerization of amino acids is what creates proteins. This condensation reaction yields the newly formed peptide bond and a molecule of water. In cells, this reaction does not occur directly; instead, the amino acid is first activated by attachment to a transfer RNA molecule through an ester bond. This aminoacyl-tRNA is produced in an ATP-dependent reaction carried out by an aminoacyl tRNA synthetase.

This aminoacyl-tRNA is then a substrate for the ribosome, which catalyzes the attack of the amino group of the elongating protein chain on the ester bond. As a result of this mechanism, all proteins made by ribosomes are synthesized starting at their N-terminus and moving toward their C-terminus.

However, not all peptide bonds are formed in this way. In a few cases, peptides are synthesized by specific enzymes. For example, the tripeptide glutathione is an essential part of the defenses of cells against oxidative stress. This peptide is synthesized in two steps from free amino acids. In the first step, gamma-glutamylcysteine synthetase condenses cysteine and glutamic acid through a peptide bond formed between the side chain carboxyl of the glutamate (the gamma carbon of this side chain) and the amino group of the cysteine. This dipeptide is then condensed with glycine by glutathione synthetase to form glutathione.

In chemistry, peptides are synthesized by a variety of reactions. One of the most-used in solid-phase peptide synthesis uses the aromatic oxime derivatives of amino acids as activated units. These are added in sequence onto the growing peptide chain, which is attached to a solid resin support. The ability to easily synthesize vast numbers of different peptides by varying the types and order of amino acids (using combinatorial chemistry) has made peptide synthesis particularly important in creating libraries of peptides for use in drug discovery through high-throughput screening.

Biosynthesis

In plants, nitrogen is first assimilated into organic compounds in the form of glutamate, formed from alpha-ketoglutarate and ammonia in the mitochondrion. In order to form other amino acids, the plant uses transaminases to move the amino group to another alpha-keto carboxylic acid. For example, aspartate aminotransferase converts glutamate and oxaloacetate to alpha-ketoglutarate and aspartate. Other organisms use transaminases for amino acid synthesis, too.

Nonstandard amino acids are usually formed through modifications to standard amino acids. For example, homocysteine is formed through the transsulfuration pathway or by the demethylation of methionine via the intermediate metabolite S-adenosyl methionine, while hydroxyproline is made by a posttranslational modification of proline.

Microorganisms and plants can synthesize many uncommon amino acids. For example, some microbes make 2-aminoisobutyric acid and lanthionine, which is a sulfide-bridged derivative of alanine. Both of these amino acids are found in peptidic lantibiotics such as alamethicin. However, in plants, 1-aminocyclopropane-1-carboxylic acid is a small disubstituted cyclic amino acid that is a key intermediate in the production of the plant hormone ethylene.

Catabolism

Amino acids can be classified according to the properties of their main products as either of the following:

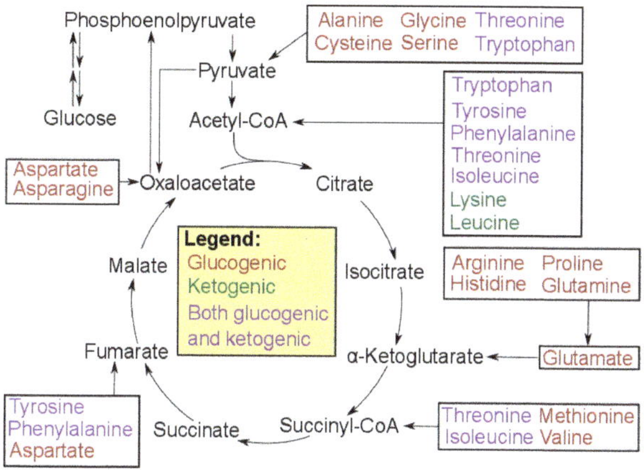

Catabolism of proteinogenic amino acids

- *Glucogenic,* with the products having the ability to form glucose by gluconeogenesis.
- *Ketogenic,* with the products not having the ability to form glucose. These products may still be used for ketogenesis or lipid synthesis.
- Amino acids catabolized into both glucogenic and ketogenic products.

Amino acids must first pass out of organelles and cells into blood circulation via amino acid transporters, since the amine and carboxylic acid groups are typically ionized. Degradation of an amino acid, occurring in the liver and kidneys, often involves deamination by moving its amino group to alpha-ketoglutarate, forming glutamate. This process involves transaminases, often the same as those used in amination during synthesis. In many vertebrates, the amino group is then removed through the urea cycle and is excreted in the form of urea. However, amino acid degradation can produce uric acid or ammonia instead. For example, serine dehydratase converts serine to pyruvate and ammonia. After removal of one or more amino groups, the remainder of the molecule can sometimes be used to synthesize new amino acids, or it can be used for energy by entering glycolysis or the citric acid cycle, as detailed in image at right.

Physicochemical Properties of Amino Acids

The 20 amino acids encoded directly by the genetic code can be divided into several groups based on their properties. Important factors are charge, hydrophilicity or hydrophobicity, size, and functional groups. These properties are important for protein structure and protein–protein interactions. The water-soluble proteins tend to have their hydrophobic residues (Leu, Ile, Val, Phe, and Trp) buried in the middle of the protein, whereas hydrophilic side chains are exposed to the aqueous solvent. (Note that in biochemistry, a residue refers to a specific monomer within the polymeric chain of a polysaccharide, protein or nucleic acid.) The integral membrane proteins tend to have outer rings of exposed hydrophobic amino acids that anchor them into the lipid bilayer. In the case part-way between these two extremes, some peripheral membrane proteins have a patch of hydrophobic amino acids on their surface that locks onto the membrane. In similar fashion, proteins that have to bind to positively charged molecules have surfaces rich with negatively charged amino acids like glutamate and aspartate, while proteins binding to negatively charged molecules have surfaces rich with positively charged chains like lysine and arginine. There are different hydrophobicity scales of amino acid residues.

Some amino acids have special properties such as cysteine, that can form covalent disulfide bonds to other cysteine residues, proline that forms a cycle to the polypeptide backbone, and glycine that is more flexible than other amino acids.

Many proteins undergo a range of posttranslational modifications, when additional chemical groups are attached to the amino acids in proteins. Some modifications can produce hydrophobic lipoproteins, or hydrophilic glycoproteins. These type of modification allow the reversible targeting of a protein to a membrane. For example, the addition and removal of the fatty acid palmitic acid to cysteine residues in some signaling proteins causes the proteins to attach and then detach from cell membranes.

Fat

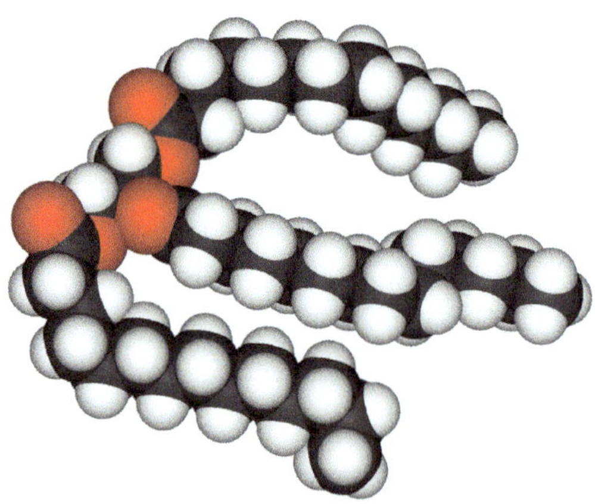

A fat, or triglyceride, molecule. Note the three fatty acid chains attached to the central glycerol portion of the molecule.

Fat is one of the three main macronutrients, along with carbohydrate and protein. Fats, also known as triglycerides, are esters of three fatty acid chains and the alcohol glycerol. The terms "oil", "fat", and "lipid" are often confused. "Oil" normally refers to a fat with short or unsaturated fatty acid chains that is liquid at room temperature, while "fat" may specifically refer to fats that are solids at room temperature. "Lipid" is the general term, though a lipid is not necessarily a triglyceride. Fats, like other lipids, are generally hydrophobic, and are soluble in organic solvents and insoluble in water.

Fat is an important foodstuff for many forms of life, and fats serve both structural and metabolic functions. They are a necessary part of the diet of most heterotrophs (including humans). Some fatty acids that are set free by the digestion of fats are called essential because they cannot be synthesized in the body from simpler constituents. There are two essential fatty acids (EFAs) in human nutrition: alpha-linolenic acid (an omega-3 fatty acid) and linoleic acid (an omega-6 fatty acid). Other lipids needed by the body can be synthesized from these and other fats. Fats and other lipids are broken down in the body by enzymes called lipases produced in the pancreas.

Fats and oils are categorized according to the number and bonding of the carbon atoms in the aliphatic chain. Fats that are saturated fats have no double bonds between the carbons in the chain. Unsaturated fats have one or more double bonded carbons in the chain. The nomenclature is based on the non-acid (non-carbonyl) end of the chain. This end is called the omega end or the n-end. Thus alpha-linolenic acid is called an omega-3 fatty acid because the 3rd carbon from that end is the first double bonded carbon in the chain counting from that end. Some oils and fats have multiple double bonds and are therefore called polyunsaturated fats. Unsaturated fats can be further divided into cis fats, which are the most common in nature, and trans fats, which are rare in nature. Unsaturated fats can be altered by reaction with hydrogen effected by a catalyst. This action, called hydrogenation, tends to break all the double bonds and makes a fully saturated fat. To make vegetable shortening, then, liquid *cis*-unsaturated fats such as vegetable oils are hydrogenated to produce saturated fats, which have more desirable physical properties e.g., they melt at a desirable temperature (30–40 °C), and store well, whereas polyunsaturated oils go rancid when they react with oxygen in the air. However, trans fats are generated during hydrogenation as contaminants created by an unwanted side reaction on the catalyst during partial hydrogenation.

Saturated fats can stack themselves in a closely packed arrangement, so they can solidify easily and are typically solid at room temperature. For example, animal fats tallow and lard are high in saturated fatty acid content and are solids. Olive and linseed oils on the other hand are unsaturated and liquid. Fats serve both as energy sources for the body, and as stores for energy in excess of what the body needs immediately. Each gram of fat when burned or metabolized releases about 9 food calories (37 kJ = 8.8 kcal). Fats are broken down in the healthy body to release their constituents, glycerol and fatty acids. Glycerol itself can be converted to glucose by the liver and so become a source of energy.

Chemical Structure

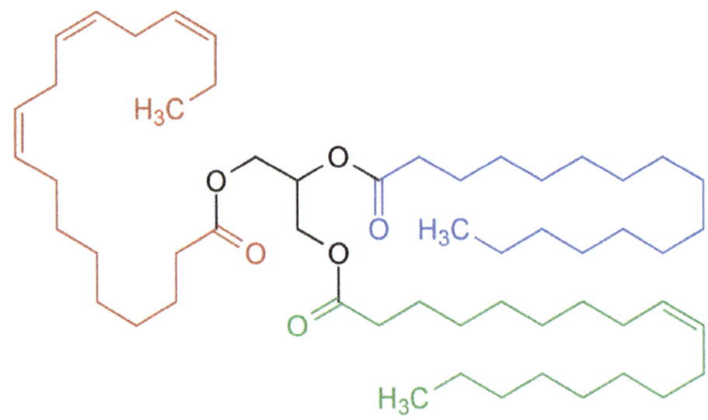

Example of a natural triglyceride with three different fatty acids. One fatty acid is saturated (blue highlighted), another contains one double bond within the carbon chain (green highlighted). The third fatty acid (a polyunsaturated fatty acid, highlighted in red) contains three double bonds within the carbon chain. All carbon-carbon double bonds shown are cis isomers.

There are many different kinds of fats, but each is a variation on the same chemical structure. All fats are derivatives of fatty acids and glycerol. Most fats are glycerides, particularly triglycerides (triesters of glycerol). One chain of fatty acid is bonded to each of the three -OH groups of the glycerol by the reaction of the carboxyl end of the fatty acid (-COOH) with the alcohol; I.e. three chains per molecule. Water is eliminated and the carbons are linked by an -O- bond through dehydration synthesis. This process is called esterification and fats are therefore esters. As a simple visual illustration, if the kinks and angles of these chains were straightened out, the molecule would have the shape of a capital letter E. The fatty acids would each be a horizontal line; the glycerol "backbone" would be the vertical line that joins the horizontal lines. Fats therefore have "ester" bonds.

Examples of fatty acids.		
***trans* Unsaturated (Example shown: Elaidic acid)**	***cis* Unsaturated (Example shown: Oleic acid)**	**Saturated (Example shown: Stearic acid)**
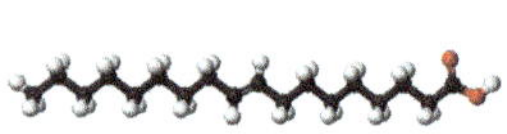	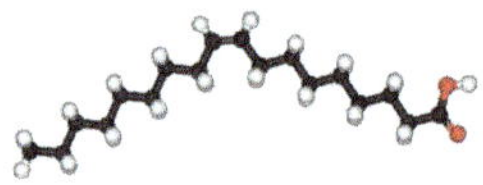	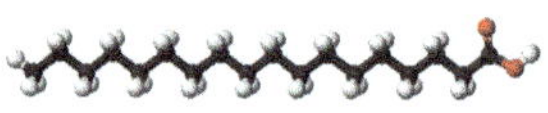
Elaidic acid is the principal *trans* unsaturated fatty acid often found in partially hydrogenated vegetable oils.	Oleic acid is a *cis* unsaturated fatty acid making up 55–80% of olive oil.	Stearic acid is a saturated fatty acid found in animal fats and is the intended product in full hydrogenation. Stearic acid is neither *cis* nor *trans* because it has no carbon-carbon double bonds.

The properties of any specific fat molecule depend on the particular fatty acids that constitute it. Fatty acids form a family of compounds that are composed of increasing numbers of carbon atoms linked into a zig-zag chain (hydrogen atoms to the side). The more carbon atoms there are in any fatty acid, the longer its chain will be. Long chains are more susceptible to intermolecular forces of attraction (in this case, van der Waals forces), and so the longer ones melt at a higher temperature (melting point).

Fatty acid chains may also differ by length, often categorized as short to very long.

- Short-chain fatty acids (SCFA) are fatty acids with aliphatic tails of fewer than six carbons (i.e. butyric acid).
- Medium-chain fatty acids (MCFA) are fatty acids with aliphatic tails of 6–12 carbons, which can form medium-chain triglycerides.
- Long-chain fatty acids (LCFA) are fatty acids with aliphatic tails 13 to 21 carbons.
- Very long chain fatty acids (VLCFA) are fatty acids with aliphatic tails longer than 22 carbons.

Any of these aliphatic fatty acid chains may be glycerated and the resultant fats may have tails of different lengths from very short triformin to very long, e.g., cerotic acid, or *hexacosanoic acid*, a 26-carbon long-chain saturated fatty acid. Long chain fats are exemplified by tallow (lard) whose chains are 17 carbons long. Most fats found in food, whether vegetable or animal, are made up of medium to long-chain fatty acids, usually of equal or nearly equal length. Many cell types can use either glucose or fatty acids for this energy. In particular, heart and skeletal muscle prefer fatty acids. Despite long-standing assertions to the contrary, fatty acids can also be used as a source of fuel for brain cells.

Importance for Living Organisms

Fats are also sources of essential fatty acids, an important dietary requirement. They provide energy as noted above. Vitamins A, D, E, and K are fat-soluble, meaning they can only be digested, absorbed, and transported in conjunction with fats. Fats play a vital role in maintaining healthy skin and hair, insulating body organs against shock, maintaining body temperature, and promoting healthy cell function. Fat also serves as a useful buffer against a host of diseases. When a particular substance, whether chemical or biotic, reaches unsafe levels in the bloodstream, the body can effectively dilute—or at least maintain equilibrium of—the offending substances by storing it in new fat tissue. This helps to protect vital organs, until such time as the offending substances can be metabolized or removed from the body by such means as excretion, urination, accidental or intentional bloodletting, sebum excretion, and hair growth.

Adipose Tissue

In animals, adipose, or fatty tissue is the body's means of storing metabolic energy over extended periods of time. Adipocytes (fat cells) store fat derived from the diet and from liver metabolism. Under energy stress these cells may degrade their stored fat to supply fatty acids and also glycerol to the circulation. These metabolic activities are regulated by several hormones (e.g., insulin, glucagon and epinephrine).

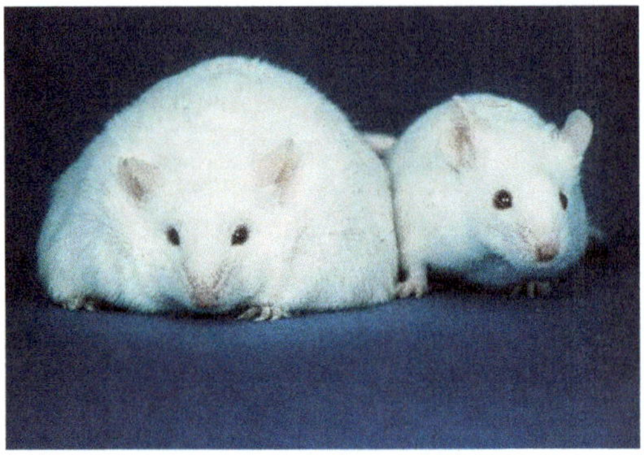

The obese mouse on the left has large stores of adipose tissue. For comparison, a mouse with a normal amount of adipose tissue is shown on the right.

The location of the tissue determines its metabolic profile: visceral fat is located within the abdominal wall (i.e., beneath the wall of abdominal muscle) whereas "subcutaneous fat" is located beneath the skin (and includes fat that is located in the abdominal area beneath the skin but *above* the abdominal muscle wall). Visceral fat was recently discovered to be a significant producer of signaling chemicals (i.e., hormones), among which several are involved in inflammatory tissue responses. One of these is resistin which has been linked to obesity, insulin resistance, and Type 2 diabetes. This latter result is currently controversial, and there have been reputable studies supporting all sides on the issue.

Fatty Acids and Human Health

Dietary consumption of fatty acids has effects on human health. Studies have found that replacing saturated fats with *cis* unsaturated fats in the diet reduces risk of cardiovascular disease. For example, a 2015 systematic review of randomized control trials by the Cochrane Library concluded: "Lifestyle advice to all those at risk of cardiovascular disease and to lower risk population groups should continue to include permanent reduction of dietary saturated fat and partial replacement by unsaturated fats."

Numerous studies have also found that consumption of *trans* fats increases risk of cardiovascular disease. The Harvard School of Public Health advises that replacing *trans* fats and saturated fats with *cis* monounsaturated and polyunsaturated fats is beneficial for health.

Saturated Fat

A saturated fat is a type of fat in which the fatty acids all have single bonds.

A fat is made of two kinds of smaller molecules: monoglyceride and fatty acids. Fats are made of long chains of carbon (C) atoms. Some carbon atoms are linked by single bonds (-C-C-) and others are linked by double bonds (-C=C-). Double bonds can react with hydrogen to form single bonds. They are called saturated, because the second bond is broken up and each half of the bond is attached to (saturated with) a hydrogen atom. Most animal fats are saturated. The fats of plants and fish are generally unsaturated. Saturated fats tend to have higher melting points than their corresponding unsaturated fats, leading to the popular understanding that saturated fats tend to be solids at room temperatures, while unsaturated fats tend to be liquid at room temperature with varying degrees of viscosity (meaning both saturated and unsaturated fats are found to be liquid at body temperature).

Various fats contain different proportions of saturated and unsaturated fat. Examples of foods containing a high proportion of saturated fat include animal fat products such as cream, cheese, butter, other whole milk dairy products and fatty meats which also contain dietary cholesterol. Certain vegetable products have high saturated fat content, such as coconut oil and palm kernel oil. Many prepared foods are high in saturated fat content, such as pizza, dairy desserts, and sausage.

The effect of saturated fat on risk of disease is controversial. Many reviews recommend a diet low in saturated fat and argue it will lower risks of cardiovascular diseases, diabetes, or death. However, other reviews have rejected those arguments or advocated for examining the proportion of saturated to unsaturated fat in the diet.

Fat Profiles

While nutrition labels regularly combine them, the saturated fatty acids appear in different proportions among food groups. Lauric and myristic acids are most commonly found in "tropical" oils (e.g., palm kernel, coconut) and dairy products. The saturated fat in meat, eggs, cacao, and nuts is primarily the triglycerides of palmitic and stearic acids.

Saturated Fat Profile of Common Foods; Esterified Fatty Acids as Percentage of Total Fat

Food	Lauric acid	Myristic acid	Palmitic acid	Stearic acid
Coconut oil	47%	18%	9%	3%
Palm kernel oil	48%	1%	44%	5%
Butter	3%	11%	29%	13%
Ground beef	0%	4%	26%	15%
Salmon	0%	1%	29%	3%
Egg yolks	0%	0.3%	27%	10%
Cashews	2%	1%	10%	7%
Soybean oil	0%	0%	11%	4%

Association with Diseases

Since the 1950s, it has been demonstrated that consumption of foods containing high amounts of saturated fatty acids (including meat fats, milk fat, butter, lard, coconut oil, palm oil, and palm kernel oil) is potentially less healthy than consuming fats with a lower proportion of saturated fatty acids. Sources of lower saturated fat but higher proportions of unsaturated fatty acids include olive oil, peanut oil, canola oil, avocados, corn, sunflower, soy, and cottonseed oils.

Cardiovascular Disease

The effect of saturated fat on cardiovascular disease is controversial.

Many health authorities such as the American Dietetic Association, the British Dietetic Association, American Heart Association, the World Heart Federation, the British National Health Service, among others, advise that saturated fat is a risk factor for cardiovascular disease. The World Health Organization in May 2015 recommends switching from saturated to unsaturated fats.

A number of systematic reviews have examined the relationship between saturated fat and cardiovascular disease and have come to different conclusions:

A 2015 systematic review found no association between consumption and risk of heart disease, stroke, diabetes, or death.

A 2014 systematic review looking at observational studies of dietary intake of fatty acids, observational studies of measured fatty acid levels in the blood, and intervention studies of polyunsaturated fat supplementation concludes that the findings "do not support cardiovascular guidelines that promote high consumption of long-chain omega-3 and omega-6 and polyunsaturated fatty acids and suggest reduced consumption of total saturated fatty acids." Researchers acknowledged that despite their results, further research is necessary, especially in people who are initially healthy. Until the picture becomes clearer, experts recommend people stick to the current guidelines on fat consumption.

Harcombe, 2015	No reduction in CHD and all-cause mortality were observed when replacing saturated fat with polyunsaturated fat, even though reductions in serum cholesterol were observed.
Schwab, 2014	There was convincing evidence that partial replacement of saturated fat with polyunsaturated fat decreases the risk of cardiovascular diseases, especially in men.
Hooper, 2012	Reducing saturated fat in diets did not reduce mortality, despite reducing the risk of having a cardiovascular event by 14 percent.
Micha, 2010	Based on consistent evidence from human studies, replacing saturated fatty acids with polyunsaturated fat modestly lowers coronary heart disease risk, with ~10% risk reduction for a 5% energy substitution; whereas replacing SFA with carbohydrate has no benefit and replacing SFA with monounsaturated fat has uncertain effects.

Mozaffarian, 2010	These findings provide evidence that consuming polyunsaturated fats (PUFA) in place of SFA reduces Coronary Heart Disease (CHD) events in randomized controlled trials (RCT). Replacing saturated fats with PUFAs as percentage of calories strongly reduced CHD mortality.
Siri-Tarino, 2010	5–23 years of follow-up of 347,747 subjects, 11,006 developed CHD or stroke. A meta-analysis of prospective epidemiologic studies showed that there is no significant evidence for concluding that dietary saturated fat is associated with an increased risk of CHD or CVD.
Danaei, 2009	Low PUFA intake has an 1-5% Increased risk of ischemic heart disease: Low dietary PUFA (in replacement of SFA). age 30–44 Increase in RR 1.05.
Mente, 2009	Single-nutrient RCTs have yet to evaluate whether reducing saturated fatty acid intake lowers the risk of CHD events. For polyunsaturated fatty acid intake, most of the RCTs have not been adequately powered and did not find a significant reduction in CHD outcomes.
Skeaff, 2009	Intake of SFA was not significantly associated with CHD mortality, with a RR of 1.14. Moreover, there was no significant association with CHD death. Intake of PUFA was strongly significantly associated with CHD mortality, with a RR of 1.25. The Health Professionals Follow-up Study and the EUROASPIRE study results mirrored those of total PUFA; intake of linoleic acid was significantly associated with CHD mortality.
Jakobsen, 2009	"The associations suggest that replacing saturated fatty acids with polyunsaturated fatty acids rather than monounsaturated fatty acids or carbohydrates prevents CHD over a wide range of intakes."
Van Horn, 2008	25-35% fats but <7% SFA and TFA reduces risk.

While many studies have found that including polyunsaturated fats in the diet in place of saturated fats produces more beneficial CVD outcomes, the effects of substituting monounsaturated fats or carbohydrates are unclear.

Dyslipidemia

The consumption of saturated fat is generally considered a risk factor for dyslipidemia, which in turn is a risk factor for some types of cardiovascular disease.

There are strong, consistent, and graded relationships between saturated fat intake, blood cholesterol levels, and the mass occurrence of cardiovascular disease. The relationships are accepted as causal. Abnormal blood lipid levels, that is high total cholesterol, high levels of triglycerides, high levels of low-density lipoprotein (LDL, "bad" cholesterol) or low levels of high-density lipoprotein (HDL, "good" cholesterol) cholesterol are all associated with increased risk of heart disease and stroke.

Meta-analyses have found a significant relationship between saturated fat and serum cholesterol levels. High total cholesterol levels, which may be caused by many factors, are associated with an increased risk of cardiovascular disease. However, other indicators measuring cholesterol such as high total/HDL cholesterol ratio are more predictive than total serum cholesterol. In a study of myocardial infarction in 52 countries, the ApoB/ApoA1 (related to LDL and HDL, respectively) ratio was the strongest predictor of CVD among all risk factors. There are other pathways involving obesity, triglyceride levels, insulin sensitivity, endothelial function, and thrombogenicity, among others, that play a role in CVD, although it seems, in the absence of an adverse blood lipid profile, the other known risk factors have only a weak atherogenic effect. Different saturated fatty acids have differing effects on various lipid levels.

Cancer

Breast Cancer

A meta-analysis published in 2003 found a significant positive relationship in both control and cohort studies between saturated fat and breast cancer. However two subsequent reviews have found weak or insignificant associations of saturated fat intake and breast cancer risk, and note the prevalence of confounding factors.

Colorectal Cancer

One review found limited evidence for a positive relationship between consuming animal fat and incidence of colorectal cancer.

Ovarian Cancer

A meta-analysis of eight observational studies published in 2001 found a statistically significant positive relationship between saturated fat and ovarian cancer. However, a 2013 study found that a pooled analysis of 12 cohort studies observed no association between total fat intake and ovarian cancer risk. Further analysis revealed that omega-3 fatty acids were protective against ovarian cancer and that trans fats were a risk factor. This study revealed that histological subtypes should be examined in determining the impact of dietary fat on ovarian cancer, rather than an oversimplified focus on total fat intake.

Prostate Cancer

Some researchers have indicated that serum myristic acid and palmitic acid and dietary myristic and palmitic saturated fatty acids and serum palmitic combined with alpha-tocopherol supplementation are associated with increased risk of prostate cancer in a dose-dependent manner. These associations may, however, reflect differences in intake or metabolism of these fatty acids between the precancer cases and controls, rather than being an actual cause.

Bones

Mounting evidence indicates that the amount and type of fat in the diet can have important effects on bone health. Most of this evidence is derived from animal studies. The data from one study indicated that bone mineral density is negatively associated with saturated fat intake, and that men may be particularly vulnerable.

Dietary Recommendations

Recommendations to reduce or limit dietary intake of saturated fats are made by the World Health Organization, Health Canada, the US Department of Health and Human Services, the UK Food Standards Agency, the Australian Department of Health and Aging, the Singapore Government Health Promotion Board, the Indian Government Citizens Health Portal, the New Zealand Ministry of Health, the Food and Drugs Board Ghana, the Republic of Guyana Ministry of Health, and Hong Kong's Centre for Food Safety.

In 2003, the World Health Organization (WHO) and Food and Agriculture Organization (FAO) expert consultation report concluded that "intake of saturated fatty acids is directly related to cardiovascular risk. The traditional target is to restrict the intake of saturated fatty acids to less than 10% of daily energy intake and less than 7% for high-risk groups. If populations are consuming less than 10%, they should not increase that level of intake. Within these limits, intake of foods rich in myristic and palmitic acids should be replaced by fats with a lower content of these particular fatty acids. In developing countries, however, where energy intake for some population groups may be inadequate, energy expenditure is high and body fat stores are low (BMI <18.5 kg/m^2). The amount and quality of fat supply has to be considered keeping in mind the need to meet energy requirements. Specific sources of saturated fat, such as coconut and palm oil, provide low-cost energy and may be an important source of energy for the poor."

A 2004 statement released by the Centers for Disease Control (CDC) determined that "Americans need to continue working to reduce saturated fat intake..." In addition, reviews by the American Heart Association led the Association to recommend reducing saturated fat intake to less than 7% of total calories according to its 2006 recommendations. This concurs with similar conclusions made by the US Department of Health and Human Services, which determined that reduction in saturated fat consumption would positively affect health and reduce the prevalence of heart disease.

The United Kingdom, National Health Service claims the majority of UK people eat too much saturated fat. The British Heart Foundation also advises people to cut down on saturated fat. People are advised to cut down on saturated fat and read labels on food they buy.

Dr. German and Dr. Dillard of University of California and Nestle Research Center in Switzerland, in their 2004 review, pointed out that "no lower safe limit of specific saturated fatty acid intakes has been identified" and recommended that the influence of varying saturated fatty acid intakes against a background of different individual lifestyles and genetic backgrounds should be the focus in future studies.

Blanket recommendations to lower saturated fat were criticized at a 2010 conference debate of the American Dietetic Association for focusing too narrowly on reducing saturated fats rather than emphasizing increased consumption of healthy fats and unrefined carbohydrates. Concern was expressed over the health risks of replacing saturated fats in the diet with refined carbohydrates, which carry a high risk of obesity and heart disease, particularly at the expense of polyunsaturated fats which may have health benefits. None of the panelists recommended heavy consumption of saturated fats, emphasizing instead the importance of overall dietary quality to cardiovascular health.

Molecular Description

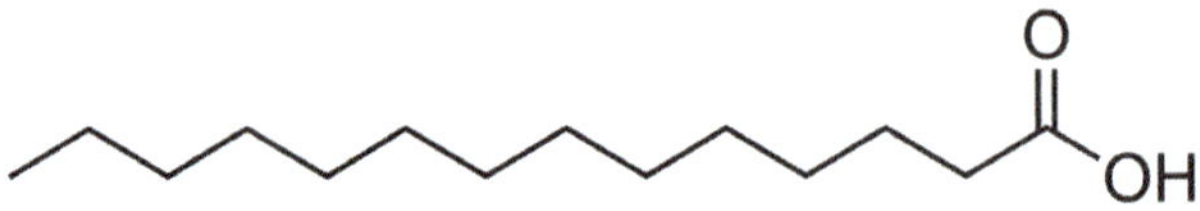

Two-dimensional representation of the saturated fatty acid myristic acid

It should be noted, as this is the defining factor of saturated fats, that the two-dimensional illustration has implicit hydrogen atoms bonded to each of the carbon atoms in the polycarbon tail of the myristic acid molecule (there are 13 carbon atoms in the tail; 14 carbon atoms in the entire molecule).

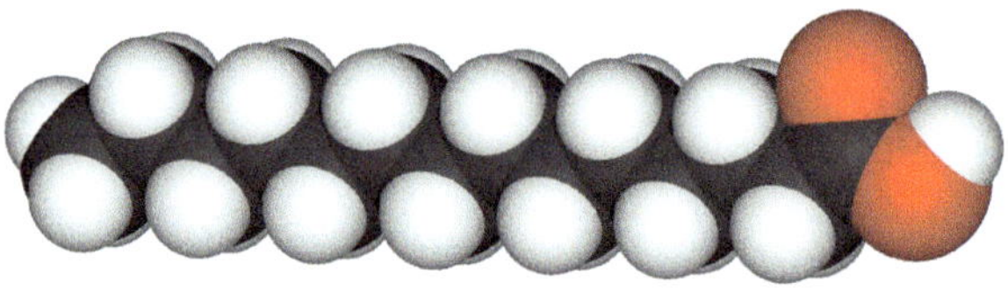

A space-filling model of the saturated fatty acid myristic acid

Carbon atoms are also implicitly drawn, as they are portrayed as intersections between two straight lines. "Saturated," in general, refers to a maximum number of hydrogen atoms bonded to each carbon of the polycarbon tail as allowed by the Octet Rule. This also means that only single bonds (sigma bonds) will be present between adjacent carbon atoms of the tail.

Monounsaturated Fat

In biochemistry and nutrition, monounsaturated fatty acids (abbreviated MUFAs, or more plainly monounsaturated fats) are fatty acids that have one double bond in the fatty acid chain with all of the remainder carbon atoms being single-bonded. By contrast, polyunsaturated fatty acids (PUFAs) have more than one double bond.

Fatty acids are long-chained molecules having an alkyl group at one end and a carboxylic acid group at the other end. Fatty acid viscosity (thickness) and melting temperature increases with decreasing number of double bonds; therefore, monounsaturated fatty acids have a higher melting point than polyunsaturated fatty acids (more double bonds) and a lower melting point than saturated fatty acids (no double bonds). Monounsaturated fatty acids are liquids at room temperature and semisolid or solid when refrigerated.

Molecular Description of Monounsaturated Fatty Acids

Common monounsaturated fatty acids are palmitoleic acid (16:1 n−7), cis-vaccenic acid (18:1 n−7) and oleic acid (18:1 n−9). Palmitoleic acid has 16 carbon atoms with the first double bond occurring 7 carbon atoms away from the methyl group (and 9 carbons from the carboxyl end). It can be lengthened to the 18-carbon cis-vaccenic acid. Oleic acid has 18 carbon atoms with the first double bond occurring 9 carbon atoms away from the carboxylic acid group. The illustrations below show a molecule of oleic acid in Lewis formula and as a space-filling model.

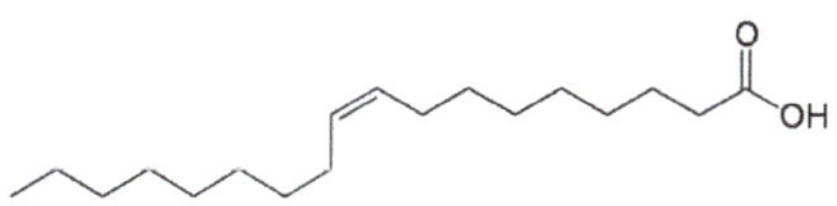

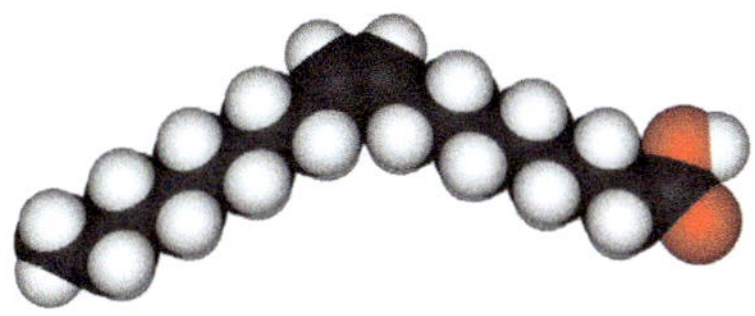

Relation to Health

Polyunsaturated fats protect against cardiovascular disease by providing more membrane fluidity than monounsaturated fats, but they are more vulnerable to lipid peroxidation (rancidity). The large scale KANWU study found that increasing monounsaturated fat and decreasing saturated fat intake could improve insulin sensitivity, but only when the overall fat intake of the diet was low. However, some monounsaturated fatty acids (in the same way as saturated fats) may promote insulin resistance, whereas polyunsaturated fatty acids may be protective against insulin resistance. Studies have shown that substituting dietary monounsaturated fat for saturated fat is associated with increased daily physical activity and resting energy expenditure. More physical activity was associated with a higher-oleic acid diet than one of a palmitic acid diet. From the study, it is shown that more monounsaturated fats lead to less anger and irritability.

Foods containing monounsaturated fats reduce low-density lipoprotein (LDL) cholesterol, while possibly increasing high-density lipoprotein (HDL) cholesterol. However, their true ability to raise HDL is still in debate.

Levels of oleic along with other monounsaturated fatty acids in red blood cell membranes were positively associated with breast cancer risk. The saturation index (SI) of the same membranes was inversely associated with breast cancer risk. Monounsaturated fats and low SI in erythrocyte membranes are predictors of postmenopausal breast cancer. Both of these variables depend on the activity of the enzyme delta-9 desaturase (Δ9-d).

In children, consumption of monounsaturated oils is associated with healthier serum lipid profiles.

The Mediterranean Diet is one heavily influenced by monounsaturated fats. People in Mediterranean countries consume more total fat than Northern European countries, but most of the fat is in the form of monounsaturated fatty acids from olive oil and omega-3 fatty acids from fish, vegetables, and certain meats like lamb, while consumption of saturated fat is minimal in comparison. The diet in Crete is fairly high in total fat (40% of total calories, almost exclusively provided by olive oil) yet affords a remarkable protection from coronary heart disease (and probably colon cancer) , but unlikely from breast cancer due to a very high oleic acid content.

Natural Sources

Monounsaturated fats are found in natural foods such as red meat, whole milk products, nuts and high fat fruits such as olives and avocados. Olive oil is about 75% monounsaturated fat. The high oleic variety sunflower oil contains as much as 85% monounsaturated fat. Canola oil and Cashews are both about 58% monounsaturated fat. Tallow (beef fat) is about 50% monounsaturated fat and lard is about 40% monounsaturated fat. Other sources include avocado oil, macadamia nut oil, grapeseed oil, groundnut oil (peanut oil), sesame oil, corn oil, popcorn, whole grain wheat, cereal, oatmeal, almond oil, sunflower oil, hemp oil, and tea-oil Camellia.

Polyunsaturated Fat

Polyunsaturated fats are lipids in which the constituent hydrocarbon chain possesses two or more carbon–carbon double bonds. Polyunsaturated fat can be found mostly in nuts, seeds, fish, seed oils, and oysters. "Unsaturated" refers to the fact that the molecules contain less than the maximum amount of hydrogen (if there were no double bonds). These materials exist as *cis* or *trans* isomers depending on the geometry of the double bond.

Saturated fats have hydrocarbon chains which can be most readily aligned. The hydrocarbon chains in trans fats align more readily than those in cis fats, but less well than those in saturated fats. This means that, in general, the melting points of fats increase from cis to trans unsaturated and then to saturated.

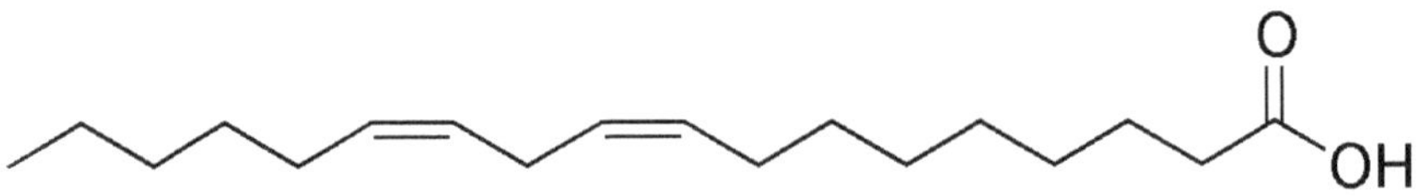

Chemical structure of the polyunsaturated fat linoleic acid.

The position of the carbon-carbon double bonds in carboxylic acid chains in fats is designated by Greek letters. The carbon atom closest to the carboxyl group is the *alpha* carbon, the next carbon is the *beta* carbon and so on. In fatty acids the carbon atom of the methyl group at the end of the hydrocarbon chain is called the *omega* carbon because *omega* is the last letter of the Greek alphabet. Omega-3 fatty acids have a double bond three carbons away from the methyl carbon, whereas omega-6 fatty acids have a double bond six carbons away from the methyl carbon. The illustration below shows the omega-6 fatty acid, linoleic acid.

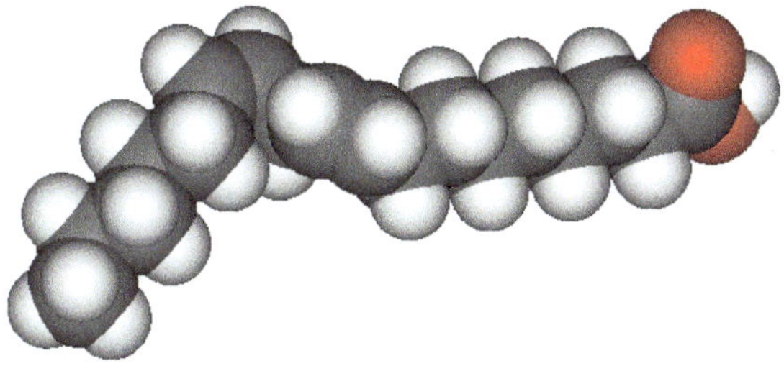

Representation of linoleic acid in a bent conformation.

While it is the *nutritional* aspects of polyunsaturated fats that are generally of greatest interest, these materials do also have non-food applications. Drying oils, which polymerize on exposure to oxygen to form solid films, are polyunsaturated fats. The most common ones are linseed (flax seed) oil, tung oil, poppy seed oil, perilla oil, and walnut oil. These oils are used to make paints and varnishes.

Health

Potential Benefits

In preliminary research, omega-3 fatty acids in algal oil, fish oil, fish and seafood have been shown to lower the risk of heart attacks. Other preliminary research indicates that omega-6 fatty acids in sunflower oil and safflower oil may also reduce the risk of cardiovascular disease.

Among n-3 fatty acids [Omega-3], neither long-chain nor short-chain forms were consistently associated with breast cancer risk. High levels of docosahexaenoic acid (DHA), however, the most abundant n-3 PUFA [Omega-3] in erythrocyte (red blood cell) membranes, were associated with a reduced risk of breast cancer. The DHA obtained through the consumption of polyunsaturated fatty acids is positively associated with cognitive and behavioral performance. In addition DHA is vital for the grey matter structure of the human brain, as well as retinal stimulation and neurotransmission.

Dietary intake of polyunsaturated fatty acids is under preliminary research to assess the risk of developing amyotrophic lateral sclerosis (ALS, Lou Gehrig's Disease).

The importance of the ratio of omega-6/omega-3 essential fatty acids as established by comparative studies shows an Omega-6:Omega-3 ratio under 4:1 may contribute to health.

Contrary to conventional advice, an evaluation of evidence from 1966-1973 pertaining to the health impacts of replacing dietary saturated fat with linoleic acid found that participants in the group doing so had *increased* rates of death from all causes, coronary heart disease, and cardiovascular disease. Although this evaluation was disputed by many scientists, it fueled debate over worldwide dietary advice to substitute polyunsaturated fats for saturated fats.

Pregnancy

Polyunsaturated fat supplementation does not decrease the incidence of pregnancy-related disorders, such as hypertension or preeclampsia, but may increase the length of gestation slightly and decreased the incidence of early premature births.

Expert panels in the United States and Europe recommend that pregnant and lactating women consume higher amounts of polyunsaturated fats than the general population to enhance the DHA status of the fetus and newborn.

Cancer

Results from observational clinical trials on polyunsaturated fat intake and cancer have been inconsistent and vary by numerous factors of cancer incidence, including gender and genetic risk. Some studies have shown associations between higher intakes and/or blood levels of polyunsaturated fat omega-3s and a decreased risk of certain cancers, including breast and colorectal cancer, while other studies found no associations with cancer risk.

Food Sources

Food sources of polyunsaturated fats include:

Food Source (100g)	Polyunsaturated Fat (g)
Walnuts	47
Canola Oil	34
Sunflower seeds	33
Sesame Seeds	26
Chia Seeds	23.7
Unsalted Peanuts	16
Peanut Butter	14.2
Avocado Oil	13.5
Olive Oil	11
Safflower Oil	12.82
Seaweed	11
Sardines	5
Soybeans	7
Tuna	14
Wild Salmon	17.3
Whole Grain Wheat	9.7

Fatty Acid

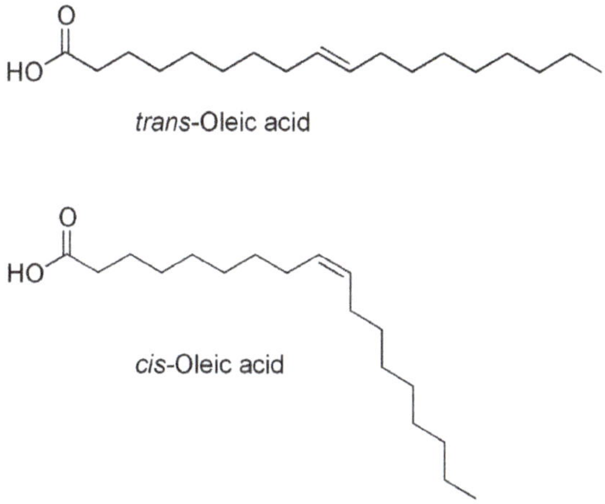

Comparison of the *trans* isomer Elaidic acid (top) and the *cis* isomer oleic acid (bottom).

In chemistry, particularly in biochemistry, a fatty acid is a carboxylic acid with a long aliphatic chain, which is either saturated or unsaturated. Most naturally occurring fatty acids have an unbranched chain of an even number of carbon atoms, from 4 to 28. Fatty acids are usually derived from triglycerides or phospholipids. Fatty acids are important dietary sources of fuel for animals because, when metabolized, they yield large quantities of ATP. Many cell types can use either glucose or fatty acids for this purpose. Long-chain fatty acids cannot cross the blood–brain barrier (BBB) and so cannot be used as fuel by the cells of the central nervous system; however, free short-chain fatty acids and medium-chain fatty acids can cross the BBB, in addition to glucose and ketone bodies.

Types of Fatty Acids

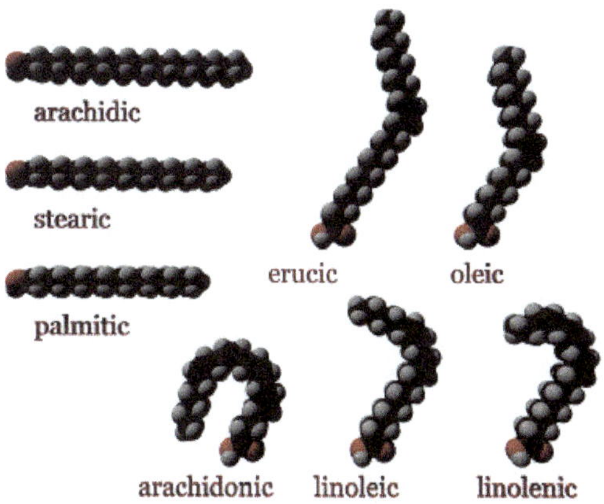

Three-dimensional representations of several fatty acids

Fatty acids that have carbon–carbon double bonds are known as unsaturated. Fatty acids without double bonds are known as saturated. They differ in length as well.

Length of Free Fatty Acid Chains

Fatty acid chains differ by length, often categorized as short to very long.

- Short-chain fatty acids (SCFA) are fatty acids with aliphatic tails of five or fewer carbons (e.g. butyric acid).
- Medium-chain fatty acids (MCFA) are fatty acids with aliphatic tails of 6 to 12 carbons, which can form medium-chain triglycerides.
- Long-chain fatty acids (LCFA) are fatty acids with aliphatic tails of 13 to 21 carbons.
- Very long chain fatty acids (VLCFA) are fatty acids with aliphatic tails of 22 or more carbons.

Unsaturated Fatty Acids

Unsaturated fatty acids have one or more double bonds between carbon atoms. (Pairs of carbon atoms connected by double bonds can be saturated by adding hydrogen atoms to them, converting the double bonds to single bonds. Therefore, the double bonds are called unsaturated.)

The two carbon atoms in the chain that are bound next to either side of the double bond can occur in a *cis* or *trans* configuration.

cis

A *cis* configuration means that the two hydrogen atoms adjacent to the double bond stick out on the same side of the chain. The rigidity of the double bond freezes its conformation and, in the case of the *cis* isomer, causes the chain to bend and restricts the conformational freedom of the fatty acid. The more double bonds the chain has in the *cis* configuration, the less flexibility it has. When a chain has many *cis* bonds, it becomes quite curved in its most accessible conformations. For example, oleic acid, with one double bond, has a "kink" in it, whereas linoleic acid, with two double bonds, has a more pronounced bend. α-Linolenic acid, with three double bonds, favors a hooked shape. The effect of this is that, in restricted environments, such as when fatty acids are part of a phospholipid in a lipid bilayer, or triglycerides in lipid droplets, cis bonds limit the ability of fatty acids to be closely packed, and therefore can affect the melting temperature of the membrane or of the fat.

trans

A *trans* configuration, by contrast, means that the adjacent two hydrogen atoms lie on *opposite* sides of the chain. As a result, they do not cause the chain to bend much, and their shape is similar to straight saturated fatty acids.

In most naturally occurring unsaturated fatty acids, each double bond has three *n* carbon atoms after it, for some n, and all are cis bonds. Most fatty acids in the *trans* configuration (trans fats) are not found in nature and are the result of human processing (e.g., hydrogenation).

The differences in geometry between the various types of unsaturated fatty acids, as well as between saturated and unsaturated fatty acids, play an important role in biological processes, and in the construction of biological structures (such as cell membranes).

Examples of Unsaturated Fatty Acids				
Common name	**Chemical structure**	**Δ^x**	***C:D***	***n−x***
Myristoleic acid	$CH_3(CH_2)_3$**CH=CH**$(CH_2)_7COOH$	*cis*-Δ^9	14:1	*n*−5
Palmitoleic acid	$CH_3(CH_2)_5$**CH=CH**$(CH_2)_7COOH$	*cis*-Δ^9	16:1	*n*−7
Sapienic acid	$CH_3(CH_2)_8$**CH=CH**$(CH_2)_4COOH$	*cis*-Δ^6	16:1	*n*−10
Oleic acid	$CH_3(CH_2)_7$**CH=CH**$(CH_2)_7COOH$	*cis*-Δ^9	18:1	*n*−9
Elaidic acid	$CH_3(CH_2)_7$**CH=CH**$(CH_2)_7COOH$	*trans*-Δ^9	18:1	*n*−9
Vaccenic acid	$CH_3(CH_2)_5$**CH=CH**$(CH_2)_9COOH$	*trans*-Δ^{11}	18:1	*n*−7
Linoleic acid	$CH_3(CH_2)_4$**CH=CH**CH_2 **CH=CH**$(CH_2)_7COOH$	*cis,cis*-Δ^9,Δ^{12}	18:2	*n*−6
Linoelaidic acid	$CH_3(CH_2)_4$**CH=CH**CH_2 **CH=CH**$(CH_2)_7COOH$	*trans,trans*-Δ^9,Δ^{12}	18:2	*n*−6
α-Linolenic acid	CH_3CH_2**CH=CH**CH_2**CH=CH**CH_2 **CH=CH**$(CH_2)_7COOH$	*cis,cis,cis*-Δ^9,Δ^{12},Δ^{15}	18:3	*n*−3
Arachidonic acid	$CH_3(CH_2)_4$**CH=CH**CH_2**CH=CH**CH_2 **CH=CH**CH_2**CH=CH**$(CH_2)_3COOH$NIST	*cis,cis,cis,cis*-Δ^{5}Δ^8, Δ^{11}, Δ^{14}	20:4	*n*−6
Eicosapentaenoic acid	CH_3CH_2**CH=CH**CH_2**CH=CH**CH_2 **CH=CH**CH_2**CH=CH**CH_2 **CH=CH**$(CH_2)_3COOH$	*cis,cis,cis,cis,cis*-Δ^5,Δ^8, Δ^{11},Δ^{14},Δ^{17}	20:5	*n*−3
Erucic acid	$CH_3(CH_2)_7$**CH=CH**$(CH_2)_{11}COOH$	*cis*-Δ^{13}	22:1	*n*−9
Docosahexaenoic acid	CH_3CH_2**CH=CH**CH_2**CH=CH**CH_2 **CH=CH**CH_2**CH=CH**CH_2**CH=CH**CH_2 **CH=CH**$(CH_2)_2COOH$	*cis,cis,cis,cis,cis,cis*-Δ^4, Δ^7,Δ^{10},Δ^{13},Δ^{16},Δ^{19}	22:6	*n*−3

Essential Fatty Acids

Fatty acids that are required by the human body but cannot be made in sufficient quantity from other substrates, and therefore must be obtained from food, are called essential fatty acids. There are two series of essential fatty acids: one has a double bond three carbon atoms away from the methyl end; the other has a double bond six carbon atoms away from the methyl end. Humans lack the ability to introduce double bonds in fatty acids beyond carbons 9 and 10, as counted from the carboxylic acid side. Two essential fatty acids are linoleic acid (LA) and alpha-linolenic acid (ALA). They are widely distributed in plant oils. The human body has a limited ability to convert ALA into the longer-chain omega-3 fatty acids — eicosapentaenoic acid (EPA) and docosahexaenoic acid (DHA), which can also be obtained from fish.

Saturated Fatty Acids

Saturated fatty acids have no double bonds. Thus, saturated fatty acids are saturated with hydrogen (since double bonds reduce the number of hydrogens on each carbon). Because saturated fatty acids have only single bonds, each carbon atom within the chain has 2 hydrogen atoms (except for the omega carbon at the end that has 3 hydrogens).

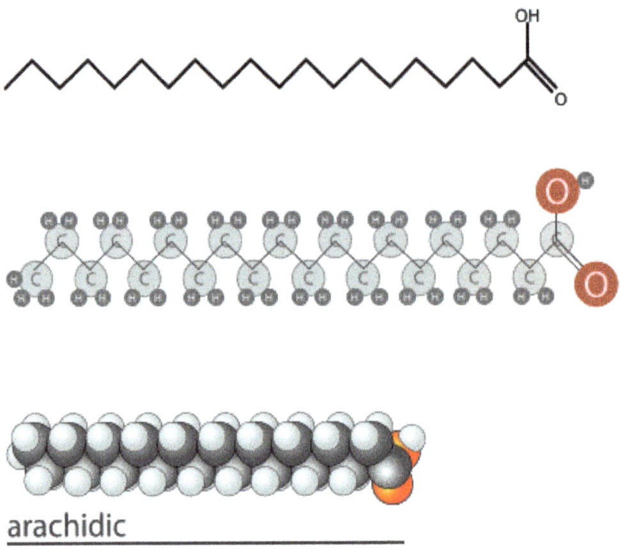

Arachidic acid, a saturated fatty acid.

Examples of Saturated Fatty Acids		
Common name	**Chemical structure**	***C:D***
Caprylic acid	$CH_3(CH_2)_6COOH$	8:0
Capric acid	$CH_3(CH_2)_8COOH$	10:0
Lauric acid	$CH_3(CH_2)_{10}COOH$	12:0
Myristic acid	$CH_3(CH_2)_{12}COOH$	14:0
Palmitic acid	$CH_3(CH_2)_{14}COOH$	16:0
Stearic acid	$CH_3(CH_2)_{16}COOH$	18:0
Arachidic acid	$CH_3(CH_2)_{18}COOH$	20:0
Behenic acid	$CH_3(CH_2)_{20}COOH$	22:0

Lignoceric acid	$CH_3(CH_2)_{22}COOH$	24:0
Cerotic acid	$CH_3(CH_2)_{24}COOH$	26:0

Nomenclature

Numbering of the Carbon Atoms in A Fatty Acid

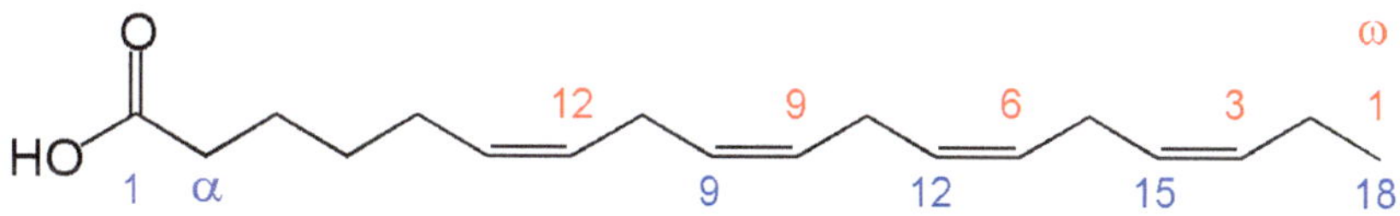

Numbering of carbon atoms

The position of the carbon atoms in a fatty acid can be indicated from the COOH- (or carboxy) end, or from the $-CH_3$ (or methyl) end. If indicated from the -COOH end, then the C-1, C-2, C-3, ...(etc.) notation is used (blue numerals in the diagram, where C-1 is the –COOH carbon). If the position is counted from the other, $-CH_3$, end then the position is indicated by the ω-*n* notation (numerals in red, where ω-1 refers to the methyl carbon).

The positions of the double bonds in a fatty acid chain can, therefore, be indicated in two ways, using the C-*n* or the ω-*n* notation. Thus, in an 18 carbon fatty acid, a double bond between C-12 (or ω-7) and C-13 (or ω-6) is reported either as Δ^{12} if counted from the –COOH end (indicating only the "beginning" of the double bond), or as ω-6 (or omega-6) if counting from the $-CH_3$ end. The "Δ" is the Greek letter "delta", which translates into "D" (for Double bond) in the Roman alphabet. Omega (ω) is the last letter in the Greek alphabet, and is therefore used to indicate the "last" carbon atom in the fatty acid chain. Since the ω-*n* notation is used almost exclusively to indicate the positions of the double bonds close to the $-CH_3$ end in essential fatty acids, there is no necessity for an equivalent "Δ"-like notation - the use of the "ω-*n*" notation always refers to the position of a double bond.

Fatty acids with an odd number of carbon atoms are called odd-chain fatty acids, whereas the rest are even-chain fatty acids. The difference is relevant to gluconeogenesis.

Naming of Fatty Acids

The following table describes the most common systems of naming fatty acids.

System	Example	Explanation
Trivial nomenclature	Palmitoleic acid	Trivial names (or common names) are non-systematic historical names, which are the most frequent naming system used in literature. Most common fatty acids have trivial names in addition to their *systematic names*. These names frequently do not follow any pattern, but they are concise and often unambiguous.

Systematic nomenclature	(9Z)-octadecenoic acid	Systematic names (or IUPAC names) derive from the standard *IUPAC Rules for the Nomenclature of Organic Chemistry*, published in 1979, along with a recommendation published specifically for lipids in 1977. Counting begins from the carboxylic acid end. Double bonds are labelled with *cis-/trans-* notation or *E-/Z-* notation, where appropriate. This notation is generally more verbose than common nomenclature, but has the advantage of being more technically clear and descriptive.
Δ^x *nomenclature*	*cis,cis-*Δ^9,Δ^{12} *octadecadienoic acid*	In Δ^x (or delta-x) nomenclature, each double bond is indicated by Δ^x, where the double bond is located on the xth carbon–carbon bond, counting from the carboxylic acid end. Each double bond is preceded by a *cis-* or *trans-* prefix, indicating the configuration of the molecule around the bond. For example, linoleic acid is designated "*cis-*Δ^9, *cis-*Δ^{12} octadecadienoic acid". This nomenclature has the advantage of being less verbose than systematic nomenclature, but is no more technically clear or descriptive.
n−x nomenclature	*n*−3	n−x (n minus x; also ω−x or omega-x) nomenclature both provides names for individual compounds and classifies them by their likely biosynthetic properties in animals. A double bond is located on the xth carbon–carbon bond, counting from the terminal methyl carbon (designated as *n* or ω) toward the carbonyl carbon. For example, α-Linolenic acid is classified as a *n*−3 or omega-3 fatty acid, and so it is likely to share a biosynthetic pathway with other compounds of this type. The ω−*x*, omega-*x*, or "omega" notation is common in popular nutritional literature, but IUPAC has deprecated it in favor of *n*−*x* notation in technical documents. The most commonly researched fatty acid biosynthetic pathways are *n*−3 and *n*−6.
Lipid numbers	18:3 18:3ω6 18:3, *cis,cis,* *cis-*Δ^9,Δ^{12},Δ^{15}	Lipid numbers take the form *C:D*, where *C* is the number of carbon atoms in the fatty acid and *D* is the number of double bonds in the fatty acid (if more than one, the double bonds are assumed to be interrupted by CH 2 units, *i.e.*, at intervals of 3 carbon atoms along the chain). This notation can be ambiguous, as some different fatty acids can have the same numbers. Consequently, when ambiguity exists this notation is usually paired with either a Δ^x or *n*−*x* term.

Esterified, Free, Unsaturated, Conjugated

When fatty acids circulating in the plasma (plasma fatty acids) are not in their glycerol ester form (glycerides), they are known as non-esterified fatty acids (NEFAs) or free fatty acids (FFAs). The latter term can be viewed as a misnomer because they are transported complexed with a transport protein, such as albumin, as opposed to being unattached to any other molecule. But the term conveys the idea that they are circulating and available for metabolism.

Fatty acids can exist in various states of saturation. Unsaturated fatty acids include monounsaturated fatty acids (MUFAs) and polyunsaturated fatty acids (PUFAs). Conjugated fatty acids are a subset of PUFAs.

Production

Industrial

Fatty acids are usually produced industrially by the hydrolysis of triglycerides, with the removal of glycerol. Phospholipids represent another source. Some fatty acids are produced synthetically by hydrocarboxylation of alkenes.

By Animals

In animals, fatty acids are formed from carbohydrates predominantly in the liver, adipose tissue, and the mammary glands during lactation.

Carbohydrates are converted into pyruvate by glycolysis as the first important step in the conversion of carbohydrates into fatty acids. Pyruvate is then dehydrogenated to form acetyl-CoA in the mitochondrion. However, this acetyl CoA needs to be transported into cytosol where the synthesis of fatty acids occurs. This cannot occur directly. To obtain cytosolic acetyl-CoA, citrate (produced by the condensation of acetyl-CoA with oxaloacetate) is removed from the citric acid cycle and carried across the inner mitochondrial membrane into the cytosol. There it is cleaved by ATP citrate lyase into acetyl-CoA and oxaloacetate. The oxaloacetate is returned to the mitochondrion as malate. The cytosolic acetyl-CoA is carboxylated by acetyl CoA carboxylase into malonyl-CoA, the first committed step in the synthesis of fatty acids.

Malonyl-CoA is then involved in a repeating series of reactions that lengthens the growing fatty acid chain by two carbons at a time. Almost all natural fatty acids, therefore, have even numbers of carbon atoms. When synthesis is complete the free fatty acids are nearly always combined with glycerol (three fatty acids to one glycerol molecule) to form triglycerides, the main storage form of fatty acids, and thus of energy in animals. However, fatty acids are also important components of the phospholipids that form the phospholipid bilayers out of which all the membranes of the cell are constructed (the cell wall, and the membranes that enclose all the organelles within the cells, such as the nucleus, the mitochondria, endoplasmic reticulum, and the Golgi apparatus).

The "uncombined fatty acids" or "free fatty acids" found in the circulation of animals come from the breakdown (or lipolysis) of stored triglycerides. Because they are insoluble in water, these fatty acids are transported bound to plasma albumin. The levels of "free fatty acids" in the blood are limited by the availability of albumin binding sites. They can be taken up from the blood by all cells that have mitochondria (with the exception of the cells of the central nervous system). Fatty acids can only be broken down to CO_2 and water in mitochondria, by means of beta-oxidation, followed by further combustion in the citric acid cycle. Cells in the central nervous system, which, although they possess mitochondria, cannot take free fatty acids up from the blood, as the blood-brain barrier is impervious to most free fatty acids, excluding short-chain fatty acids and medium-chain fatty acids. These cells have to manufacture their own fatty acids from carbohydrates, as described above, in order to produce and maintain the phospholipids of their cell membranes, and those of their organelles.

Fatty Acids in Dietary Fats

The following table gives the fatty acid, vitamin E and cholesterol composition of some common dietary fats.

	Saturated	Monounsaturated	Polyunsaturated	Cholesterol	Vitamin E
	g/100g	g/100g	g/100g	mg/100g	mg/100g
		Animal fats			
Lard	40.8	43.8	9.6	93	0.60
Duck fat	33.2	49.3	12.9	100	2.70
Butter	54.0	19.8	2.6	230	2.00
		Vegetable Fats			
Coconut oil	85.2	6.6	1.7	0	.66
Cocoa butter	60.0	32.9	3.0	0	1.8
Palm kernel oil	81.5	11.4	1.6	0	3.80
Palm oil	45.3	41.6	8.3	0	33.12
Cottonseed oil	25.5	21.3	48.1	0	42.77
Wheat germ oil	18.8	15.9	60.7	0	136.65
Soybean oil	14.5	23.2	56.5	0	16.29
Olive oil	14.0	69.7	11.2	0	5.10
Corn oil	12.7	24.7	57.8	0	17.24
Sunflower oil	11.9	20.2	63.0	0	49.00
Safflower oil	10.2	12.6	72.1	0	40.68
Hemp oil	10	15	75	0	12.34
Canola/Rapeseed oil	5.3	64.3	24.8	0	22.21

Reactions of Fatty Acids

Fatty acids exhibit reactions like other carboxylic acids, i.e. they undergo esterification and acid-base reactions.

Acidity

Fatty acids do not show a great variation in their acidities, as indicated by their respective pK_a. Nonanoic acid, for example, has a pK_a of 4.96, being only slightly weaker than acetic acid (4.76). As the chain length increases, the solubility of the fatty acids in water decreases very rapidly, so that the longer-chain fatty acids have minimal effect on the pH of an aqueous solution. Even those fatty acids that are insoluble in water will dissolve in warm ethanol, and can be titrated with sodium hydroxide solution using phenolphthalein as an indicator. This analysis is used to determine the free fatty acid content of fats; i.e., the proportion of the triglycerides that have been hydrolyzed.

Hydrogenation and Hardening

Hydrogenation of unsaturated fatty acids is widely practiced, typical conditions involving 2.0–3.0 MPa of H2 pressure, 150 °C, and nickel supported on silica. This treatment affords saturated fatty acids, as reflected in their iodine number. Hydrogenated fatty acids are less prone toward rancidification. Since the saturated fatty acids are higher melting than the unsaturated precursors, the process is called hardening. Related technology is used to convert vegetable oils into margarine. The hydrogenation of triglycerides is advantageous because the carboxylic acids degrade the nickel catalysts, affording nickel soaps. During partial hydrogenation, unsaturated fatty acids can be isomerized from *cis* to *trans* configuration.

More forcing hydrogenation, i.e. using higher pressures of H_2 and higher temperatures, converts fatty acids into fatty alcohols. Fatty alcohols are, however, more easily produced from fatty acid esters.

In the Varrentrapp reaction certain unsaturated fatty acids are cleaved in molten alkali, a reaction at one time of relevance to structure elucidation.

Auto-oxidation and Rancidity

Unsaturated fatty acids undergo a chemical change known as auto-oxidation. The process requires oxygen (air) and is accelerated by the presence of trace metals. Vegetable oils resist this process because they contain antioxidants, such as tocopherol. Fats and oils often are treated with chelating agents such as citric acid to remove the metal catalysts.

Ozonolysis

Unsaturated fatty acids are susceptible to degradation by ozone. This reaction is practiced in the production of azelaic acid ($(CH_2)_7(CO_2H)_2$) from oleic acid.

Analysis

In chemical analysis, fatty acids are separated by gas chromatography of methyl esters; additionally, a separation of unsaturated isomers is possible by argentation thin-layer chromatography.

Circulation

Digestion and Intake

Short- and medium-chain fatty acids are absorbed directly into the blood via intestine capillaries and travel through the portal vein just as other absorbed nutrients do. However, long-chain fatty acids are not directly released into the intestinal capillaries. Instead they are absorbed into the fatty walls of the intestine villi and reassembled again into triglycerides. The triglycerides are coated with cholesterol and protein (protein coat) into a compound called a chylomicron.

From within the cell, the chylomicron is released into a lymphatic capillary called a lacteal, which merges into larger lymphatic vessels. It is transported via the lymphatic system and the thoracic duct up to a location near the heart (where the arteries and veins are larger). The thoracic duct empties the chylomicrons into the bloodstream via the left subclavian vein. At this point the chylomicrons can transport the triglycerides to tissues where they are stored or metabolized for energy.

Metabolism

Fatty acids (provided either by ingestion or by drawing on triglycerides stored in fatty tissues) are distributed to cells to serve as a fuel for muscular contraction and general metabolism. They are broken down to CO_2 and water by the intra-cellular mitochondria, releasing large amounts of energy, captured in the form of ATP through beta oxidation and the citric acid cycle.

Distribution

Blood fatty acids are in different forms in different stages in the blood circulation. They are taken in through the intestine in chylomicrons, but also exist in very low density lipoproteins (VLDL) and low density lipoproteins (LDL) after processing in the liver. In addition, when released from adipocytes, fatty acids exist in the blood as free fatty acids.

It is proposed that the blend of fatty acids exuded by mammalian skin, together with lactic acid and pyruvic acid, is distinctive and enables animals with a keen sense of smell to differentiate individuals.

Carbohydrate

A carbohydrate is a biological molecule consisting of carbon (C), hydrogen (H) and oxygen (O) atoms, usually with a hydrogen–oxygen atom ratio of 2:1 (as in water); in other words, with the empirical formula $C_m(H_2O)_n$ (where *m* could be different from *n*). This formula holds true for monosaccharides. Some exceptions exist; for example, deoxyribose, a sugar component of DNA, has the empirical formula $C_5H_{10}O_4$. Carbohydrates are technically hydrates of carbon; structurally it is more accurate to view them as polyhydroxy aldehydes and ketones.

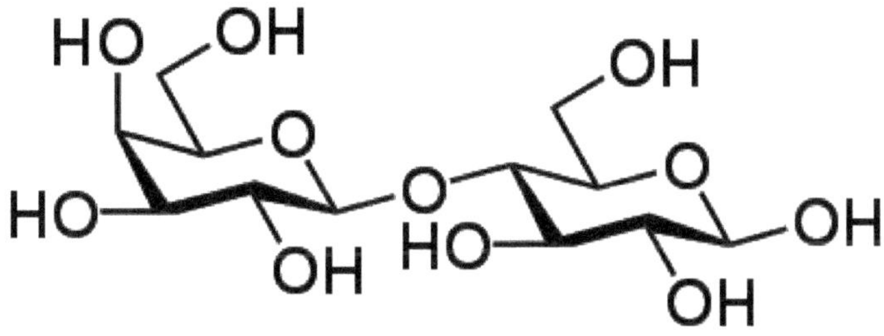

Lactose is a disaccharide found in animal milk. It consists of a molecule of D-galactose and a molecule of D-glucose bonded by beta-1-4 glycosidic linkage. It has a formula of $C_{12}H_{22}O_{11}$.

The term is most common in biochemistry, where it is a synonym of 'saccharide', a group that includes sugars, starch, and cellulose. The saccharides are divided into four chemical groups: monosaccharides, disaccharides, oligosaccharides, and polysaccharides. Monosaccharides and disaccharides, the smallest (lower molecular weight) carbohydrates, are commonly referred to as sugars. The word *saccharide* comes from the Greek word (*sákkharon*), meaning "sugar". While the scientific nomenclature of carbohydrates is complex, the names of the monosaccharides and disaccharides very often end in the suffix -ose. For example, grape sugar is the monosaccharide glucose, cane sugar is the disaccharide sucrose, and milk sugar is the disaccharide lactose.

Carbohydrates perform numerous roles in living organisms. Polysaccharides serve for the storage of energy (e.g. starch and glycogen) and as structural components (e.g. cellulose in plants and chitin in arthropods). The 5-carbon monosaccharide ribose is an important component of coenzymes (e.g. ATP, FAD and NAD) and the backbone of the genetic molecule known as RNA. The related deoxyribose is a component of DNA. Saccharides and their derivatives include many other important biomolecules that play key roles in the immune system, fertilization, preventing pathogenesis, blood clotting, and development.

In food science and in many informal contexts, the term carbohydrate often means any food that is particularly rich in the complex carbohydrate starch (such as cereals, bread and pasta) or simple carbohydrates, such as sugar (found in candy, jams, and desserts).

Often in lists of nutritional information, such as the USDA National Nutrient Database, the term "carbohydrate" (or "carbohydrate by difference") is used for everything other than water, protein, fat, ash, and ethanol. This will include chemical compounds such as acetic or lactic acid, which are not normally considered carbohydrates. It also includes "dietary fiber" which is a carbohydrate but which does not contribute much in the way of food energy (calories), even though it is often included in the calculation of total food energy just as though it were a sugar.

Carbohydrates are found in wide variety of foods. The important sources are cereals (wheat, maize, rice), potatoes, sugarcane, fruits, table sugar(sucrose), bread, milk, etc. Starch and sugar are the important carbohydrates in our diet. Starch is abundant in potatoes, maize, rice and other cereals. Sugar appears in our diet mainly as sucrose(table sugar) which is added to drinks and many prepared foods such as jam, biscuits and cakes. Glucose and fructose are found naturally in many fruits and some vegetables. Glycogen is carbohydrate found in the liver and muscles (as animal source). Cellulose in the cell wall of all plant tissue is a carbohydrate. It is important in our diet as fibre which helps to maintain a healthy digestive system.

Structure

Formerly the name "carbohydrate" was used in chemistry for any compound with the formula $C_m (H_2O)_n$. Following this definition, some chemists considered formaldehyde (CH_2O) to be the simplest carbohydrate, while others claimed that title for glycolaldehyde. Today, the term is generally understood in the biochemistry sense, which excludes compounds with only one or two carbons and includes many biological carbohydrates which deviate from this formula. For example, while the above representative formulas would seem to capture the commonly known carbohydrates, ubiquitous and abundant carbohydrates often deviate from this. For example, carbohydrates often display chemical groups such as: *N*-acetyl (e.g. chitin), sulphate (e.g. glycosaminoglycans), carboxylic acid (e.g. sialic acid) and deoxy modifications (e.g. fucose and sialic acid).

Natural saccharides are generally built of simple carbohydrates called monosaccharides with general formula $(CH_2O)_n$ where n is three or more. A typical monosaccharide has the structure $H–(CHOH)_x(C=O)–(CHOH)_y–H$, that is, an aldehyde or ketone with many hydroxyl groups added, usually one on each carbon atom that is not part of the aldehyde or ketone functional group. Examples of monosaccharides are glucose, fructose, and glyceraldehydes. However, some biological substances commonly called "monosaccharides" do not conform to this formula (e.g. uronic acids and deoxy-sugars such as fucose) and there are many chemicals that do conform to this formula but are not considered to be monosaccharides (e.g. formaldehyde CH_2O and inositol $(CH_2O)_6$).

The open-chain form of a monosaccharide often coexists with a closed ring form where the aldehyde/ketone carbonyl group carbon (C=O) and hydroxyl group (–OH) react forming a hemiacetal with a new C–O–C bridge.

Monosaccharides can be linked together into what are called polysaccharides (or oligosaccharides) in a large variety of ways. Many carbohydrates contain one or more modified monosaccharide units that have had one or more groups replaced or removed. For example, deoxyribose, a component of DNA, is a modified version of ribose; chitin is composed of repeating units of N-acetyl glucosamine, a nitrogen-containing form of glucose.

Division

Carbohydrates are polyhydroxy aldehydes, ketones, alcohols, acids, their simple derivatives and their polymers having linkages of the acetal type. They may be classified according to their degree of polymerization and may be divided initially into three principal groups, namely sugars, oligosaccharides and polysaccharides.

The major dietary carbohydrates		
Class (DP*)	**Subgroup**	**Components**
Sugars (1–2)	Monosaccharides	Glucose, galactose, fructose, xylose
	Disaccharides	Sucrose, lactose, maltose, trehalose
	Polyols	Sorbitol, mannitol
Oligosaccharides (3–9)	Malto-oligosaccharides	Maltodextrins
	Other oligosaccharides	Raffinose, stachyose, fructo-oligosaccharides
Polysaccharides (>9)	Starch	Amylose, amylopectin, modified starches
	Non-starch polysaccharides	Cellulose, hemicellulose, pectins, hydrocolloids

DP * = Degree of polymerization

Monosaccharides

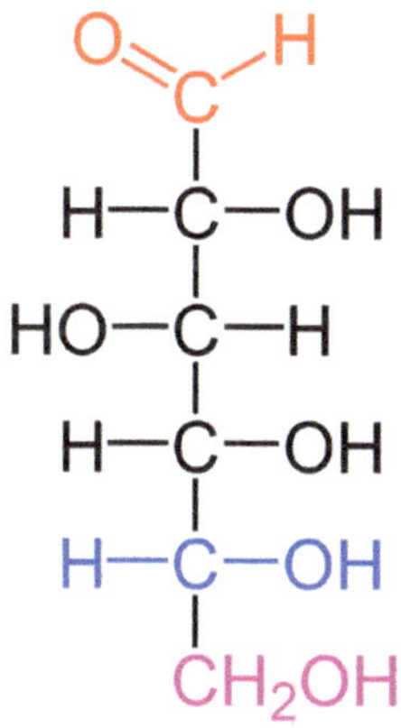

D-glucose is an aldohexose with the formula $(C \cdot H_2O)_6$. The red atoms highlight the aldehyde group and the blue atoms highlight the asymmetric center furthest from the aldehyde; because this -OH is on the right of the Fischer projection, this is a D sugar.

Monosaccharides are the simplest carbohydrates in that they cannot be hydrolyzed to smaller carbohydrates. They are aldehydes or ketones with two or more hydroxyl groups. The general chemical formula of an unmodified monosaccharide is $(C \cdot H_2O)_n$, literally a "carbon hydrate". Monosaccharides are important fuel molecules as well as building blocks for nucleic acids. The smallest monosaccharides, for which n=3, are dihydroxyacetone and D- and L-glyceraldehydes.

Classification of Monosaccharides

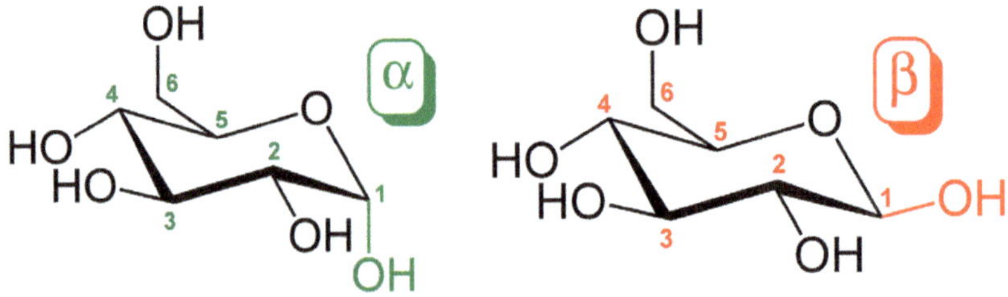

The α and β anomers of glucose. Note the position of the hydroxyl group (red or green) on the anomeric carbon relative to the CH_2OH group bound to carbon 5: they either have identical absolute configurations (R,R or S,S) (α), or opposite absolute configurations (R,S or S,R) (β).

Monosaccharides are classified according to three different characteristics: the placement of its carbonyl group, the number of carbon atoms it contains, and its chiral handedness. If the carbonyl group is an aldehyde, the monosaccharide is an aldose; if the carbonyl group is a ketone, the monosaccharide is a ketose. Monosaccharides with three carbon atoms are called trioses, those with four are called tetroses, five are called pentoses, six are hexoses, and so on. These two systems of classification are often combined. For example, glucose is an aldohexose (a six-carbon aldehyde), ribose is an aldopentose (a five-carbon aldehyde), and fructose is a ketohexose (a six-carbon ketone).

Each carbon atom bearing a hydroxyl group (-OH), with the exception of the first and last carbons, are asymmetric, making them stereo centers with two possible configurations each (R or S). Because of this asymmetry, a number of isomers may exist for any given monosaccharide formula. Using Le Bel-van't Hoff rule, the aldohexose D-glucose, for example, has the formula $(C{\cdot}H_2O)_6$, of which four of its six carbons atoms are stereogenic, making D-glucose one of 2^4=16 possible stereoisomers. In the case of glyceraldehydes, an aldotriose, there is one pair of possible stereoisomers, which are enantiomers and epimers. 1, 3-dihydroxyacetone, the ketose corresponding to the aldose glyceraldehydes, is a symmetric molecule with no stereo centers. The assignment of D or L is made according to the orientation of the asymmetric carbon furthest from the carbonyl group: in a standard Fischer projection if the hydroxyl group is on the right the molecule is a D sugar, otherwise it is an L sugar. The "D-" and "L-" prefixes should not be confused with "d-" or "l-", which indicate the direction that the sugar rotates plane polarized light. This usage of "d-" and "l-" is no longer followed in carbohydrate chemistry.

Ring-straight Chain Isomerism

The aldehyde or ketone group of a straight-chain monosaccharide will react reversibly with a hydroxyl group on a different carbon atom to form a hemiacetal or hemiketal, forming a heterocyclic ring with an oxygen bridge between two carbon atoms. Rings with five and six atoms are called furanose and pyranose forms, respectively, and exist in equilibrium with the straight-chain form.

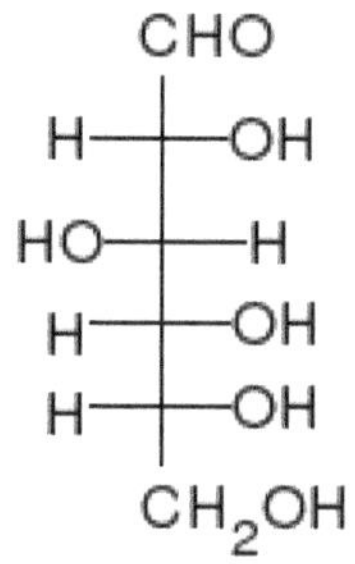

Glucose can exist in both a straight-chain and ring form.

During the conversion from straight-chain form to the cyclic form, the carbon atom containing the carbonyl oxygen, called the anomeric carbon, becomes a stereogenic center with two possible configurations: The oxygen atom may take a position either above or below the plane of the ring. The resulting possible pair of stereoisomers is called anomers. In the *α anomer*, the -OH substituent on the anomeric carbon rests on the opposite side (trans) of the ring from the CH_2OH side branch. The alternative form, in which the CH_2OH substituent and the anomeric hydroxyl are on the same side (cis) of the plane of the ring, is called the *β anomer*.

Use in Living Organisms

Monosaccharides are the major source of fuel for metabolism, being used both as an energy source (glucose being the most important in nature) and in biosynthesis. When monosaccharides are not immediately needed by many cells they are often converted to more space-efficient forms, often polysaccharides. In many animals, including humans, this storage form is glycogen, especially in liver and muscle cells. In plants, starch is used for the same purpose. The most abundant carbohydrate, cellulose, is a structural component of the cell wall of plants and many forms of algae. Ribose is a component of RNA. Deoxyribose is a component of DNA. Lyxose is a component of lyxoflavin found in the human heart. Ribulose and xylulose occur in the pentose phosphate pathway. Galactose, a component of milk sugar lactose, is found in galactolipids in plant cell membranes and in glycoproteins in many tissues. Mannose occurs in human metabolism, especially in the glycosylation of certain proteins. Fructose, or fruit sugar, is found in many plants and in humans, it is metabolized in the liver, absorbed directly into the intestines during digestion, and found in semen. Trehalose, a major sugar of insects, is rapidly hydrolyzed into two glucose molecules to support continuous flight.

Disaccharides

Two joined monosaccharides are called a disaccharide and these are the simplest polysaccharides. Examples include sucrose and lactose. They are composed of two monosaccharide units bound together by a covalent bond known as a glycosidic linkage formed via a dehydration reaction, resulting in the loss of a hydrogen atom from one monosaccharide and a hydroxyl group from the other. The formula of unmodified disaccharides is $C_{12}H_{22}O_{11}$. Although there are numerous kinds of disaccharides, a handful of disaccharides are particularly notable.

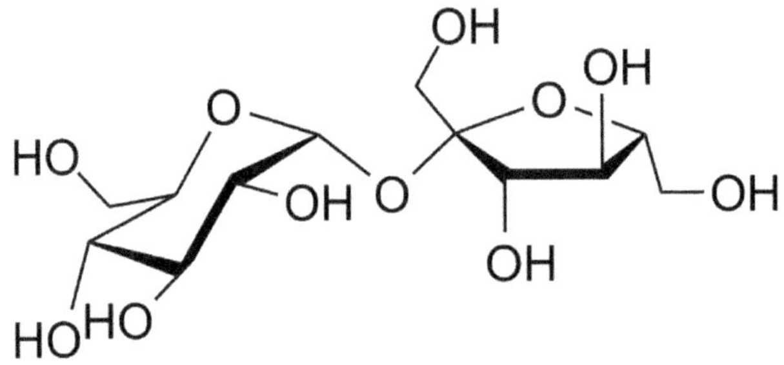

Sucrose, also known as table sugar, is a common disaccharide. It is composed of two monosaccharides: D-glucose (left) and D-fructose (right).

Sucrose, pictured to the right, is the most abundant disaccharide, and the main form in which carbohydrates are transported in plants. It is composed of one D-glucose molecule and one D-fructose molecule. The systematic name for sucrose, *O*-α-D-glucopyranosyl-(1→2)-D-fructofuranoside, indicates four things:

- Its monosaccharides: glucose and fructose.
- Their ring types: glucose is a pyranose and fructose is a furanose.
- How they are linked together: the oxygen on carbon number 1 (C1) of α-D-glucose is linked to the C2 of D-fructose.
- The *-oside* suffix indicates that the anomeric carbon of both monosaccharides participates in the glycosidic bond.

Lactose, a disaccharide composed of one D-galactose molecule and one D-glucose molecule, occurs naturally in mammalian milk. The systematic name for lactose is *O*-β-D-galactopyranosyl-(1→4)-D-glucopyranose. Other notable disaccharides include maltose (two D-glucoses linked α-1,4) and cellulobiose (two D-glucoses linked β-1,4). Disaccharides can be classified into two types: reducing and non-reducing disaccharides. If the functional group is present in bonding with another sugar unit, it is called a reducing disaccharide or biose.

Nutrition

Carbohydrate consumed in food yields 3.87 calories of energy per gram for simple sugars, and 3.57 to 4.12 calories per gram for complex carbohydrate in most other foods. Relatively high levels of carbohydrate are associated with processed foods or refined foods made from plants, including sweets, cookies and candy, table sugar, honey, soft drinks, breads and crackers, jams and fruit products, pastas and breakfast cereals. Lower amounts of carbohydrate are usually associated with unrefined foods, including beans, tubers, rice, and unrefined fruit. Animal-based foods generally have the lowest carbohydrate levels, although milk does contain a high proportion of lactose.

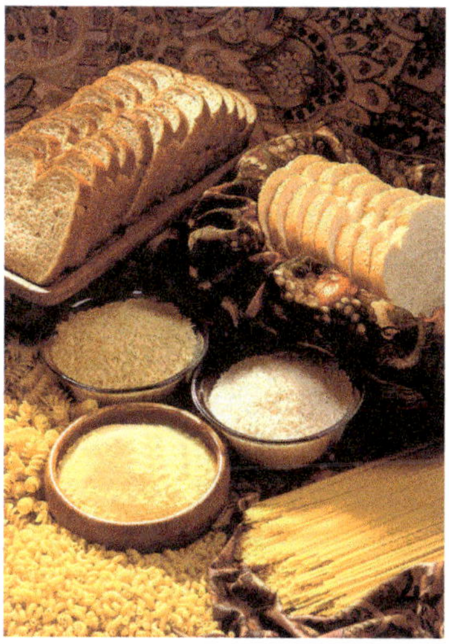

Grain products: rich sources of carbohydrates

Carbohydrates are a common source of energy in living organisms; however, no carbohydrate is an essential nutrient in humans. Humans are able to obtain all of their energy requirement from protein and fats, though the potential for some negative health effects of extreme carbohydrate restriction remains, as the issue has not been studied extensively yet. However, in the case of dietary fiber – indigestible carbohydrates which are not a source of energy – inadequate intake can lead to significant increases in mortality.

Following a diet consisting of very low amounts of daily carbohydrate for several days will usually result in higher levels of blood ketone bodies than an isocaloric diet with similar protein content. This relatively high level of ketone bodies is commonly known as ketosis and is very often confused with the potentially fatal condition often seen in type 1 diabetics known as diabetic ketoacidosis. Somebody suffering ketoacidosis will have much higher levels of blood ketone bodies along with high blood sugar, dehydration and electrolyte imbalance.

Long-chain fatty acids cannot cross the blood–brain barrier, but the liver can break these down to produce ketones. However, the medium-chain fatty acids octanoic and heptanoic acids can cross the barrier and be used by the brain, which normally relies upon glucose for its energy. Gluconeogenesis allows humans to synthesize some glucose from specific amino acids: from the glycerol backbone in triglycerides and in some cases from fatty acids.

Organisms typically cannot metabolize all types of carbohydrate to yield energy. Glucose is a nearly universal and accessible source of energy. Many organisms also have the ability to metabolize other monosaccharides and disaccharides but glucose is often metabolized first. In *Escherichia coli,* for example, the lac operon will express enzymes for the digestion of lactose when it is present, but if both lactose and glucose are present the *lac* operon is repressed, resulting in the glucose being used first. Polysaccharides are also common sources of energy. Many organisms can easily break down starches into glucose; most organisms, however, cannot metabolize cellulose or other polysaccharides like chitin and arabinoxylans. These carbohydrate types can be metabolized by some bacteria and protists. Ruminants and termites, for example, use microorganisms to process cellulose. Even though these complex carbohydrates are not very digestible, they represent an important dietary element for humans, called dietary fiber. Fiber enhances digestion, among other benefits.

Based on the effects on risk of heart disease and obesity in otherwise healthy middle-aged adults, the Institute of Medicine recommends that American and Canadian adults get between 45–65% of dietary energy from whole-grain carbohydrates. The Food and Agriculture Organization and World Health Organization jointly recommend that national dietary guidelines set a goal of 55–75% of total energy from carbohydrates, but only 10% directly from sugars (their term for simple carbohydrates).

Classification

Nutritionists often refer to carbohydrates as either simple or complex. However, the exact distinction between these groups can be ambiguous. The term *complex carbohydrate* was first used in the U.S. Senate Select Committee on Nutrition and Human Needs publication *Dietary Goals for the United States* (1977) where it was intended to distinguish sugars from other carbohydrates (which were perceived to be nutritionally superior). However, the report put "fruit, vegetables and whole-grains" in the complex carbohydrate column, despite the fact that these may contain sugars as well as polysaccharides. This confusion persists as today some nutritionists use the term complex carbohydrate to refer to any sort of digestible saccharide present in a whole food, where fiber, vitamins and minerals are also found (as opposed to processed carbohydrates, which provide energy but few other nutrients). The standard usage, however, is to classify carbohydrates chemically: simple if they are sugars (monosaccharides and disaccharides) and complex if they are polysaccharides (or oligosaccharides).

In any case, the simple vs. complex chemical distinction has little value for determining the nutritional quality of carbohydrates. Some simple carbohydrates (e.g. fructose) raise blood glucose slowly, while some complex carbohydrates (starches), especially if processed, raise blood sugar rapidly. The speed of digestion is determined by a variety of factors including which other nutrients are consumed with the carbohydrate, how the food is prepared, individual differences in metabolism, and the chemistry of the carbohydrate.

The USDA's *Dietary Guidelines for Americans 2010* call for moderate- to high-carbohydrate consumption from a balanced diet that includes six one-ounce servings of grain foods each day, at least half from whole grain sources and the rest from enriched.

The glycemic index (GI) and glycemic load concepts have been developed to characterize food behavior during human digestion. They rank carbohydrate-rich foods based on the rapidity and magnitude of their effect on blood glucose levels. Glycemic index is a measure of how quickly food glucose is absorbed, while glycemic load is a measure of the total absorbable glucose in foods. The insulin index is a similar, more recent classification method that ranks foods based on their effects on blood insulin levels, which are caused by glucose (or starch) and some amino acids in food.

Metabolism

Carbohydrate metabolism denotes the various biochemical processes responsible for the formation, breakdown and interconversion of carbohydrates in living organisms.

The most important carbohydrate is glucose, a simple sugar (monosaccharide) that is metabolized by nearly all known organisms. Glucose and other carbohydrates are part of a wide variety of metabolic pathways across species: plants synthesize carbohydrates from carbon dioxide and water by photosynthesis storing the absorbed energy internally, often in the form of starch or lipids. Plant components are consumed by animals and fungi, and used as fuel for cellular respiration. Oxidation of one gram of carbohydrate yields approximately 4 kcal of energy, while the oxidation of one gram of lipids yields about 9 kcal. Energy obtained from metabolism (e.g., oxidation of glucose) is usually stored temporarily within cells in the form of ATP. Organisms capable of aerobic respiration metabolize glucose and oxygen to release energy with carbon dioxide and water as byproducts.

Catabolism

Catabolism is the metabolic reaction which cells undergo to extract energy. There are two major metabolic pathways of monosaccharide catabolism: glycolysis and the citric acid cycle.

In glycolysis, oligo/polysaccharides are cleaved first to smaller monosaccharides by enzymes called glycoside hydrolases. The monosaccharide units can then enter into monosaccharide catabolism. In some cases, as with humans, not all carbohydrate types are usable as the digestive and metabolic enzymes necessary are not present.

Carbohydrate Chemistry

Carbohydrate chemistry is a large and economically important branch of organic chemistry. Some of the main organic reactions that involve carbohydrates are:

- Carbohydrate acetalisation
- Cyanohydrin reaction
- Lobry de Bruyn–van Ekenstein transformation

- Amadori rearrangement
- Nef reaction
- Wohl degradation
- Koenigs–Knorr reaction
- Carbohydrate digestion

Dietary Fiber

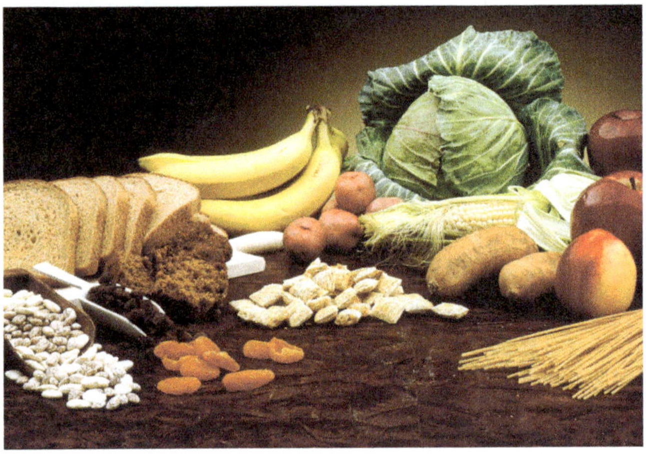

Foods rich in fibers: fruits, vegetables and grains.

Dietary fiber or roughage is the indigestible portion of food derived from plants. It has two main components:

- Soluble fiber, which dissolves in water, is readily fermented in the colon into gases and physiologically active byproducts, and can be prebiotic and viscous. It delays gastric emptying which in turn can cause an extended feeling of fullness.
- Insoluble fiber, which does not dissolve in water, is metabolically inert and provides bulking, or it can be prebiotic and metabolically ferment in the large intestine. Bulking fibers absorb water as they move through the digestive system, easing defecation.

Dietary fibers can act by changing the nature of the contents of the gastrointestinal tract and by changing how other nutrients and chemicals are absorbed. Some types of soluble fiber absorb water to become a gelatinous, viscous substance which is fermented by bacteria in the digestive tract. Some types of insoluble fiber have bulking action and are not fermented. Lignin, a major dietary insoluble fiber source, may alter the rate and metabolism of soluble fibers. Other types of insoluble fiber, notably resistant starch, are fully fermented. Some but not all soluble plant fibers block intestinal mucosal adherence and translocation of potentially pathogenic bacteria and may therefore modulate intestinal inflammation, an effect that has been termed contrabiotic.

Chemically, dietary fiber consists of non-starch polysaccharides such as arabinoxylans, cellulose, and many other plant components such as resistant starch, resistant dextrins, inulin, lignin, chitins, pectins, beta-glucans, and oligosaccharides. A novel position has been adopted by the US Department of Agriculture to include *functional fibers* as isolated fiber sources that may be included in the diet. The term "fiber" is something of a misnomer, since many types of so-called dietary fiber are not actually fibrous.

Food sources of dietary fiber are often divided according to whether they provide (predominantly) soluble or insoluble fiber. Plant foods contain both types of fiber in varying degrees, according to the plant's characteristics.

Advantages of consuming fiber are the production of healthful compounds during the fermentation of soluble fiber, and insoluble fiber's ability (via its passive hygroscopic properties) to increase bulk, soften stool, and shorten transit time through the intestinal tract. A disadvantage of a diet high in fiber is the potential for significant intestinal gas production and bloating.

Definition

Originally, fiber was defined to be the components of plants that resist human digestive enzymes, a definition that includes lignin and polysaccharides. The definition was later changed to also include resistant starch, along with inulin and other oligosaccharides.

Official definition of dietary fiber differs a little among different institutions:

Organization (reference)	Definition
Institute of Medicine	Dietary fiber consists of nondigestible carbohydrates and lignin that are intrinsic and intact in plants. Functional fiber consists of isolated, nondigestible carbohydrates that have beneficial physiologic effects in humans. Total fiber is the sum of dietary fiber and functional fiber.
American Association of Cereal Chemists	Dietary fiber is the edible parts of plants or analogous carbohydrates that are resistant to digestion and absorption in the human small intestine, with complete or partial fermentation in the large intestine. Dietary fiber includes polysaccharides, oligosaccharides, lignin, and associated plant substances. Dietary fibers promote beneficial physiologic effects including laxation, and/or blood cholesterol attenuation, and/or blood glucose attenuation.
Codex Alimentarius Commission	Dietary fiber means carbohydrate polymers with ≥10 monomeric units, which are not hydrolyzed by the endogenous enzymes in the small intestine of humans.

Types and Sources of Dietary Fiber

Nutrient	Food additive	appearance / preparationi
water-insoluble dietary fibers		
β-glucans (a few of which are water-soluble)		
Cellulose	E 460	cereals, fruit, vegetables (in all plants in general)
Chitin	–	in fungi, exoskeleton of insects and crustaceans
Hemicellulose		cereals, bran, timber, legumes
Hexoses	–	wheat, barley
Pentose	–	rye, oat
Lignin	–	stones of fruits, vegetables (filaments of the garden bean), cereals
Xanthan gum	E 415	production with Xanthomonas-bacteria from sugar substrates
Resistant starch		Can be starch protected by seed or shell (type RS1), granular starch (type RS2) or retrograded starch (type RS3)
Resistant starch	–	high amylose corn, barley, high amylose wheat, legumes, bananas, etc.
water-soluble dietary fibers		
Arabinoxylan (a hemicellulose)	–	psyllium
Fructans		replace or complement in some plant taxa the starch as storage carbohydrate
Inulin	–	in diverse plants, e.g. topinambour, chicory, etc.
Polyuronide		
Pectin	E 440	in the fruit skin (mainly apples, quinces), vegetables
Alginic acids (Alginates)	E 400–E 407	in Algae
Sodium alginate	E 401	
Potassium alginate	E 402	
Ammonium alginate	E 403	
Calcium alginate	E 404	
Propylene glycol alginate (PGA)	E 405	
agar	E 406	
carrageen	E 407	red algae
Raffinose	–	legumes
Xylose	–	monosacharide, pentose
Polydextrose	E 1200	synthetic polymer, ca. 1kcal/g
Lactulose	–	synthetic disaccharide

Fiber Contents in Food

Dietary fibers are found in fruits, vegetables and whole grains. The exact amount of fiber contained in the food can be seen in the following table of expected fiber in USDA food groups/subgroups

Food Group	Serving Mean	Fiber g/Serving
Fruit	0.5 cup	1.1
Dark-green vegetables	0.5 cup	6.4
Orange vegetables	0.5 cup	2.1
Cooked dry beans (legumes)	0.5 cup	8.0
Starchy vegetables	0.5 cup	1.7
Other vegetables	0.5 cup	1.1
Whole grains	28 g (1 oz)	2.4
Meat	28 g (1 oz)	0.1

Dietary fiber is found in plants. While all plants contain some fiber, plants with high fiber concentrations are generally the most practical source.

Fiber-rich plants can be eaten directly. Or, alternatively, they can be used to make supplements and fiber-rich processed foods.

The Academy of Nutrition and Dietetics (AND), formerly the American Dietetic Association, recommends consuming a variety of fiber-rich foods.

Plant Sources of fiber

Some plants contain significant amounts of soluble and insoluble fiber. For example, plums and prunes have a thick skin covering a juicy pulp. The skin is a source of insoluble fiber, whereas soluble fiber is in the pulp. Grapes also contain a fair amount of fiber.

The root of the konjac plant, or glucomannan, produces results similar to fiber and may also be used to relieve constipation. Glucomannan is sold in various forms, and while safe in some forms, it can be unsafe in others, possibly leading to throat or intestinal blockage.

Soluble fiber is found in varying quantities in all plant foods, including:

- legumes (peas, soybeans, lupins and other beans)
- oats, rye, chia, and barley
- some fruits (including figs, avocados, plums, prunes, berries, ripe bananas, and the skin of apples, quinces and pears)
- certain vegetables such as broccoli, carrots, and Jerusalem artichokes

- root tubers and root vegetables such as sweet potatoes and onions (skins of these are sources of insoluble fiber also)
- psyllium seed husks (a mucilage soluble fiber) and flax seeds
- nuts, with almonds being the highest in dietary fiber

Sources of insoluble fiber include:

- whole grain foods
- wheat and corn bran
- legumes such as beans and peas
- nuts and seeds
- potato skins
- lignans
- vegetables such as green beans, cauliflower, zucchini (courgette), celery, and nopal
- some fruits including avocado, and unripe bananas
- the skins of some fruits, including kiwifruit, grapes and tomatoes

Fiber Supplements

These are a few example forms of fiber that have been sold as supplements or food additives. These may be marketed to consumers for nutritional purposes, treatment of various gastrointestinal disorders, and for such possible health benefits as lowering cholesterol levels, reducing risk of colon cancer, and losing weight.

Soluble fiber supplements may be beneficial for alleviating symptoms of irritable bowel syndrome, such as diarrhea or constipation and abdominal discomfort. Prebiotic soluble fiber products, like those containing inulin or oligosaccharides, may contribute to relief from inflammatory bowel disease, as in Crohn's disease, ulcerative colitis, and *Clostridium difficile*, due in part to the short-chain fatty acids produced with subsequent anti-inflammatory actions upon the bowel. Fiber supplements may be effective in an overall dietary plan for managing irritable bowel syndrome by modification of food choices.

One insoluble fiber, resistant starch from high-amylose corn, has been used as a supplement and may contribute to improving insulin sensitivity and glycemic management as well as promoting regularity and possibly relief of diarrhea. One preliminary finding indicates that resistant corn starch may reduce symptoms of ulcerative colitis.

Inulins

Chemically defined as oligosaccharides occurring naturally in most plants, inulins have nutritional value as carbohydrates, or more specifically as fructans, a polymer of the natural plant sugar, fructose. Inulin is typically extracted by manufacturers from enriched plant sources such as chicory roots or Jerusalem artichokes for use in prepared foods. Subtly sweet, it can be used to replace sugar, fat, and flour, is often used to improve the flow and mixing qualities of powdered nutritional supplements, and has significant potential health value as a prebiotic fermentable fiber.

Inulin is advantageous because it contains 25–30% the food energy of sugar or other carbohydrates and 10–15% the food energy of fat. As a prebiotic fermentable fiber, its metabolism by gut flora yields short-chain fatty acids which increase absorption of calcium, magnesium, and iron, resulting from upregulation of mineral-transporting genes and their membrane transport proteins within the colon wall. Among other potential beneficial effects noted above, inulin promotes an increase in the mass and health of intestinal *Lactobacillus* and *Bifidobacterium* populations.

Inulin's primary disadvantage is its tolerance. As a soluble fermentable fiber, it is quickly and easily fermented within the intestinal tract, which may cause gas and digestive distress at doses higher than 15 grams/day in most people. Individuals with digestive diseases have benefited from removing fructose and inulin from their diet. While clinical studies have shown changes in the microbiota at lower levels of inulin intake, some of the health effects require higher than 15 grams per day to achieve the benefits.

Vegetable Gums

Vegetable gum fiber supplements are relatively new to the market. Often sold as a powder, vegetable gum fibers dissolve easily with no aftertaste. In preliminary clinical trials, they have proven effective for the treatment of irritable bowel syndrome. Examples of vegetable gum fibers are guar gum and acacia Senegal gum.

Mechanisms of Action

Many molecules that are considered to be "dietary fiber" are so because humans lack the necessary enzymes to split the glycosidic bond and they reach the large intestine. Many foods contain varying types of dietary fibers, all of which contribute to health in different ways.

Dietary fibers have three primary mechanisms: bulking, viscosity and fermentation. Different fibers have different effects, suggesting that a variety of dietary fibers contribute to overall health. Some fibers contribute through one primary mechanism. For instance, cellulose and wheat bran provide excellent bulking effects, but are minimally fermented. Alternatively, many dietary fibers can contribute to health through more than one of these mechanisms. For instance, psyllium provides bulking as well as viscosity.

Bulking fibers can be soluble (i.e., psyllium) or insoluble (i.e., cellulose and hemicellulose). They absorb water and can significantly increase stool weight and regularity. Most bulking fibers are not fermented or are minimally fermented throughout the intestinal tract.

Viscous fibers thicken the contents of the intestinal tract and may attenuate the absorption of sugar, reduce sugar response after eating, and reduce lipid absorption (notably shown with cholesterol absorption). Their use in food formulations is often limited to low levels, due to their viscosity and thickening effects. Some viscous fibers may also be partially or fully fermented within the intestinal tract (guar gum, beta-glucan, glucomannan and pectins), but some viscous fibers are minimally or not fermented (modified cellulose such as methylcellulose and psyllium).

Fermentable fibers are consumed by the microbiota within the large intestines, mildly increasing fecal bulk and producing short-chain fatty acids as byproducts with wide-ranging physiological activities (discussion below). Resistant starch, inulin, fructooligosaccharide and galactooligosaccharide are dietary fibers which are fully fermented. These include insoluble as well as soluble fibers. This fermentation impacts the expression of many genes within the large intestine, which impact digestive function and lipid and glucose metabolism, as well as the immune system, inflammation and more.

Dietary fibers can change the nature of the contents of the gastrointestinal tract and can change how other nutrients and chemicals are absorbed through bulking and viscosity. Some types of soluble fibers bind to bile acids in the small intestine, making them less likely to re-enter the body; this in turn lowers cholesterol levels in the blood from the actions of cytochrome P450-mediated oxidation of cholesterol.

Insoluble fiber is associated with reduced diabetes risk, but the mechanism by which this occurs is unknown. One type of insoluble dietary fiber, resistant starch has been shown to directly increase insulin sensitivity in healthy people, in type 2 diabetics, and in individuals with insulin resistance, possibly contributing to reduced risk of type 2 diabetes.

Not yet formally proposed as an essential macro-nutrient, dietary fiber is nevertheless regarded as important for the diet, with regulatory authorities in many developed countries recommending increases in fiber intake.

Physicochemical Properties

Dietary fiber has distinct physicochemical properties. Most semi-solid foods, fiber and fat are a combination of gel matrices which are hydrated or collapsed with microstructural elements, globules, solutions or encapsulating walls. Fresh fruit and vegetables are cellular materials.

- The cells of cooked potatoes and legumes are gels filled with gelatinized starch granules. The cellular structures of fruits and vegetables are foams with a closed cell geometry filled with a gel, surrounded by cell walls which are composites with an amorphous matrix strengthened by complex carbohydrate fibers.

- Particle size and interfacial interactions with adjacent matrices affect the mechanical properties of food composites.
- Food polymers may be soluble in and/or plasticized by water. Water is the most important plasticizer, particularly in biological systems thereby changing mechanical properties.
- The variables include chemical structure, polymer concentration, molecular weight, degree of chain branching, the extent of ionization (for electrolytes), solution pH, ionic strength and temperature.
- Cross-linking of different polymers, protein and polysaccharides, either through chemical covalent bonds or cross-links through molecular entanglement or hydrogen or ionic bond cross-linking.
- Cooking and chewing food alters these physicochemical properties and hence absorption and movement through the stomach and along the intestine.

Dietary Fiber and the Upper Gastrointestinal Tract

A slowly eaten meal will enter the absorptive phase of the gastrointestinal tract more slowly than a rapidly eaten meal of similar composition. Many of the differences between low and high glycemic foods would disappear if a meal was eaten slowly.

The chemical and physico-chemical nature (lipid, protein, carbohydrate) of the meal will also influence the gastric emptying of the food multiphase system. Fatty foods and hypertonic solutions empty slowly. The movement of food, i.e., chyme, along the gastrointestinal tract is typical of flow in a disperse system. As chyme moves along the gastrointestinal tract, polymer flow and diffusion becomes important.

Following a meal, the stomach and upper gastrointestinal contents consist of

- food compounds
- complex lipids/micellar/aqueous/hydrocolloid and hydrophobic phases
- hydrophilic phases
- solid, liquid, colloidal and gas bubble phases.

Micelles are colloid-sized clusters of molecules which form in conditions as those above, similar to the critical micelle concentration of detergents. In the upper gastrointestinal tract, these detergents consist of bile acids and di- and monoacyl glycerols which solubilize triacylglycerols and cholesterol.

Two mechanisms bring nutrients into contact with the epithelium:

1. intestinal contractions create turbulence; and
2. convection currents direct contents from the lumen to the epithelial surface.

The multiple physical phases in the intestinal tract slow the rate of absorption compared to that of the suspension solvent alone.

1. Nutrients diffuse through the thin, relatively unstirred layer of fluid adjacent to the epithelium.
2. Immobilizing of nutrients and other chemicals within complex polysaccharide molecules affects their release and subsequent absorption from the small intestine, an effect influential on the glycemic index.
3. Molecules begin to interact as their concentration increases. During absorption, water must be absorbed at a rate commensurate with the absorption of solutes. The transport of actively and passively absorbed nutrients across epithelium is affected by the unstirred water layer covering the microvillus membrane.
4. The presence of mucus or fiber, e.g., pectin or guar, in the unstirred layer may alter the viscosity and solute diffusion coefficient.

Adding viscous polysaccharides to carbohydrate meals can reduce post-prandial blood glucose concentrations. Wheat and maize but not oats modify glucose absorption, the rate being dependent upon the particle size. The reduction in absorption rate with guar gum may be due to the increased resistance by viscous solutions to the convective flows created by intestinal contractions.

Dietary fiber interacts with pancreatic and enteric enzymes and their substrates. Human pancreatic enzyme activity is reduced when incubated with most fiber sources. Fiber may affect amylase activity and hence the rate of hydrolysis of starch. The more viscous polysaccharides extend the mouth-to-cecum transit time; guar, tragacanth and pectin being slower than wheat bran.

Fiber in the Colon

The colon may be regarded as two organs,

1. the right side (cecum and ascending colon), a fermenter. The right side of the colon is involved in nutrient salvage so that dietary fiber, resistant starch, fat and protein are utilized by bacteria and the end-products absorbed for use by the body.
2. the left side (transverse, descending, and sigmoid colon), affecting continence.

The presence of bacteria in the colon produces an 'organ' of intense, mainly reductive, metabolic activity, whereas the liver is oxidative. The substrates utilized by the cecum have either passed along the entire intestine or are biliary excretion products. The effects of dietary fiber in the colon are on

1. bacterial fermentation of some dietary fibers
2. thereby an increase in bacterial mass
3. an increase in bacterial enzyme activity
4. changes in the water-holding capacity of the fiber residue after fermentation

Enlargement of the cecum is a common finding when some dietary fibers are fed and this is now believed to be normal physiological adjustment. Such an increase may be due to a number of factors, prolonged cecal residence of the fiber, increased bacterial mass, or increased bacterial end-products. Some non-absorbed carbohydrates, e.g. pectin, gum arabic, oligosaccharides and resistant starch, are fermented to short-chain fatty acids (chiefly acetic, propionic and n-butyric), and carbon dioxide, hydrogen and methane. The cecal fermentation of 40–50 g of complex polysaccharides will yield 400–500 mmol total short-chain fatty acids, 240–300 mmol acetate, and 80–100 mmol of both propionate and butyrate. Almost all of these short-chain fatty acids will be absorbed from the colon. This means that fecal short-chain fatty acid estimations do not reflect cecal and colonic fermentation, only the efficiency of absorption, the ability of the fiber residue to sequestrate short-chain fatty acids, and the continued fermentation of fiber around the colon, which presumably will continue until the substrate is exhausted. The production of short-chain fatty acids has several possible actions on the gut mucosa. All of the short-chain fatty acids are readily absorbed by the colonic mucosa, but only acetic acid reaches the systemic circulation in appreciable amounts. Butyric acid appears to be used as a fuel by the colonic mucosa as the preferred energy source for colonic cells.

Dietary Fiber and Cholesterol Metabolism

Dietary fiber may act on each phase of ingestion, digestion, absorption and excretion to affect cholesterol metabolism, such as the following:

1. Caloric energy of foods through a bulking effect
2. Slowing of gastric emptying time
3. A glycemic index type of action on absorption
4. A slowing of bile acid absorption in the ileum so bile acids escape through to the cecum
5. Altered or increased bile acid metabolism in the cecum
6. Indirectly by absorbed short-chain fatty acids, especially propionic acid, resulting from fiber fermentation affecting the cholesterol metabolism in the liver.

7. Binding of bile acids to fiber or bacteria in the cecum with increased fecal loss from the entero-hepatic circulation.

An important action of some fibers is to reduce the reabsorption of bile acids in the ileum and hence the amount and type of bile acid and fats reaching the colon. A reduction in the reabsorption of bile acid from the ileum has several direct effects.

1. Bile acids may be trapped within the lumen of the ileum either because of a high luminal viscosity or because of binding to a dietary fiber.
2. Lignin in fiber adsorbs bile acids, but the unconjugated form of the bile acids are adsorbed more than the conjugated form. In the ileum where bile acids are primarily absorbed the bile acids are predominantly conjugated.
3. The enterohepatic circulation of bile acids may be altered and there is an increased flow of bile acids to the cecum, where they are deconjugated and 7alpha-dehydroxylated.
4. These water-soluble form, bile acids e.g., deoxycholic and lithocholic are adsorbed to dietary fiber and an increased fecal loss of sterols, dependent in part on the amount and type of fiber.
5. A further factor is an increase in the bacterial mass and activity of the ileum as some fibers e.g., pectin are digested by bacteria. The bacterial mass increases and cecal bacterial activity increases.
6. The enteric loss of bile acids results in increased synthesis of bile acids from cholesterol which in turn reduces body cholesterol.

The fibers that are most effective in influencing sterol metabolism (e.g. pectin) are fermented in the colon. It is therefore unlikely that the reduction in body cholesterol is due to adsorption to this fermented fiber in the colon.

1. There might be alterations in the end-products of bile acid bacterial metabolism or the release of short chain fatty acids which are absorbed from the colon, return to the liver in the portal vein and modulate either the synthesis of cholesterol or its catabolism to bile acids.
2. The prime mechanism whereby fiber influences cholesterol metabolism is through bacteria binding bile acids in the colon after the initial deconjugation and dehydroxylation.
3. Fermentable fibers e.g., pectin will by virtue of their providing a medium for bacterial growth increase the bacterial mass in the colon. The sequestrated bile acids are then excreted in feces.
4. Other fibers, e.g., gum arabic, act as stabilizers and cause a significant decrease in serum cholesterol without increasing fecal bile acid excretion.

Dietary Fiber and Fecal Weight

Feces consist of plasticine-like material, made up of water, bacteria, lipids, sterols, mucus and fiber.

1. Feces are 75% water; bacteria make a large contribution to the dry weight, the residue being unfermented fiber and excreted compounds.
2. Fecal output may vary over a range of between 20 and 280 g over 24 hours. The amount of feces egested a day varies for any one individual over a period of time.
3. Of dietary constituents, only dietary fiber increases fecal weight.

Water is distributed in the colon in three ways:

1. Free water which can be absorbed from the colon.
2. Water that is incorporated into bacterial mass.
3. Water that is bound by fiber.

Fecal weight is dictated by:

1. the holding of water by the residual dietary fiber after fermentation.
2. the bacterial mass.
3. There may also be an added osmotic effect of products of bacterial fermentation on fecal mass.

Wheat bran is minimally fermented and binds water and when added to the diet increases fecal weight in a predictable linear manner and decreases intestinal transit time. The particle size of the fiber is all-important, coarse wheat bran being more effective than fine wheat bran. The greater the water-holding capacity of the bran, the greater the effect on fecal weight. For most healthy individuals, an increase in wet fecal weight, depending on the particle size of the bran, is generally of the order of 3–5 g/g fiber. The fermentation of some fibers results in an increase in the bacterial content and possibly fecal weight. Other fibers, e.g. pectin, are fermented and have no effect on stool weight.

Effects of Fiber Intake

Research has shown that fiber may benefit health in several different ways. Lignin and probably related materials that are resistant to enzymatic degradation, diminish the nutritional value of foods.

Table Legend

Color coding of table entries:

- Both Applies to both soluble and insoluble fiber

- Soluble Applies to soluble fiber only
- Insoluble Applies to insoluble fiber only

Effects
Increases food volume without increasing caloric content to the same extent as digestible carbohydrates, providing satiety which may reduce appetite.
Attracts water and forms a viscous gel during digestion, slowing the emptying of the stomach and intestinal transit, shielding carbohydrates from enzymes, and delaying absorption of glucose, which lowers variance in blood sugar levels
Lowers total and LDL cholesterol, which may reduce the risk of cardiovascular disease
Regulates blood sugar, which may reduce glucose and insulin levels in diabetic patients and may lower risk of diabetes
Speeds the passage of foods through the digestive system, which facilitates regular defecation
Adds bulk to the stool, which alleviates constipation
Balances intestinal pH and stimulates intestinal fermentation production of short-chain fatty acids, which may reduce risk of colorectal cancer

Fiber does not bind to minerals and vitamins and therefore does not restrict their absorption, but rather evidence exists that fermentable fiber sources improve absorption of minerals, especially calcium. Some plant foods can reduce the absorption of minerals and vitamins like calcium, zinc, vitamin C, and magnesium, but this is caused by the presence of phytate (which is also thought to have important health benefits), not by fiber.

Research

An experiment designed with a large sample and conducted by NIH-AARP Diet and Health Study studied the correlation between fiber intake and colorectal cancer. The analytic cohort consisted of 291 988 men and 197 623 women aged 50–71 y. Diet was assessed with a self-administered food-frequency questionnaire at baseline in 1995-1996; 2974 incident colorectal cancer cases were identified during 5 y of follow-up. The result was that total fiber intake was not associated with colorectal cancer. But on the other hand, the analyses of fiber from different food sources showed that fiber from grains was associated with a lower risk of colorectal cancer.

Although many researchers believe that dietary fiber intake reduces risk of colon cancer, one study conducted by researchers at the Harvard School of Medicine of over 88,000 women did not show a statistically significant relationship between higher fiber consumption and lower rates of colorectal cancer or adenomas. Similarly, a 2010 study of 58,279 men found no relationship between dietary fiber and colorectal cancer.

Dietary Fiber and Obesity

Dietary fiber has many functions in diet, one of which may be to aid in energy intake control and reduced risk for development of obesity. The role of dietary fiber in energy intake regulation and obesity development is related to its unique physical and chemical properties that aid in early signals of satiation and enhanced or prolonged signals of satiety. Early signals of satiation may be induced through cephalic- and gastric-phase responses related to the bulking effects of dietary fiber on energy density and palatability, whereas the viscosity-producing effects of certain fibers may enhance satiety through intestinal-phase events related to modified gastrointestinal function and subsequent delay in fat absorption. In general, fiber-rich diets, whether achieved through fiber supplementation or incorporation of high fiber foods into meals, have a reduced energy density compared with high fat diets. This is related to fiber's ability to add bulk and weight to the diet. There are also indications that women may be more sensitive to dietary manipulation with fiber than men. The relationship of body weight status and fiber effect on energy intake suggests that obese individuals may be more likely to reduce food intake with dietary fiber inclusion.

Guidelines on Fiber Intake

Current recommendations from the United States National Academy of Sciences, Institute of Medicine, suggest that adults should consume 20–35 grams of dietary fiber per day, but the average American's daily intake of dietary fiber is only 12–18 grams.

The AND (Academy of Nutrition and Dietetics, previously ADA) recommends a minimum of 20–35 g/day for a healthy adult depending on calorie intake (e.g., a 2000 Cal/8400 kJ diet should include 25 g of fiber per day). The AND's recommendation for children is that intake should equal age in years plus 5 g/day (e.g., a 4 year old should consume 9 g/day). No guidelines have yet been established for the elderly or very ill. Patients with current constipation, vomiting, and abdominal pain should see a physician. Certain bulking agents are not commonly recommended with the prescription of opioids because the slow transit time mixed with larger stools may lead to severe constipation, pain, or obstruction.

The British Nutrition Foundation has recommended a minimum fiber intake of 18 g/day for healthy adults.

Fiber Recommendations

United States

On average, North Americans consume less than 50% of the dietary fiber levels recommended for good health. In the preferred food choices of today's youth, this value may be as low as 20%, a factor considered by experts as contributing to the obesity levels seen in many developed countries.

The actual fiber intake gaps of different age groups of Americans are shown in the graph from USDA:

Recognizing the growing scientific evidence for physiological benefits of increased fiber intake, regulatory agencies such as the Food and Drug Administration (FDA) of the United States have given approvals to food products making health claims for fiber.

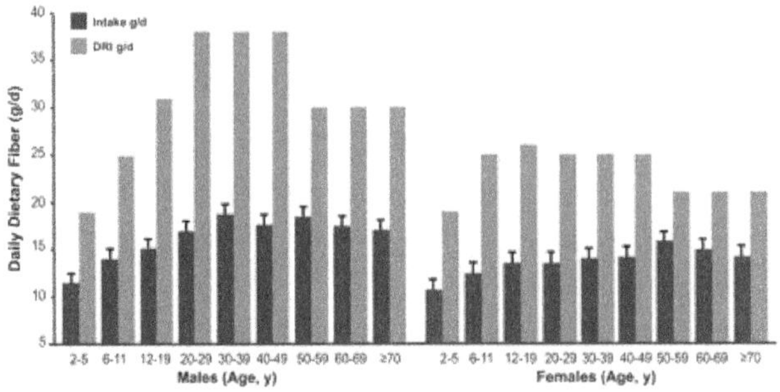

American Fiber Intake Gap

In clinical trials to date, these fiber sources were shown to significantly reduce blood cholesterol levels, an important factor for general cardiovascular health, and to lower risk of onset for some types of cancer.

Viscous fiber sources gaining FDA approval are:

- Psyllium seed husk (7 grams per day)
- Beta-glucan from oat bran, whole oats, oatrim, or rolled oats (3 grams per day)
- Beta-glucan from whole grain or dry-milled barley (3 grams per day)

Other examples of bulking fiber sources used in functional foods and supplements include cellulose, guar gum and xanthan gum.

Other examples of fermentable fiber sources (from plant foods or biotechnology) used in functional foods and supplements include resistant starch, inulin, fructans, fructooligosaccharides (FOS), and oligo- or polysaccharides, and resistant dextrins, which may be partially or fully fermented.

Consistent intake of fermentable fiber through foods like berries and other fresh fruit, vegetables, whole grains, seeds, and nuts is now known to reduce risk of some of the world's most prevalent diseases—obesity, diabetes, high blood cholesterol, cardiovascular disease, and numerous gastrointestinal disorders. In this last category are constipation, inflammatory bowel disease, ulcerative colitis, hemorrhoids, Crohn's disease, diverticulitis, and colon cancer—all disorders of the intestinal tract where fermentable fiber can provide healthful benefits.

Insufficient fiber in the diet can complicate defecation. Low-fiber feces are dehydrated and hardened, making them difficult to evacuate—defining constipation and possibly leading to development of hemorrhoids or anal fissures.

In 2014, the International Scientific Association for Probiotics and Prebiotics submitted a petition to the Food and Drug Administration expanding the physiological effects of fiber consumption to the bulleted list below.

United Kingdom

In June 2007, the British Nutrition Foundation issued a statement to define dietary fiber more concisely and list the potential health benefits established to date. Statement: 'Dietary fibre' has been used as a collective term for a complex mixture of substances with different chemical and physical properties which exert different types of physiological effects.

The use of certain analytical methods to quantify dietary fiber by nature of its indigestibility results in many other indigestible components being isolated along with the carbohydrate components of dietary fiber. These components include resistant starches and oligosaccharides along with other substances that exist within the plant cell structure and contribute to the material that passes through the digestive tract. Such components are likely to have physiological effects.

Yet, some differentiation has to be made between these indigestible plant components and other partially digested material, such as protein, that appears in the large bowel. Thus, it is better to classify fiber as a group of compounds with different physiological characteristics, rather than to be constrained by defining it chemically (end quote).

Diets naturally high in fiber can be considered to bring about several main physiological consequences:

- increases fecal bulk and helps prevent constipation by decreasing fecal transit time in the large intestine
- reduces blood pressure
- improves gastrointestinal health
- improves glucose tolerance and the insulin response following a meal
- increases colonic fermentation and short-chain fatty acid production
- positively modulates colonic microflora
- reduces hyperlipidemia, hypertension, and other coronary heart disease risk factors
- reduces the risk of developing some cancers, particularly colon cancer
- increases satiety and hence some degree of weight management

Fiber is defined by its physiological impact, with many heterogenous types of fibers.

Some fibers may primarily impact one of these benefits (i.e., cellulose increases fecal bulking and prevents constipation), but many fibers impact more than one of these benefits (i.e., resistant starch increases bulking, increases colonic fermentation, positively modulates colonic microflora as well as increases satiety and insulin sensitivity). The beneficial effects of high fiber diets are the summation of the effects of the different types of fiber present in the diet and also other components of such diets.

Defining fiber physiologically allows recognition of indigestible carbohydrates with structures and physiological properties similar to those of naturally occurring dietary fibers.

Fiber and Calories

Fiber contributes less energy—usually measured in kilojoules (kJ) or kilocalories (kcal), also known as dietary *Calories* (Cal)—than sugars and starches because it cannot be fully absorbed by the body. Sugars and starches provide 17 kJ/g (4.1 kcal/g), and the human body has specific enzymes to break them down into glucose, fructose, and galactose, which can then be absorbed by the body. The human body lacks enzymes to break down fiber. Some types of insoluble fiber do not change inside the body, so the body cannot absorb it and it provides no energy (i.e., cellulose). Fermentable fiber is partially fermented, with the degree of fermentability varying with the type of fiber, and contributes some energy when broken down and absorbed by the body. Dietitians have not reached a consensus on how much energy is actually absorbed, but some approximate 8 kJ/g (1.9 kcal/g). Regardless of the type of fiber, the body absorbs less than 17 kJ/g (4.1 kcal/g), which can create inconsistencies for actual product nutrition labels. In some countries fiber is not listed on nutrition labels and is considered to provide no energy. In other countries all fiber must be listed and is simplistically considered to provide 17 kJ/g (4.1 kcal/g) (because chemically fiber is a type of carbohydrate and other carbohydrates provide that amount of energy). In the US, soluble fiber must be counted as 4 kcal/g (17 kJ/g), but insoluble fiber may be (and usually is) treated as not providing energy and not mentioned on the label.

Fiber and Fermentation

The American Association of Cereal Chemists has defined soluble fiber this way: *"the edible parts of plants or similar carbohydrates resistant to digestion and absorption in the human small intestine with complete or partial fermentation in the large intestine."* In this definition:

edible parts of plants

> indicates that some parts of a plant we eat—skin, pulp, seeds, stems, leaves, roots—contain fiber. Both insoluble and soluble sources are in those plant components.

carbohydrates

complex carbohydrates, such as long-chained sugars also called starch, oligosaccharides, or polysaccharides, are sources of soluble fermentable fiber.

resistant to digestion and absorption in the human small intestine

foods providing nutrients are digested by gastric acid and digestive enzymes in the stomach and small intestine where the nutrients are released then absorbed through the intestinal wall for transport via the blood throughout the body. A food resistant to this process is undigested, as insoluble and soluble fibers are. They pass to the large intestine only affected by their absorption of water (insoluble fiber) or dissolution in water (soluble fiber).

complete or partial fermentation in the large intestine

the large intestine comprises a segment called the colon within which additional nutrient absorption occurs through the process of fermentation. Fermentation occurs by the action of colonic bacteria on the food mass, producing gases and short-chain fatty acids. It is these short-chain fatty acids—butyric, acetic (ethanoic), propionic, and valeric acids—that scientific evidence is revealing to have significant health properties.

As an example of fermentation, shorter-chain carbohydrates (a type of fiber found in legumes) cannot be digested, but are changed via fermentation in the colon into short-chain fatty acids and gases (which are typically expelled as flatulence).

According to a 2002 journal article, fiber compounds with partial or low fermentability include:

- cellulose, a polysaccharide
- hemicellulose, a polysaccharide
- lignans, a group of phytoestrogens
- plant waxes

fiber compounds with high fermentability include:

- resistant starches
- beta-glucans, a group of polysaccharides
- pectins, a group of heteropolysaccharides
- natural gums, a group of polysaccharides
- inulins, a group of polysaccharides
- oligosaccharides

Short-chain Fatty Acids

When fermentable fiber is fermented, short-chain fatty acids (SCFA) are produced. SCFAs are involved in numerous physiological processes promoting health, including:

- stabilize blood glucose levels by acting on pancreatic insulin release and liver control of glycogen breakdown
- stimulate gene expression of glucose transporters in the intestinal mucosa, regulating glucose absorption
- provide nourishment of colonocytes, particularly by the SCFA butyrate
- suppress cholesterol synthesis by the liver and reduce blood levels of LDL cholesterol and triglycerides responsible for atherosclerosis
- lower colonic pH (i.e., raises the acidity level in the colon) which protects the lining from formation of colonic polyps and increases absorption of dietary minerals
- stimulate production of T helper cells, antibodies, leukocytes, cytokines, and lymph mechanisms having crucial roles in immune protection
- improve barrier properties of the colonic mucosal layer, inhibiting inflammatory and adhesion irritants, contributing to immune functions

SCFAs that are absorbed by the colonic mucosa pass through the colonic wall into the portal circulation (supplying the liver), and the liver transports them into the general circulatory system.

Overall, SCFAs affect major regulatory systems, such as blood glucose and lipid levels, the colonic environment, and intestinal immune functions.

The major SCFAs in humans are butyrate, propionate, and acetate, where butyrate is the major energy source for colonocytes, propionate is destined for uptake by the liver, and acetate enters the peripheral circulation to be metabolized by peripheral tissues.

U.S. FDA-approved Health Claims

The United States FDA allows producers of foods containing 1.7 g per serving of psyllium husk soluble fiber or 0.75 g of oat or barley soluble fiber as beta-glucans to claim that reduced risk of heart disease can result from their regular consumption.

The FDA statement template for making this claim is: *Soluble fiber from foods such as [name of soluble fiber source, and, if desired, name of food product], as part of a diet low in saturated fat and cholesterol, may reduce the risk of heart disease. A serving of [name of food product] supplies __ grams of the [necessary daily dietary intake for the benefit] soluble fiber from [name of soluble fiber source] necessary per day to have this effect.*

Eligible sources of soluble fiber providing beta-glucan include:

- Oat bran
- Rolled oats
- Whole oat flour
- Oatrim
- Whole grain barley and dry milled barley
- Soluble fiber from psyllium husk with purity of no less than 95%

The allowed label may state that diets low in saturated fat and cholesterol and that include soluble fiber from certain of the above foods "may" or "might" reduce the risk of heart disease.

As discussed in FDA regulation 21 CFR 101.81, the daily dietary intake levels of soluble fiber from sources listed above associated with reduced risk of coronary heart disease are:

- 3 g or more per day of beta-glucan soluble fiber from either whole oats or barley, or a combination of whole oats and barley.
- 7 g or more per day of soluble fiber from psyllium seed husk.

Soluble fiber from consuming grains is included in other allowed health claims for lowering risk of some types of cancer and heart disease by consuming fruit and vegetables (21 CFR 101.76, 101.77, and 101.78).

Research

A study of 388,000 adults ages 50 to 71 for nine years found that the highest consumers of fiber were 22% less likely to die over this period. In addition to lower risk of death from heart disease, adequate consumption of fiber-containing foods, especially grains, was also associated with reduced incidence of infectious and respiratory illnesses, and, particularly among males, reduced risk of cancer-related death.

References

- Brosnan J (June 2003). "Interorgan amino acid transport and its regulation". Journal of Nutrition. 133 (6 Suppl 1): 2068S–72S. PMID 12771367
- Dobson CM (2000). "The nature and significance of protein folding". In Pain RH. Mechanisms of Protein Folding. Oxford, Oxfordshire: Oxford University Press. pp. 1–28. ISBN 0-19-963789-X
- EBI External Services (2010-01-20). "The Catalytic Site Atlas at The European Bioinformatics Institute". Ebi.ac.uk. Retrieved 2011-01-16

- Ritchie DW (2008). "Recent progress and future directions in protein–protein docking". Current Protein and Peptide Science. 9 (1): 1–15. PMID 18336319. doi:10.2174/138920308783565741
- Sumner JB (1926). "The isolation and crystallization of the enzyme urease. Preliminary paper" (PDF). Journal of Biological Chemistry. 69 (2): 435–41
- Sleator RD. (2012). "Prediction of protein functions". Methods in Molecular Biology. Methods in Molecular Biology. 815: 15–24. ISBN 978-1-61779-423-0. PMID 22130980. doi:10.1007/978-1-61779-424-7_2
- Elzanowski A, Ostell J (7 April 2008). "The Genetic Codes". National Center for Biotechnology Information (NCBI). Retrieved 10 March 2010
- Yuste R (2005). "Fluorescence microscopy today". Nature Methods. 2 (12): 902–904. PMID 16299474. doi:10.1038/nmeth1205-902
- Simoni RD, Hill RL, Vaughan M (September 2002). "The discovery of the amino acid threonine: the work of William C. Rose [classical article]". The Journal of Biological Chemistry. 277 (37): E25. PMID 12218068
- Walker JH, Wilson K (2000). Principles and Techniques of Practical Biochemistry. Cambridge, UK: Cambridge University Press. pp. 287–89. ISBN 0-521-65873-X
- Baumann E (1884). "Über cystin und cystein". Z Physiol Chem. 8 (4): 299–305. Archived from the original on 14 March 2011. Retrieved 28 March 2011
- Vermeer C (March 1990). "Gamma-carboxyglutamate-containing proteins and the vitamin K-dependent carboxylase". The Biochemical Journal. 266 (3): 625–36. PMC 1131186. PMID 2183788. doi:10.1042/bj2660625
- Peter Tompa; Alan Fersht (18 November 2009). Structure and Function of Intrinsically Disordered Proteins. CRC Press. ISBN 978-1-4200-7893-0
- Thombre SM, Sarwade BD (2005). "Synthesis and Biodegradability of Polyaspartic Acid: A Critical Review". Journal of Macromolecular Science, Part A. 42 (9): 1299–1315. doi:10.1080/10601320500189604
- Hatem, Salama Mohamed Ali (2006). "Gas chromatographic determination of Amino Acid Enantiomers in tobacco and bottled wines". University of Giessen. Retrieved 17 November 2008
- Bairoch A (2000). "The ENZYME database in 2000" (PDF). Nucleic Acids Research. 28 (1): 304–305. PMC 102465. PMID 10592255. doi:10.1093/nar/28.1.304. Archived from the original (PDF) on June 1, 2011
- Pollegioni L, Servi S, eds. (2012). Unnatural Amino Acids: Methods and Protocols. Methods in Molecular Biology – Volume 794. Humana Press. p. v. ISBN 978-1-61779-331-8. OCLC 756512314
- Hanf V, Gonder U (2005-12-01). "Nutrition and primary prevention of breast cancer: foods, nutrients and breast cancer risk.". European journal of obstetrics, gynecology, and reproductive biology. 123 (2)
- Creighton TH (1993). "Chapter 1". Proteins: structures and molecular properties. San Francisco: W. H. Freeman. ISBN 978-0-7167-7030-5
- Wagner I, Musso H (November 1983). "New Naturally Occurring Amino Acids". Angewandte Chemie International Edition in English. 22 (11): 816–28. doi:10.1002/anie.198308161

3

An Overview of Micronutrients

Micronutrients are essential elements that are necessarily required in small amounts by organisms. Some of the essential micronutrients are vitamins, minerals, etc. Both plants and animals can develop deficiencies in micronutrients. The chapter serves as a source to understand the major categories related to micronutrients.

Micronutrient

Micronutrients are nutrients required by organisms throughout life in small quantities to orchestrate a range of physiological functions. For people, they include dietary trace minerals in amounts generally less than 100 milligrams per day, as opposed to macrominerals, which are required in larger quantities. The microminerals or trace elements include at least iron, cobalt, chromium, copper, iodine, manganese, selenium, zinc and molybdenum. Micronutrients also include vitamins, which are organic compounds required as nutrients in trace amounts.

Public Health Initiatives for Humans

At the 1990 World Summit for Children, the gathered nations identified deficiencies in two microminerals and one micronutrient – iodine, iron, and vitamin A – as being particularly common and posing public health risks in developing countries. The Summit set goals for elimination of these deficiencies. The Ottawa-based Micronutrient Initiative was formed in response to this challenge with the mission to undertake research and fund and implement micronutrient programming.

As programming around these micronutrients grew, new research in the 1990s led to the implementation of folate and zinc supplementation programmes as well.

Priority programs include supplementation with vitamin A for children 6–59 months, zinc supplementation as a treatment for diarrhoeal disease, iron and folate supplementation for women of child-bearing age, salt iodization, staple food fortification, multiple micronutrient powders, biofortification of crops and behaviour-centred nutrition education.

Salt Iodization

Salt iodization is the recommended strategy for ensuring adequate human iodine intake. To iodize salt, potassium iodate is added to salt after it is refined and dried and before it is packed. Although large-scale iodization is most efficient, given the proliferation of small scale salt producers in developing countries, technology for small-scale iodization has also been developed. International organizations work with national governments to identify and support small salt producers in adopting iodization activity.

In 1990, less than 20 percent of households in developing countries were consuming iodized salt. By 1994, international partnerships had formed in a global campaign for Universal Salt Iodization. By 2008, it was estimated that 72 per cent of households in developing countries were consuming iodized salt and the number of countries in which iodine deficiency disorders were a public health concern reduced by more than half from 110 to 47 countries.

Vitamin A Supplementation

In 1997, national vitamin A supplementation programming received a boost when experts met to discuss rapid scale-up of supplementation activity and the Micronutrient Initiative, with support from the Government of Canada, began to ensure vitamin A supply to UNICEF.

In areas with vitamin A deficiency, it is recommended that children aged 6–59 months receive two doses annually. In many countries, vitamin A supplementation is combined with immunization and campaign-style health events.

Global vitamin A supplementation efforts have targeted 103 priority countries. In 1999, 16 per cent of children in these countries received two annual doses of vitamin A. By 2007, the rate increased to 62 percent.

The Micronutrient Initiative, with funding from the Government of Canada, supplies 75 per cent of the vitamin A required for supplementation in developing countries.

Double-fortified Salt

Double-fortified salt (DFS) is a public health tool for delivering nutritional iron. DFS is fortified with both iodine and iron. It was developed by Venkatesh Mannar, Executive Director of the Micronutrient Initiative and University of Toronto Professor Levente Diosady, who discovered a process for coating iron particles with a vegetable fat to prevent the negative interaction of iodine and iron.

In India, Tata Salt Plus, priced at an economical rate of Rs 20 per kg, is an iodine plus iron fortified salt, developed by the National Institute of Nutrition, Hyderabad through double fortification technology. This technology was offered to Tata Chemicals under a long-term MoU after due studies on bio-availability across the population strata conducted and published by NIN.

It was first used in public programming in 2004. In September 2010 DFS was produced in the Indian State of Tamil Nadu and distributed through a state school feeding program. DFS has also been used to combat Iron Deficiency Anemia (IDA) in the Indian state of Bihar. In September 2010, Venkatesh Mannar was named a Laureat of the California-based Tech Awards for his work in developing Double-Fortified Salt.

Micro-enriched Fertilization

The returns of applying micronutrient-enriched fertilizers could be huge for human health, social and economic development. Research has shown that enriching fertilizers with micronutrients had not only an impact on plant deficiencies but also on humans and animals, through the food chain. A 1994 report by the World Bank estimated that micronutrient malnutrition costs developing economies at least 5 percent of gross domestic product. The Asian Development Bank has summarized the benefits of eliminating micronutrient deficiencies as follows:

Along with a growing understanding of the extent and impact of micronutrient malnutrition, several interventions have demonstrated the feasibility and benefits of correction and prevention. Distributing inexpensive capsules, diversifying to include more micronutrient-rich foods, or fortifying commonly consumed foods can make an enormous difference. Correcting iodine, vitamin A, and iron deficiencies can improve the population-wide intelligence quotient by 10-15 points, reduce maternal deaths by one fourth, decrease infant and child mortality by 40 percent, and increase people's work capacity by almost half. The elimination of these deficiencies will reduce health care and education costs, improve work capacity and productivity, and accelerate equitable economic growth and national development. Improved nutrition is essential to sustained economic growth. Micronutrient deficiency elimination is as cost effective as the best public health interventions and fortification is the most cost-effective strategy.

Addressing Zinc Deficiencies through Zinc Fertilization

Experiments show that soil and foliar application of zinc fertilizer can effectively reduce the phytate zinc ratio in grain. People who eat bread prepared from zinc enriched wheat show a significant increase in serum zinc, suggesting that the zinc fertilizer strategy is a promising approach to address zinc deficiencies in humans.

Where zinc deficiency is a limiting factor, zinc fertilization can increase crop yields. Balanced crop nutrition supplying all essential nutrients, including zinc, is a cost effective management strategy. Even with zinc-efficient varieties, zinc fertilizers are needed when the available zinc in the topsoil becomes depleted.

Micronutrients for Plants

There are about seven nutrients essential to plant growth and health that are only needed in very small quantities. Though these are present in only small quantities, they are all necessary:

- Boron is believed to be involved in carbohydrate transport in plants; it also assists in metabolic regulation. Boron deficiency will often result in bud dieback.
- Chlorine is necessary for osmosis and ionic balance; it also plays a role in photosynthesis.
- Copper is a component of some enzymes. Symptoms of copper deficiency include browning of leaf tips and chlorosis.
- Iron is essential for chlorophyll synthesis, which is why an iron deficiency results in chlorosis.
- Manganese activates some important enzymes involved in chlorophyll formation. Manganese deficient plants will develop chlorosis between the veins of its leaves. The availability of manganese is partially dependent on soil pH.
- Molybdenum is essential to plant health. Molybdenum is used by plants to reduce nitrates into usable forms. Some plants use it for nitrogen fixation, thus it may need to be added to some soils before seeding legumes.
- Zinc participates in chlorophyll formation, and also activates many enzymes. Symptoms of zinc deficiency include chlorosis and stunted growth.

Micronutrient Deficiencies in Crops

Micronutrient deficiencies are widespread. 51% of world cereal soils are deficient in zinc and 30% of cultivated soils globally are deficient in iron. Steady growth of crop yields during recent decades (in particular through the Green Revolution) compounded the problem by progressively depleting soil micronutrient pools.

In general, farmers only apply micronutrients when crops show deficiency symptoms, while micronutrient deficiencies decrease yields before symptoms appear. Some common farming practices (such as liming acid soils) contribute to widespread occurrence of micronutrient deficiencies in crops by decreasing the availability of the micronutrients present in the soil. Also, extensive use of glyphosate is increasingly suspected to impair micronutrient uptake by crops, especially with regard to manganese, iron and zinc.

Vitamin

A vitamin is an organic compound and a vital nutrient that an organism requires in limited amounts. An organic chemical compound (or related set of compounds) is called a vitamin when the organism cannot synthesize the compound in sufficient quantities, and it must be obtained through the diet; thus, the term *vitamin* is conditional upon the circumstances and the particular organism. For example, ascorbic acid (one form of vitamin C) is a vitamin for humans, but not for most other animal organisms. Supplementation is important for the treatment of certain health problems, but there is little evidence of nutritional benefit when used by otherwise healthy people.

By convention the term *vitamin* does not include other essential nutrients, such as dietary minerals, essential fatty acids, essential amino acids (which are needed in greater amounts than vitamins) or the many other nutrients that promote health, and are required less often to maintain the health of the organism. Thirteen vitamins are universally recognized at present. Vitamins are classified by their biological and chemical activity, not their structure. Thus, each vitamin refers to a number of vitamer compounds that all show the biological activity associated with a particular vitamin. Such a set of chemicals is grouped under an alphabetized vitamin "generic descriptor" title, such as "vitamin A", which includes the compounds retinal, retinol, and four known carotenoids. Vitamers by definition are convertible to the active form of the vitamin in the body, and are sometimes inter-convertible to one another, as well.

Vitamins have diverse biochemical functions. Some, such as vitamin D, have hormone-like functions as regulators of mineral metabolism, or regulators of cell and tissue growth and differentiation (such as some forms of vitamin A). Others function as antioxidants (e.g., vitamin E and sometimes vitamin C). The largest number of vitamins, the B complex vitamins, function as enzyme cofactors (coenzymes) or the precursors for them; coenzymes help enzymes in their work as catalysts in metabolism. In this role, vitamins may be tightly bound to enzymes as part of prosthetic groups: For example, biotin is part of enzymes involved in making fatty acids. They may also be less tightly bound to enzyme catalysts as coenzymes, detachable molecules that function to carry chemical groups or electrons between molecules. For example, folic acid may carry methyl, formyl, and methylene groups in the cell. Although these roles in assisting enzyme-substrate reactions are vitamins' best-known function, the other vitamin functions are equally important.

Until the mid-1930s, when the first commercial yeast-extract vitamin B complex and semi-synthetic vitamin C supplement tablets were sold, vitamins were obtained solely through food intake, and changes in diet (which, for example, could occur during a particular growing season) usually greatly altered the types and amounts of vitamins ingested. However, vitamins have been produced as commodity chemicals and made widely available as inexpensive semisynthetic and synthetic-source multivitamin dietary and food supplements and additives, since the middle of the 20th century. Study of structural activity, function and their role in maintaining health is called vitaminology.

Health Effects

Vitamins are essential for the normal growth and development of a multicellular organism. Using the genetic blueprint inherited from its parents, a fetus begins to develop from the nutrients it absorbs. It requires certain vitamins and minerals to be present at certain times. These nutrients facilitate the chemical reactions that produce among other things, skin, bone, and muscle. If there is serious deficiency in one or more of these nutrients, a child may develop a deficiency disease. Even minor deficiencies may cause permanent damage.

For the most part, vitamins are obtained with food, but a few are obtained by other means. For example, microorganisms in the intestine — commonly known as "gut flora" — produce vitamin K and biotin, while one form of vitamin D is synthesized in the skin with the help of the natural ultraviolet wavelength of sunlight. Humans can produce some vitamins from precursors they consume. Examples include vitamin A, produced from beta carotene, and niacin, from the amino acid tryptophan.

Once growth and development are completed, vitamins remain essential nutrients for the healthy maintenance of the cells, tissues, and organs that make up a multicellular organism; they also enable a multicellular life form to efficiently use chemical energy provided by food it eats, and to help process the proteins, carbohydrates, and fats required for cellular respiration.

Supplements

In those who are otherwise healthy, there is little evidence that supplements have any benefits with respect to cancer or heart disease. Vitamin A and E supplements not only provide no health benefits for generally healthy individuals, but they may increase mortality, though the two large studies that support this conclusion included smokers for whom it was already known that beta-carotene supplements can be harmful. While other findings suggest that vitamin E toxicity is limited to only a specific form when taken in excess.

The European Union and other countries of Europe have regulations that define limits of vitamin (and mineral) dosages for their safe use as food supplements. Most vitamins that are sold as food supplements cannot exceed a maximum daily dosage. Vitamin products above these legal limits are not considered food supplements and must be registered as prescription or non-prescription (over-the-counter drugs) due to their potential side effects. As a result, most of the fat-soluble vitamins (such as the vitamins A, D, E, and K) that contain amounts above the daily allowance are drug products. The daily dosage of a vitamin supplement for example cannot exceed 300% of the recommended daily allowance, and for vitamin A, this limit is even lower (200%). Such regulations are applicable in most European countries.

Dietary supplements often contain vitamins, but may also include other ingredients, such as minerals, herbs, and botanicals. Scientific evidence supports the benefits of dietary supplements for persons with certain health conditions. In some cases, vitamin supplements may have unwanted effects, especially if taken before surgery, with other dietary supplements or medicines, or if the person taking them has certain health conditions. They may also contain levels of vitamins many times higher, and in different forms, than one may ingest through food.

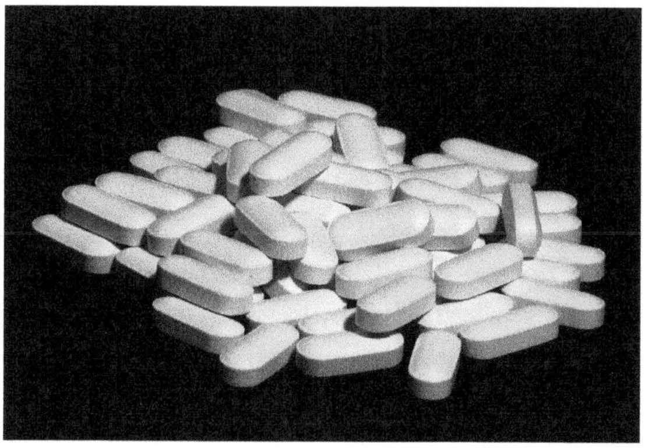

500 mg calcium supplement tablets, with vitamin D, made from calcium carbonate, maltodextrin, mineral oil, hypromellose, glycerin, cholecalciferol, polyethylene glycol, and carnauba wax.

Effect of Cooking

The USDA has conducted extensive studies on the percentage losses of various nutrients from different food types and cooking methods.

It should be noted however that some vitamins may become more "bio-available" – that is, usable by the body – when steamed or cooked.

The table below shows whether various vitamins are susceptible to loss from heat—such as heat from boiling, steaming, cooking etc.—and other agents. The effect of cutting vegetables can be seen from exposure to air and light. Water-soluble vitamins such as B and C seep into the water when a vegetable is boiled.

Vitamin	Soluble in Water	Exposure to Air	Exposure to Light	Exposure to Heat
Vitamin A	no	partially	partially	relatively stable
Vitamin C	very unstable	yes	yes	yes
Vitamin D	no	no	no	no
Vitamin E	no	yes	yes	no
Vitamin K	no	no	yes	no
Thiamine (B_1)	highly	no	?	> 100 °C
Riboflavin (B_2)	slightly	no	in solution	no
Niacin (B_3)	yes	no	no	no
Pantothenic Acid (B_5)	quite stable	?	no	yes
Vitamin B_6	yes	?	yes	?

Vitamin	Soluble in Water	Exposure to Air	Exposure to Light	Exposure to Heat
Biotin (B_7)	somewhat	?	?	no
Folic Acid (B_9)	yes	?	when dry	at high temp
Vitamin B_{12}	yes	?	yes	no

Deficiencies

Humans must consume vitamins periodically but with differing schedules, to avoid deficiency. The body's stores for different vitamins vary widely; vitamins A, D, and B_{12} are stored in significant amounts, mainly in the liver, and an adult's diet may be deficient in vitamins A and D for many months and B_{12} in some cases for years, before developing a deficiency condition. However, vitamin B_3 (niacin and niacinamide) is not stored in significant amounts, so stores may last only a couple of weeks. For vitamin C, the first symptoms of scurvy in experimental studies of complete vitamin C deprivation in humans have varied widely, from a month to more than six months, depending on previous dietary history that determined body stores.

Deficiencies of vitamins are classified as either primary or secondary. A primary deficiency occurs when an organism does not get enough of the vitamin in its food. A secondary deficiency may be due to an underlying disorder that prevents or limits the absorption or use of the vitamin, due to a "lifestyle factor", such as smoking, excessive alcohol consumption, or the use of medications that interfere with the absorption or use of the vitamin. People who eat a varied diet are unlikely to develop a severe primary vitamin deficiency. In contrast, restrictive diets have the potential to cause prolonged vitamin deficits, which may result in often painful and potentially deadly diseases.

Well-known human vitamin deficiencies involve thiamine (beriberi), niacin (pellagra), vitamin C (scurvy), and vitamin D (rickets). In much of the developed world, such deficiencies are rare; this is due to (1) an adequate supply of food and (2) the addition of vitamins and minerals to common foods (fortification). In addition to these classical vitamin deficiency diseases, some evidence has also suggested links between vitamin deficiency and a number of different disorders.

Side-effects

In large doses, some vitamins have documented side-effects that tend to be more severe with a larger dosage. The likelihood of consuming too much of any vitamin from food is remote, but overdosing (vitamin poisoning) from vitamin supplementation does occur. At high enough dosages, some vitamins cause side-effects such as nausea, diarrhea, and vomiting. When side-effects emerge, recovery is often accomplished by reducing the dosage. The doses of vitamins differ because individual tolerances can vary widely and appear to be related to age and state of health.

In 2008, overdose exposure to all formulations of vitamins and multivitamin-mineral formulations was reported by 68,911 individuals to the American Association of Poison Control Centers (nearly 80% of these exposures were in children under the age of 6), leading to 8 "major" life-threatening outcomes, but no deaths.

Pharmacology

Vitamins are classified as either water-soluble or fat-soluble. In humans there are 13 vitamins: 4 fat-soluble (A, D, E, and K) and 9 water-soluble (8 B vitamins and vitamin C). Water-soluble vitamins dissolve easily in water and, in general, are readily excreted from the body, to the degree that urinary output is a strong predictor of vitamin consumption. Because they are not as readily stored, more consistent intake is important. Many types of water-soluble vitamins are synthesized by bacteria. Fat-soluble vitamins are absorbed through the intestinal tract with the help of lipids (fats). Because they are more likely to accumulate in the body, they are more likely to lead to hypervitaminosis than are water-soluble vitamins. Fat-soluble vitamin regulation is of particular significance in cystic fibrosis.

History

The discovery dates of the vitamins and their sources

Year of discovery	**Vitamin**	**Food source**
1913	Vitamin A (Retinol)	Cod liver oil
1910	Vitamin B_1 (Thiamine)	Rice bran
1920	Vitamin C (Ascorbic acid)	Citrus, most fresh foods
1920	Vitamin D (Calciferol)	Cod liver oil
1920	Vitamin B_2 (Riboflavin)	Meat, dairy products, eggs
1922	Vitamin E (Tocopherol)	Wheat germ oil, unrefined vegetable oils
1929	Vitamin K_1 (Phylloquinone)	Leaf vegetables
1931	Vitamin B_5 (Pantothenic acid)	Meat, whole grains, in many foods
1931	Vitamin B_7 (Biotin)	Meat, dairy products, eggs
1934	Vitamin B_6 (Pyridoxine)	Meat, dairy products
1936	Vitamin B_3 (Niacin)	Meat, grains
1941	Vitamin B_9 (Folic acid)	Leaf vegetables
1948	Vitamin B_{12} (Cobalamins)	Liver, eggs, animal products

The value of eating a certain food to maintain health was recognized long before vitamins were identified. The ancient Egyptians knew that feeding liver to a person may help with night blindness, an illness now known to be caused by a vitamin A deficiency.

The advancement of ocean voyages during the Renaissance resulted in prolonged periods without access to fresh fruits and vegetables, and made illnesses from vitamin deficiency common among ships' crews.

In 1747, the Scottish surgeon James Lind discovered that citrus foods helped prevent scurvy, a particularly deadly disease in which collagen is not properly formed, causing poor wound healing, bleeding of the gums, severe pain, and death. In 1753, Lind published his *Treatise on the Scurvy,* which recommended using lemons and limes to avoid scurvy, which was adopted by the British Royal Navy. This led to the nickname *limey* for British sailors. Lind's discovery, however, was not widely accepted by individuals in the Royal Navy's Arctic expeditions in the 19th century, where it was widely believed that scurvy could be prevented by practicing good hygiene, regular exercise, and maintaining the morale of the crew while on board, rather than by a diet of fresh food. As a result, Arctic expeditions continued to be plagued by scurvy and other deficiency diseases. In the early 20th century, when Robert Falcon Scott made his two expeditions to the Antarctic, the prevailing medical theory at the time was that scurvy was caused by "tainted" canned food.

During the late 18th and early 19th centuries, the use of deprivation studies allowed scientists to isolate and identify a number of vitamins. Lipid from fish oil was used to cure rickets in rats, and the fat-soluble nutrient was called "antirachitic A". Thus, the first "vitamin" bioactivity ever isolated, which cured rickets, was initially called "vitamin A"; however, the bioactivity of this compound is now called vitamin D. In 1881, Russian surgeon Nikolai Lunin studied the effects of scurvy at the University of Tartu in present-day Estonia. He fed mice an artificial mixture of all the separate constituents of milk known at that time, namely the proteins, fats, carbohydrates, and salts. The mice that received only the individual constituents died, while the mice fed by milk itself developed normally. He made a conclusion that "a natural food such as milk must therefore contain, besides these known principal ingredients, small quantities of unknown substances essential to life." However, his conclusions were rejected by his advisor, Gustav von Bunge, even after other students reproduced his results. A similar result by Cornelius Pekelharing appeared in a Dutch medical journal in 1905, but it was not widely reported.

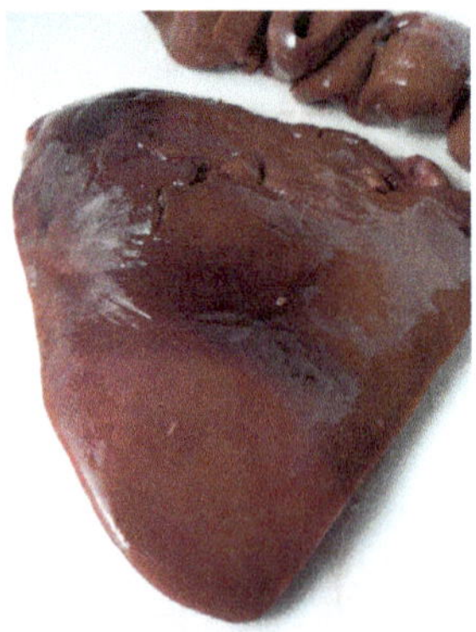

The Ancient Egyptians knew that feeding a person liver may help with night blindness.

In East Asia, where polished white rice was the common staple food of the middle class, beriberi resulting from lack of vitamin B_1 was endemic. In 1884, Takaki Kanehiro, a British trained medical doctor of the Imperial Japanese Navy, observed that beriberi was endemic among low-ranking crew who often ate nothing but rice, but not among officers who consumed a Western-style diet. With the support of the Japanese navy, he experimented using crews of two battleships; one crew was fed only white rice, while the other was fed a diet of meat, fish, barley, rice, and beans. The group that ate only white rice documented 161 crew members with beriberi and 25 deaths, while the latter group had only 14 cases of beriberi and no deaths. This convinced Takaki and the Japanese Navy that diet was the cause of beriberi, but they mistakenly believed that sufficient amounts of protein prevented it. That diseases could result from some dietary deficiencies was further investigated by Christiaan Eijkman, who in 1897 discovered that feeding unpolished rice instead of the polished variety to chickens helped to prevent beriberi in the chickens. The following year, Frederick Hopkins postulated that some foods contained "accessory factors" — in addition to proteins, carbohydrates, fats *etc.* — that are necessary for the functions of the human body. Hopkins and Eijkman were awarded the Nobel Prize for Physiology or Medicine in 1929 for their discoveries.

In 1910, the first vitamin complex was isolated by Japanese scientist Umetaro Suzuki, who succeeded in extracting a water-soluble complex of micronutrients from rice bran and named it aberic acid (later *Orizanin*). He published this discovery in a Japanese scientific journal. When the article was translated into German, the translation failed to state that it was a newly discovered nutrient, a claim made in the original Japanese article, and hence his discovery failed to gain publicity. In 1912 Polish-born biochemist Casimir Funk, working in London, isolated the same complex of micronutrients and proposed the complex be named "vitamine". It was later to be known as vitamin B_3 (niacin), though he described it as "anti-beri-beri-factor" (which would today be called thiamine or vitamin B_1). Funk proposed the hypothesis that other diseases, such as rickets, pellagra, coeliac disease, and scurvy could also be cured by vitamins. Max Nierenstein a friend and reader of Biochemistry at Bristol University reportedly suggested the "vitamine" name (from "vital amine").). The name soon became synonymous with Hopkins' "accessory factors", and, by the time it was shown that not all vitamins are amines, the word was already ubiquitous. In 1920, Jack Cecil Drummond proposed that the final "e" be dropped to deemphasize the "amine" reference, after researchers began to suspect that not all "vitamines" (in particular, vitamin A) have an amine component.

In 1930, Paul Karrer elucidated the correct structure for beta-carotene, the main precursor of vitamin A, and identified other carotenoids. Karrer and Norman Haworth confirmed Albert Szent-Györgyi's discovery of ascorbic acid and made significant contributions to the chemistry of flavins, which led to the identification of lactoflavin. For their investigations on carotenoids, flavins and vitamins A and B_2, they both received the Nobel Prize in Chemistry in 1937.

In 1931, Albert Szent-Györgyi and a fellow researcher Joseph Svirbely suspected that "hexuronic acid" was actually vitamin C, and gave a sample to Charles Glen King, who proved its anti-scorbutic activity in his long-established guinea pig scorbutic assay. In 1937, Szent-Györgyi was awarded the Nobel Prize in Physiology or Medicine for his discovery. In 1943, Edward Adelbert Doisy and Henrik Dam were awarded the Nobel Prize in Physiology or Medicine for their discovery of vitamin K and its chemical structure. In 1967, George Wald was awarded the Nobel Prize (along with Ragnar Granit and Haldan Keffer Hartline) for his discovery that vitamin A could participate directly in a physiological process.

Etymology

The term *vitamin* was derived from "vitamine", a compound word coined in 1912 by the Polish biochemist Kazimierz Funk when working at the Lister Institute of Preventive Medicine. The name is from *vital* and *amine*, meaning amine of life, because it was suggested in 1912 that the organic micronutrient food factors that prevent beriberi and perhaps other similar dietary-deficiency diseases might be chemical amines. This was true of thiamine, but after it was found that other such micronutrients were not amines the word was shortened to vitamin in English.

Society and Culture

Once discovered, vitamins were actively promoted in articles and advertisements in *McCall's*, *Good Housekeeping*, and other media outlets. Marketers enthusiastically promoted cod-liver oil, a source of Vitamin D, as "bottled sunshine", and bananas as a "natural vitality food". They promoted foods such as yeast cakes, a source of B vitamins, on the basis of scientifically-determined nutritional value, rather than taste or appearance. World War II researchers focused on the need to ensure adequate nutrition, especially in processed foods. Robert W. Yoder is credited with first using the term *vitamania*, in 1942, to describe the appeal of relying on nutritional supplements rather than on obtaining vitamins from a varied diet of foods. The continuing preoccupation with a healthy lifestyle has led to an obsessive consumption of additives the beneficial effects of which are questionable.

Governmental Regulation

Most countries place dietary supplements in a special category under the general umbrella of *foods*, not drugs. As a result, the manufacturer, and not the government, has the responsibility of ensuring that its dietary supplement products are safe before they are marketed. Regulation of supplements varies widely by country. In the United States, a dietary supplement is defined under the Dietary Supplement Health and Education Act of 1994. There is no FDA approval process for dietary supplements, and no requirement that manufacturers prove the safety or efficacy of supplements introduced before 1994. The Food and Drug Administration must rely on its Adverse Event Reporting

System to monitor adverse events that occur with supplements. In 2007, the US Code of Federal Regulations (CFR) Title 21, part III took effect, regulating GMP practices in the manufacturing, packaging, labeling, or holding operations for dietary supplements. Even though product registration is not required, these regulations mandate production and quality control standards (including testing for identity, purity and adulterations) for dietary supplements. In the European Union, the Food Supplements Directive requires that only those supplements that have been proven safe can be sold without a prescription. For most vitamins, pharmacopoeial standards have been established. In the United States, the United States Pharmacopeia (USP) sets standards for the most commonly used vitamins and preparations thereof. Likewise, monographs of the European Pharmacopoeia (Ph.Eur.) regulate aspects of identity and purity for vitamins on the European market.

Naming

Nomenclature of Reclassified Vitamins		
Previous name	**Chemical name**	**Reason for name change**
Vitamin B_4	Adenine	DNA metabolite; synthesized in body
Vitamin B_8	Adenylic acid	DNA metabolite; synthesized in body
Vitamin B_T	Carnitine	Synthesized in body
Vitamin F	Essential fatty acids	Needed in large quantities (does not fit the definition of a vitamin).
Vitamin G	Riboflavin	Reclassified as Vitamin B_2
Vitamin H	Biotin	Reclassified as Vitamin B_7
Vitamin J	Catechol, Flavin	Catechol nonessential; flavin reclassified as Vitamin B_2
Vitamin L_1	Anthranilic acid	Non essential
Vitamin L_2	Adenylthiomethylpentose	RNA metabolite; synthesized in body
Vitamin M	Folic acid	Reclassified as Vitamin B_9
Vitamin P	Flavonoids	No longer classified as a vitamin
Vitamin PP	Niacin	Reclassified as Vitamin B_3
Vitamin S	Salicylic acid	Proposed inclusion of salicylate as an essential micronutrient
Vitamin U	S-Methylmethionine	Protein metabolite; synthesized in body

The reason that the set of vitamins skips directly from E to K is that the vitamins corresponding to letters F–J were either reclassified over time, discarded as false leads, or renamed because of their relationship to vitamin B, which became a complex of vitamins.

The German-speaking scientists who isolated and described vitamin K (in addition to naming it as such) did so because the vitamin is intimately involved in the coagulation of blood following wounding (from the German word *Koagulation*). At the time, most (but not all) of the letters from F through to J were already designated, so the use of the letter K was considered quite reasonable. The table *nomenclature of reclassified vitamins* lists chemicals that had previously been classified as vitamins, as well as the earlier names of vitamins that later became part of the B-complex.

There are other missing B vitamins which were reclassified or determined not to be vitamins. For example, B_9 is folic acid and five of the folates are in the range B_{11} through B_{16}, forms of other vitamins already discovered, not required as a nutrient by the entire population (like B_{10}, PABA for internal use), biologically inactive, toxic, or with unclassifiable effects in humans, or not generally recognised as vitamins by science, such as the highest-numbered, which some naturopath practitioners call B_{21} and B_{22}. There are also nine lettered B complex vitamins (e.g. B_m). There are other D vitamins now recognised as other substances, which some sources of the same type number up to D_7. The controversial cancer treatment laetrile was at one point lettered as vitamin B_{17}. There appears to be no consensus on any vitamins Q, R, T, V, W, X, Y or Z, nor are there substances officially designated as Vitamins N or I, although the latter may have been another form of one of the other vitamins or a known and named nutrient of another type.

Anti-vitamins

Anti-vitamins are chemical compounds that inhibit the absorption or actions of vitamins. For example, avidin is a protein in egg whites that inhibits the absorption of biotin. Pyrithiamine is similar to thiamine, vitamin B_1, and inhibits the enzymes that use thiamine.

Vitamin A

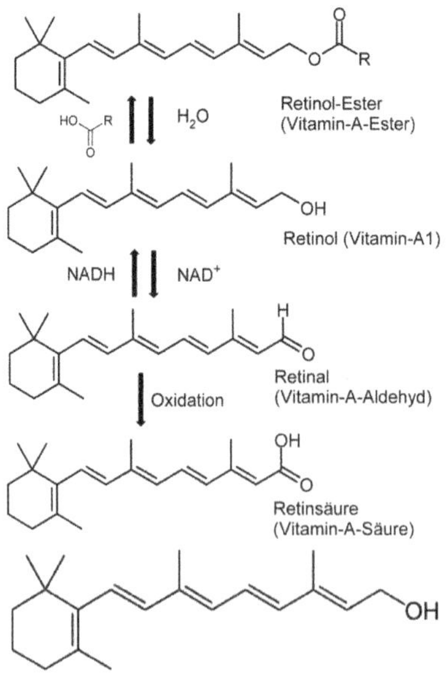

Chemical structure of retinol, one of the major forms of vitamin A

Vitamin A is a group of unsaturated nutritional organic compounds that includes retinol, retinal, retinoic acid, and several provitamin A carotenoids (most notably beta-carotene). Vitamin A has multiple functions: it is important for growth and development, for the maintenance of the immune system and good vision. Vitamin A is needed by the retina of the eye in the form of retinal, which combines with protein opsin to form rhodopsin, the light-absorbing molecule necessary for both low-light (scotopic vision) and color vision. Vitamin A also functions in a very different role as retinoic acid (an irreversibly oxidized form of retinol), which is an important hormone-like growth factor for epithelial and other cells.

In foods of animal origin, the major form of vitamin A is an ester, primarily retinyl palmitate, which is converted to retinol (chemically an alcohol) in the small intestine. The retinol form functions as a storage form of the vitamin, and can be converted to and from its visually active aldehyde form, retinal.

All forms of vitamin A have a beta-ionone ring to which an isoprenoid chain is attached, called a *retinyl group*. Both structural features are essential for vitamin activity. The orange pigment of carrots (beta-carotene) can be represented as two connected retinyl groups, which are used in the body to contribute to vitamin A levels. Alpha-carotene and gamma-carotene also have a single retinyl group, which give them some vitamin activity. None of the other carotenes have vitamin activity. The carotenoid beta-cryptoxanthin possesses an ionone group and has vitamin activity in humans.

Vitamin A can be found in two principal forms in foods:

- Retinol, the form of vitamin A absorbed when eating animal food sources, is a yellow, fat-soluble substance. Since the pure alcohol form is unstable, the vitamin is found in tissues in a form of retinyl ester. It is also commercially produced and administered as esters such as retinyl acetate or palmitate.
- The carotenes alpha-carotene, beta-carotene, gamma-carotene; and the xanthophyll beta-cryptoxanthin (all of which contain beta-ionone rings), but no other carotenoids, function as provitamin A in herbivores and omnivore animals, which possess the enzyme beta-carotene 15,15'-dioxygenase which cleaves beta-carotene in the intestinal mucosa and converts it to retinol. In general, carnivores are poor converters of ionone-containing carotenoids, and pure carnivores such as cats and ferrets lack beta-carotene 15,15'-dioxygenase and cannot convert any carotenoids to retinal (resulting in *none* of the carotenoids being forms of vitamin A for these species).

Medical Use

Deficiency

Vitamin A deficiency is estimated to affect approximately one third of children under the age of five around the world. It is estimated to claim the lives of 670,000 children under five annually. Approximately 250,000–500,000 children in developing countries become blind each year owing to vitamin A deficiency, with the highest prevalence in Southeast Asia and Africa. Vitamin A deficiency is "the leading cause of preventable childhood blindness," according to UNICEF. It also increases the risk of death from common childhood conditions such as diarrhea. UNICEF regards addressing vitamin A deficiency as critical to reducing child mortality, the fourth of the United Nations' Millennium Development Goals.

Vitamin A deficiency can occur as either a primary or a secondary deficiency. A primary vitamin A deficiency occurs among children and adults who do not consume an adequate intake of provitamin A carotenoids from fruits and vegetables or preformed vitamin A from animal and dairy products. Early weaning from breastmilk can also increase the risk of vitamin A deficiency.

Secondary vitamin A deficiency is associated with chronic malabsorption of lipids, impaired bile production and release, and chronic exposure to oxidants, such as cigarette smoke, and chronic alcoholism. Vitamin A is a fat-soluble vitamin and depends on micellar solubilization for dispersion into the small intestine, which results in poor use of vitamin A from low-fat diets. Zinc deficiency can also impair absorption, transport, and metabolism of vitamin A because it is essential for the synthesis of the vitamin A transport proteins and as the cofactor in conversion of retinol to retinal. In malnourished populations, common low intakes of vitamin A and zinc increase the severity of vitamin A deficiency and lead physiological signs and symptoms of deficiency. A study in Burkina Faso showed major reduction of malaria morbidity with combined vitamin A and zinc supplementation in young children.

Due to the unique function of retinal as a visual chromophore, one of the earliest and specific manifestations of vitamin A deficiency is impaired vision, particularly in reduced light – night blindness. Persistent deficiency gives rise to a series of changes, the most devastating of which occur in the eyes. Some other ocular changes are referred to as xerophthalmia. First there is dryness of the conjunctiva (xerosis) as the normal lacrimal and mucus-secreting epithelium is replaced by a keratinized epithelium. This is followed by the build-up of keratin debris in small opaque plaques (Bitot's spots) and, eventually, erosion of the roughened corneal surface with softening and destruction of the cornea (keratomalacia) and leading to total blindness. Other changes include impaired immunity (increased risk of ear infections, urinary tract infections, Meningococcal disease), hyperkeratosis (white lumps at hair follicles), keratosis pilaris and squamous metaplasia of the epithelium lining the upper respiratory passages and urinary bladder to a keratinized epithelium. In relation to dentistry, a deficiency in vitamin A may lead to enamel hypoplasia.

Adequate supply, but not excess vitamin A, is especially important for pregnant and breastfeeding women for normal fetal development and in breastmilk. Deficiencies cannot be compensated by postnatal supplementation. Excess vitamin A, which is most common with high dose vitamin supplements, can cause birth defects and therefore should not exceed recommended daily values.

Vitamin A metabolic inhibition as a result of alcohol consumption during pregnancy is the elucidated mechanism for fetal alcohol syndrome and is characterized by teratogenicity closely matching maternal vitamin A deficiency.

Vitamin A Supplementation

Global efforts to support national governments in addressing vitamin A deficiency are led by the Global Alliance for Vitamin A (GAVA), which is an informal partnership between A2Z, the Canadian International Development Agency, Helen Keller International, the Micronutrient Initiative, UNICEF, USAID, and the World Bank. Joint GAVA activity is coordinated by the Micronutrient Initiative.

While strategies include intake of vitamin A through a combination of breast feeding and dietary intake, delivery of oral high-dose supplements remain the principal strategy for minimizing deficiency. A meta-analysis of 43 studies showed that vitamin A supplementation of children under five who are at risk of deficiency reduces mortality by up to 24%. About 75% of the vitamin A required for supplementation activity by developing countries is supplied by the Micronutrient Initiative with support from the Canadian International Development Agency. Food fortification approaches are becoming increasingly feasible but cannot yet ensure coverage levels.

The World Health Organization estimates that Vitamin A supplementation has averted 1.25 million deaths due to vitamin A deficiency in 40 countries since 1998. In 2008 it was estimated that an annual investment of US$60 million in vitamin A and zinc supplementation combined would yield benefits of more than US$1 billion per year, with every dollar spent generating benefits of more than US$17. These combined interventions were ranked by the Copenhagen Consensus 2008 as the world's best development investment.

Observational studies of pregnant women in sub-Saharan Africa have shown that low serum vitamin A levels are associated with an increased risk of mother-to-child transmission (MTCT) of HIV. Vitamin A is cheap and easily provided through existing health services in low-income settings. It is thus important to determine the effect of routine supplementation of H levels, and because low blood vitamin A levels have been associated with rapid HIV infection and deaths, To identify randomised controlled trials comparing vitamin A supplementation with placebo in known HIV-infected pregnant women, authors searched the Cochrane Library, PubMed, EMBASE, AIDSearch and GATEWAY; checked reference lis,. Authoritative reviews of more recent and better-designed studies have found no relationship between the level of serum maternal and/ or infant vitamin A and the likelihood of vertical (MTCT) HIV transmission. of HIV, our trials which enrolled 3033 HIV-infected pregnant women met inclusion criteria. Authors found significant statistical heterogeneity between the three trials with information on MTCT of HIV. Overall, there was no evidence of an effect of antenatal vitamin A supplementation on the risk of MTCT of HIV. However, antenatal vitamin A supplementation significantly improved birth weight, but there was no evidence of an effect on preterm births, stillbirths, deaths by 24 months. Evidence is also lacking on whether vitamin A supplementation for infants up to six months of age reduces infant mortality or morbidity in low- and middle-income countries.

Side Effects

Since vitamin A is fat-soluble, disposing of any excesses taken in through diet takes much longer than with water-soluble B vitamins and vitamin C. This allows for toxic levels of vitamin A to accumulate. These toxicities only occur with preformed (retinoid) vitamin A (such as from liver). The carotenoid forms (such as beta-carotene as found in carrots), give no such symptoms, except with supplements and chronic alcoholism, but excessive dietary intake of beta-carotene can lead to carotenodermia, a harmless but cosmetically displeasing orange-yellow discoloration of the skin.

In general, acute toxicity occurs at doses of 25,000 IU/kg of body weight, with chronic toxicity occurring at 4,000 IU/kg of body weight daily for 6–15 months. However, liver toxicities can occur at levels as low as 15,000 IU (4500 micrograms) per day to 1.4 million IU per day, with an average daily toxic dose of 120,000 IU, particularly with excessive consumption of alcohol. In people with renal failure, 4000 IU can cause substantial damage. Children can reach toxic levels at 1,500 IU/kg of body weight.

Excessive vitamin A consumption can lead to nausea, irritability, anorexia (reduced appetite), vomiting, blurry vision, headaches, hair loss, muscle and abdominal pain and weakness, drowsiness, and altered mental status. In chronic cases, hair loss, dry skin, drying of the mucous membranes, fever, insomnia, fatigue, weight loss, bone fractures, anemia, and diarrhea can all be evident on top of the symptoms associated with less serious toxicity. Some of these symptoms are also common to acne treatment with Isotretinoin. Chronically high doses of vitamin A, and also pharmaceutical retinoids such as 13-cis retinoic acid, can produce the syndrome of pseudotumor cerebri. This syndrome includes headache, blurring of vision and confusion, associated with increased intracerebral pressure. Symptoms begin to resolve when intake of the offending substance is stopped.

Chronic intake of 1500 RAE of preformed vitamin A may be associated with osteoporosis and hip fractures because it suppresses bone building while simultaneously stimulating bone breakdown.

High vitamin A intake has been associated with spontaneous bone fractures in animals. Cell culture studies have linked increased bone resorption and decreased bone formation with high intakes. This interaction may occur because vitamins A and D may compete for the same receptor and then interact with parathyroid hormone, which regulates calcium. Indeed, a study by Forsmo *et al.* shows a correlation between low bone mineral density and too high intake of vitamin A. Sufficiently high levels of vitamin D may be protective against the bone density lowering effects of high vitamin A, while inadequate levels of vitamin D may exacerbate those effects.

Toxic effects of vitamin A have been shown to significantly affect developing fetuses. Therapeutic doses used for acne treatment have been shown to disrupt cephalic neural cell activity. The fetus is particularly sensitive to vitamin A toxicity during the period of organogenesis.

Hepatic (liver) injury has been found in human and animal studies where consumption of alcohol is paired with high dose vitamin A and beta-carotene supplementation.

Researchers have succeeded in creating water-miscible vitamin A, but one human trial reported water-miscible vitamin A was approximately 10 times as toxic as fat-soluble vitamin. A 2006 study found children given water-miscible vitamin A and D, which are typically fat-soluble, suffer from asthma twice as much as a control group supplemented with the fat-soluble vitamins.

In some studies, the use of Vitamin A supplements has been linked to an increased rate of mortality.

History

The discovery of vitamin A may have stemmed from research dating back to 1816, when physiologist François Magendie observed that dogs deprived of nutrition developed corneal ulcers and had a high mortality rate. In 1912, Frederick Gowland Hopkins demonstrated that unknown accessory factors found in milk, other than carbohydrates, proteins, and fats were necessary for growth in rats. Hopkins received a Nobel Prize for this discovery in 1929. By 1913, one of these substances was independently discovered by Elmer McCollum and Marguerite Davis at the University of Wisconsin–Madison, and Lafayette Mendel and Thomas Burr Osborne at Yale University who studied the role of fats in the diet. McCollum and Davis ultimately received credit because they submitted their paper three weeks before Mendel and Osborne. Both papers appeared in the same issue of the *Journal of Biological Chemistry* in 1913. The "accessory factors" were termed "fat soluble" in 1918 and later "vitamin A" in 1920. In 1919, Harry Steenbock (University of Wisconsin–Madison) proposed a relationship between yellow plant pigments (beta-carotene) and vitamin A. In 1931, Swiss chemist Paul Karrer described the chemical structure of vitamin A. Vitamin A was first synthesized in 1947 by two Dutch chemists, David Adriaan van Dorp and Jozef Ferdinand Arens.

Equivalencies of Retinoids and Carotenoids (IU)

As some carotenoids can be converted into vitamin A, attempts have been made to determine how much of them in the diet is equivalent to a particular amount of retinol, so that comparisons can be made of the benefit of different foods. The situation can be confusing because the accepted equivalences have changed. For many years, a system of equivalencies in which an international unit (IU) was equal to 0.3 μg of retinol, 0.6 μg of β-carotene, or 1.2 μg of other provitamin-A carotenoids was used. Later, a unit called retinol equivalent (RE) was introduced. Prior to 2001, one RE corresponded to 1 μg retinol, 2 μg β-carotene dissolved in oil (it is only partly dissolved in most supplement pills, due to very poor solubility in any medium), 6 μg β-carotene in normal food (because it is not absorbed as well as when in oils), and 12 μg of either α-carotene, γ-carotene, or β-cryptoxanthin in food.

Newer research has shown that the absorption of provitamin-A carotenoids is only half as much as previously thought. As a result, in 2001 the US Institute of Medicine recommended a new unit, the retinol activity equivalent (RAE). Each μg RAE corresponds to 1 μg retinol, 2 μg of β-carotene in oil, 12 μg of "dietary" beta-carotene, or 24 μg of the three other dietary provitamin-A carotenoids.

Substance and its chemical environment	Micrograms of retinol equivalent per microgram of the substance
retinol	1
beta-carotene, dissolved in oil	1/2
beta-carotene, common dietary	1/12
alpha-carotene, common dietary	1/24
gamma-carotene, common dietary	1/24
beta-cryptoxanthin, common dietary	1/24

Because the conversion of retinol from provitamin carotenoids by the human body is actively regulated by the amount of retinol available to the body, the conversions apply strictly only for vitamin A-deficient humans. The absorption of provitamins depends greatly on the amount of lipids ingested with the provitamin; lipids increase the uptake of the provitamin.

The conclusion that can be drawn from the newer research is that fruits and vegetables are not as useful for obtaining vitamin A as was thought; in other words, the IUs that these foods were reported to contain were worth much less than the same number of IUs of fat-dissolved oils and (to some extent) supplements. This is important for vegetarians, as night blindness is prevalent in countries where little meat or vitamin A-fortified foods are available.

A sample vegan diet for one day that provides sufficient vitamin A has been published by the Food and Nutrition Board (page 120). On the other hand, reference values for retinol or its equivalents, provided by the National Academy of Sciences, have decreased. The RDA (for men) of 1968 was 5000 IU (1500 μg retinol). In 1974, the RDA was set to 1000 RE (1000 μg retinol), whereas now the Dietary Reference Intake is 900 RAE (900 μg or 3000 IU retinol). This is equivalent to 1800 μg of β-carotene supplement (3000 IU) or 10800 μg of β-carotene in food (18000 IU).

Recommended Dietary Allowance

Vitamin A

Dietary Reference Intakes:

Life stage group	RDAs or Adequate intakes (AI*) μg/day	Upper limits (UL*) μg/day
Infants		
0–6 months	400*	600
7–12 months	500*	600
Children		
1–3 years	300	600
4–8 years	400	900
Males		
9–13 years	600	1700
14–18 years	900	2800
19 – >70 years	900	3000
Females		
9–13 years	600	1700
14–18 years	700	2800
19 – >70 years	700	3000
Pregnancy		
<19 years	750	2800
19 – >50 years	770	3000
Lactation		
<19 years	1200	2800
19 – >50 years	1300	3000

- Adequate Intakes (AIs) are established when there is not sufficient information to set RDAs. For healthy breastfed infants, the AI was set to the mean intake."
- For U.S. food and dietary supplement labeling purposes the amount in a serving is expressed as a percent of Daily Value (%DV). For vitamin A labeling purposes 100% of the Daily Value was set at 5,000 IU, but as of May 2016 it has been revised to 900 μg RAE. A table of the pre-change adult Daily Values is provided at Reference Daily Intake. Food and supplement companies have until July 28, 2018 to comply with the change.

- Upper Limits (ULs) are for synthetic and natural retinol ester forms of vitamin A. Carotene forms from dietary sources are not toxic and are not added when calculating total vitamin A intake for safety purposes.

Sources

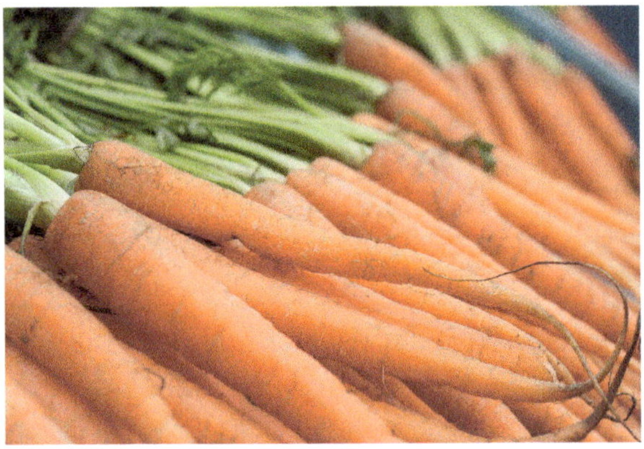

Carrots

Vitamin A is found in many foods:

- cod liver oil (30000 µg 3333%)
- liver (turkey) (8058 µg 895%)
- liver (beef, pork, fish) (6500 µg 722%)
- liver (chicken) (3296 µg 366%)
- capsicum, red (2081 µg 231%)
- sweet potato (961 µg 107%)
- carrot (835 µg 93%)
- broccoli leaf (800 µg 89%)
- butter (684 µg 76%)
- kale (681 µg 76%)
- collard greens (frozen then boiled) (575 µg 64%)
- Butternut squash (532 µg vit-A per 100 g, (532/900) * 100% = 59% daily value per 100 g)
- dandelion greens (508 µg 56%)
- spinach (469 µg 52%)
- pumpkin (426 µg 43%)

- collard greens (333 μg 37%)
- cheddar cheese (265 μg 29%)
- cantaloupe melon (169 μg 19%)
- egg (140 μg 16%)
- apricot (96 μg 11%)
- papaya (55 μg 6%)
- tomatoes (42 μg 5%)
- mango (38 μg 4%)
- pea (38 μg 4%)
- broccoli florets (31 μg 3%)
- milk (28 μg 3%)
- bell pepper, green (18 μg 2%)
- spirulina (3 μg 0.3%)

Bracketed values are retinol activity equivalences (RAEs) and percentage of the adult male RDA, per 100 grams of the foodstuff (average). Conversion of carotene to retinol varies from person to person and bioavailability of carotene in food varies.

Metabolic Functions

Vitamin A plays a role in a variety of functions throughout the body, such as:

- Vision
- Gene transcription
- Immune function
- Embryonic development and reproduction
- Bone metabolism
- Haematopoiesis
- Skin and cellular health
- Antioxidant activity
- Teeth
- Mucous membrane

Vision

The role of vitamin A in the visual cycle is specifically related to the retinal form. Within the eye, 11-*cis*-retinal is bound to the protein "opsin" to form rhodopsin in rods and iodopsin (cones) at conserved lysine residues. As light enters the eye, the 11-*cis*-retinal is isomerized to the all-"trans" form. The all-"trans" retinal dissociates from the opsin in a series of steps called photo-bleaching. This isomerization induces a nervous signal along the optic nerve to the visual center of the brain. After separating from opsin, the all-"trans"-retinal is recycled and converted back to the 11-"cis"-retinal form by a series of enzymatic reactions. In addition, some of the all-"trans" retinal may be converted to all-"trans" retinol form and then transported with an interphotoreceptor retinol-binding protein (IRBP) to the pigment epithelial cells. Further esterification into all-"trans" retinyl esters allow for storage of all-trans-retinol within the pigment epithelial cells to be reused when needed. The final stage is conversion of 11-*cis*-retinal will rebind to opsin to reform rhodopsin (visual purple) in the retina. Rhodopsin is needed to see in low light (contrast) as well as for night vision. Kühne showed that rhodopsin in the retina is only regenerated when the retina is attached to retinal pigmented epithelium, which provides retinal. It is for this reason that a deficiency in vitamin A will inhibit the reformation of rhodopsin and lead to one of the first symptoms, night blindness.

Gene Transcription

Vitamin A, in the retinoic acid form, plays an important role in gene transcription. Once retinol has been taken up by a cell, it can be oxidized to retinal (retinaldehyde) by retinol dehydrogenases and then retinaldehyde can be oxidized to retinoic acid by retinaldehyde dehydrogenases. The conversion of retinaldehyde to retinoic acid is an irreversible step, meaning that the production of retinoic acid is tightly regulated, due to its activity as a ligand for nuclear receptors. The physiological form of retinoic acid (all-trans-retinoic acid) regulates gene transcription by binding to nuclear receptors known as retinoic acid receptors (RARs) which are bound to DNA as heterodimers with retinoid "X" receptors (RXRs). RAR and RXR must dimerize before they can bind to the DNA. RAR will form a heterodimer with RXR (RAR-RXR), but it does not readily form a homodimer (RAR-RAR). RXR, on the other hand, may form a homodimer (RXR-RXR) and will form heterodimers with many other nuclear receptors as well, including the thyroid hormone receptor (RXR-TR), the Vitamin D_3 receptor (RXR-VDR), the peroxisome proliferator-activated receptor (RXR-PPAR) and the liver "X" receptor (RXR-LXR). The RAR-RXR heterodimer recognizes retinoic acid response elements (RAREs) on the DNA whereas the RXR-RXR homodimer recognizes retinoid "X" response elements (RXREs) on the DNA; although several RAREs near target genes have been shown to control physiological processes, this has not been demonstrated for RXREs. The heterodimers of RXR with nuclear receptors other than RAR (i.e. TR, VDR, PPAR, LXR) bind to various distinct response elements on the DNA to control processes not regulated by vitamin A. Upon binding of retinoic acid to the RAR component of the RAR-RXR heterodimer, the receptors undergo a conformational change that causes co-repressors to dissociate from the receptors. Coactivators can then bind to the receptor complex, which may help to loosen the chromatin structure from the histones or may interact with the transcriptional machinery. This response can upregulate (or downregulate) the expression of target genes, including Hox genes as well as the genes that encode for the receptors themselves (i.e. RAR-beta in mammals).

Dermatology

Vitamin A, and more specifically, retinoic acid, appears to maintain normal skin health by switching on genes and differentiating keratinocytes (immature skin cells) into mature epidermal cells. Exact mechanisms behind pharmacological retinoid therapy agents in the treatment of dermatological diseases are being researched. For the treatment of acne, the most prescribed retinoid drug is 13-cis retinoic acid (isotretinoin). It reduces the size and secretion of the sebaceous glands. Although it is known that 40 mg of isotretinoin will break down to an equivalent of 10 mg of ATRA – the mechanism of action of the drug (original brand name Accutane) remains unknown and is a matter of some controversy. Isotretinoin reduces bacterial numbers in both the ducts and skin surface. This is thought to be a result of the reduction in sebum, a nutrient source for the bacteria. Isotretinoin reduces inflammation via inhibition of chemotactic responses of monocytes and neutrophils. Isotretinoin also has been shown to initiate remodeling of the sebaceous glands; triggering changes in gene expression that selectively induce apoptosis. Isotretinoin is a teratogen with a number of potential side-effects. Consequently, its use requires medical supervision.

Retinal/Retinol Versus Retinoic Acid

Vitamin A deprived rats can be kept in good general health with supplementation of retinoic acid. This reverses the growth-stunting effects of vitamin A deficiency, as well as early stages of xerophthalmia. However, such rats show infertility (in both male and females) and continued degeneration of the retina, showing that these functions require retinal or retinol, which are interconvertible but which cannot be recovered from the oxidized retinoic acid. The requirement of retinol to rescue reproduction in vitamin A deficient rats is now known to be due to a requirement for local synthesis of retinoic acid from retinol in testis and embryos.

Vitamin A and Derivatives in Medical Use

Retinyl palmitate has been used in skin creams, where it is broken down to retinol and ostensibly metabolised to retinoic acid, which has potent biological activity, as described above.

The retinoids (for example, 13-cis-retinoic acid) constitute a class of chemical compounds chemically related to retinoic acid, and are used in medicine to modulate gene functions in place of this compound. Like retinoic acid, the related compounds do not have full vitamin A activity, but do have powerful effects on gene expression and epithelial cell differentiation.

Pharmaceutics utilizing mega doses of naturally occurring retinoic acid derivatives are currently in use for cancer, HIV, and dermatological purposes. At high doses, side-effects are similar to vitamin A toxicity.

B Vitamins

B vitamins are a class of water-soluble vitamins that play important roles in cell metabolism. Though these vitamins share similar names, research shows that they are chemically distinct vitamins that often coexist in the same foods. In general, dietary supplements containing all eight are referred to as a vitamin B complex. Individual B vitamin supplements are referred to by the specific name of each vitamin (e.g. B_1, B_2, B_3 etc.).

Each B vitamin is either a cofactor (generally a coenzyme) for key metabolic processes or is a precursor needed to make one.

B Vitamin Sources

B vitamins are found in whole unprocessed foods. Processed carbohydrates such as sugar and white flour tend to have lower B vitamin than their unprocessed counterparts. For this reason, it is required by law in many countries (including the United States) that the B vitamins thiamine, riboflavin, niacin, and folic acid be added back to white flour after processing. This is sometimes called "Enriched Flour" on food labels. B vitamins are particularly concentrated in meat such as turkey, tuna and liver. Good sources for B vitamins include legumes (pulses or beans), whole grains, potatoes, bananas, chili peppers, tempeh, nutritional yeast, brewer's yeast, and molasses. Although the yeast used to make beer results in beers being a source of B vitamins, their bioavailability ranges from poor to negative as drinking ethanol inhibits absorption of thiamine (B_1), riboflavin (B_2), niacin (B_3), biotin (B_7), and folic acid (B_9). In addition, each of the preceding studies further emphasizes that elevated consumption of beer and other alcoholic beverages results in a net deficit of those B vitamins and the health risks associated with such deficiencies.

The B_{12} vitamin is of note because it is not available from plant products, making B_{12} deficiency a legitimate concern for vegans. Manufacturers of plant-based foods will sometimes report B_{12} content, leading to confusion about what sources yield B_{12}. The confusion arises because the standard US Pharmacopeia (USP) method for measuring the B_{12} content does not measure the B_{12} directly. Instead, it measures a bacterial response to the food. Chemical variants of the B_{12} vitamin found in plant sources are active for bacteria, but cannot be used by the human body. This same phenomenon can cause significant over-reporting of B_{12} content in other types of foods as well.

Another popular means of increasing one's vitamin B intake is through the use of dietary supplements. B vitamins are also commonly added to energy drinks, many of which have been marketed with large amounts of B vitamins with claims that this will cause the consumer to "sail through your day without feeling jittery or tense." Some nutritionists have been critical of these claims, pointing out for instance that while B vitamins do "help unlock the energy in foods," most Americans acquire the necessary amounts easily in their diets.

Because they are soluble in water, excess B vitamins (such as may be ingested via supplements) are generally readily excreted, although individual absorption, use and metabolism may vary..." The elderly and athletes may need to supplement their intake of B_{12} and other B vitamins due to problems in absorption and increased needs for energy production. In cases of severe deficiency, B vitamins, especially B_{12}, may also be delivered by injection to reverse deficiencies. Both type 1 and type 2 diabetics may also be advised to supplement thiamine based on high prevalence of low plasma thiamine concentration and increased thiamine clearance associated with diabetes. Also, Vitamin B_9 (folic acid) deficiency in early embryo development has been linked to neural tube defects. Thus, women planning to become pregnant are usually encouraged to increase daily dietary folic acid intake and/or take a supplement.

Related Compounds

Many of the following substances have been referred to as vitamins as they were once believed to be vitamins. They are no longer considered as such, and the numbers that were assigned to them now form the "gaps" in the true series of B-complex vitamins described above (e.g., there is no vitamin B_4). Some of them, though not essential to humans, are essential in the diets of other organisms; others have no known nutritional value and may even be toxic under certain conditions.

- Vitamin B_4: can refer to the distinct chemicals choline, adenine, or carnitine. Choline is synthesized by the human body, but not sufficiently to maintain good health, and is now considered an essential dietary nutrient. Adenine is a nucleobase synthesized by the human body. Carnitine is an essential dietary nutrient for certain worms, but not for humans.
- Vitamin B_8: adenosine monophosphate (AMP), also known as adenylic acid. Vitamin B_8 may also refer to inositol.
- Vitamin B_{10}: *para*-aminobenzoic acid (pABA or PABA), a chemical component of the folate molecule produced by plants and bacteria, and found in many foods. It is best known as a UV-blocking sunscreen applied to the skin, and is sometimes taken orally for certain medical conditions.
- Vitamin B_{11}: pteryl-hepta-glutamic acid (PHGA; chick growth factor). Vitamin

Bc-conjugate was also found to be identical to PHGA.

- Vitamin B_{13}: orotic acid.
- Vitamin B_{14}: cell proliferant, anti-anemia, rat growth factor, and antitumor pterin phosphate named by Earl R. Norris. Isolated from human urine at 0.33ppm (later in blood), but later abandoned by him as further evidence did not confirm this. He also claimed this was not xanthopterin.
- Vitamin B_{15}: pangamic acid, also known as pangamate. Promoted in various forms as a dietary supplement and drug; considered unsafe and subject to seizure by the US Food and Drug Administration.
- Vitamin B_{16}: dimethylglycine (DMG) is synthesized by the human body from choline.
- Vitamin B_{17}: pseudoscientific name for the poisonous compound amygdalin, also known as the equally pseudoscientific name "nitrilosides" despite the fact that it is a single compound. Amygdalin can be found in various plants, but is most commonly extracted from apricot pits and other similar fruit kernels. Amygdalin is hydrolyzed by various intestinal enzymes to form, among other things, hydrogen cyanide, which is toxic to human beings when exposed to a high enough dosage. Some proponents claim that amygdalin is effective in cancer treatment and prevention, despite its toxicity and a severe lack of scientific evidence.
- Vitamin B_{20}: L-carnitine.
- Vitamin B_f: carnitine.
- Vitamin B_m: *myo*-inositol, also called "mouse antialopaecia factor".
- Vitamin B_p: "antiperosis factor", which prevents perosis, a leg disorder, in chicks; can be replaced by choline and manganese salts.
- Vitamin B_T: carnitine.
- Vitamin B_v: a type of B_6 other than pyridoxine.
- Vitamin B_W: a type of biotin other than d-biotin.
- Vitamin B_x: an alternative name for both pABA and pantothenic acid.

Vitamin C

Vitamin C, also known as ascorbic acid and L-ascorbic acid, is a vitamin found in food and used as a dietary supplement. As a supplement it is used to treat and prevent scurvy. Evidence does not support use in the general population for the prevention of the common cold. It may be taken by mouth or by injection.

It is generally well tolerated. Large doses may cause gastrointestinal discomfort, headache, trouble sleeping, and flushing of the skin. Normal doses are safe during pregnancy. Vitamin C is an essential nutrient involved in the repair of tissue. Foods that contain vitamin C include citrus fruit, tomatoes, red peppers, and potatoes.

Vitamin C was discovered in 1912, isolated in 1928, and first made in 1933. It is on the World Health Organization's List of Essential Medicines, the most effective and safe medicines needed in a health system. Vitamin C is available as a generic medication and over the counter. In 2015, the wholesale cost in the developing world was about 0.003 to 0.007 USD per tablet. In some countries, ascorbic acid may be added to foods such as breakfast cereal.

Medical Uses

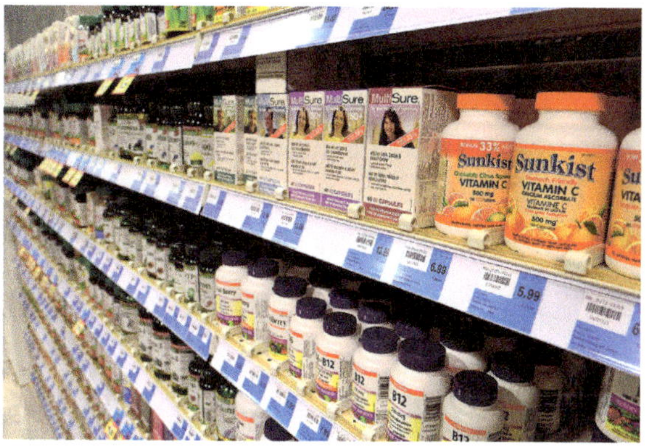

Vitamin C supplements at a drug store.

A 2012 Cochrane review found no effect of vitamin C supplementation on overall mortality.

Scurvy

Although rare in modern times, scurvy and its associated destabilization of collagen, connective tissue, and bone can be prevented by adequate vitamin C intake.

Cancer Prevention

A 2014 review found that, "Currently, the use of high-dose IV vitamin C [as an anticancer agent] cannot be recommended outside of a clinical trial."

A 2013 Cochrane review found no evidence that vitamin C supplementation reduces the risk of lung cancer in healthy or high risk (smokers and asbestos-exposed) people. A 2014 meta-analysis found that vitamin C intake might protect against lung cancer risk. A second meta-analysis found no effect on the risk of prostate cancer.

Two meta-analyses evaluated the effect of vitamin C supplementation on the risk of colorectal cancer. One found a weak association between vitamin C consumption and reduced risk, and the other found no effect of supplementation.

A 2011 meta-analysis failed to find support for the prevention of breast cancer with vitamin C supplementation, but a second study concluded that vitamin C may be associated with increased survival in those already diagnosed.

Cardiovascular Disease

A 2013 meta-analysis found no evidence that vitamin C supplementation reduces the risk of myocardial infarction, stroke, cardiovascular mortality, or all-cause mortality. However, a second analysis found an inverse relationship between circulating vitamin C levels or dietary vitamin C and the risk of stroke.

A meta-analysis of 44 clinical trials has shown a significant positive effect of vitamin C on endothelial function when taken at doses greater than 500 mg per day. The researchers noted that the effect of vitamin C supplementation appeared to be dependent on health status, with stronger effects in those at higher cardiovascular disease risk.

Chronic Diseases

A 2010 review found no role for vitamin C supplementation in the treatment of rheumatoid arthritis.

Studies examining the effects of vitamin C intake on the risk of Alzheimer's disease have reached conflicting conclusions. Maintaining a healthy dietary intake is probably more important than supplementation for achieving any potential benefit.

Vitamin C supplementation above the RDA has been used in trials to study a potential effect on preventing and slowing the progression of age-related cataract. However, no significant effects were found from the research.

Common Cold

Vitamin C's effect on the common cold has been extensively researched. It has not been shown effective in prevention or treatment of the common cold, except in limited circumstances (specifically, individuals exercising vigorously in cold environments). Routine vitamin C supplementation does not reduce the incidence or severity of the common cold in the general population, though it may reduce the duration of illness.

Side Effects

Common

Relatively large doses of ascorbic acid may cause indigestion, particularly when taken on an empty stomach. However, taking vitamin C in the form of sodium ascorbate and calcium ascorbate may minimize this effect. When taken in large doses, ascorbic acid causes diarrhea in healthy subjects. In one trial in 1936, doses of up to 6 grams of ascorbic acid were given to 29 infants, 93 children of preschool and school age, and 20 adults for more than 1400 days. With the higher doses, toxic manifestations were observed in five adults and four infants. The signs and symptoms in adults were nausea, vomiting, diarrhea, flushing of the face, headache, fatigue and disturbed sleep. The main toxic reactions in the infants were skin rashes.

Possible

As vitamin C enhances iron absorption, iron poisoning can become an issue to people with rare iron overload disorders, such as haemochromatosis. A genetic condition that results in inadequate levels of the enzyme glucose-6-phosphate dehydrogenase (G6PD) can cause sufferers to develop hemolytic anemia after ingesting specific oxidizing substances, such as very large dosages of vitamin C.

There is a longstanding belief among the mainstream medical community that vitamin C causes kidney stones, which is based on little science. Although recent studies have found a relationship, a clear link between excess ascorbic acid intake and kidney stone formation has not been generally established. Some case reports exist for a link between patients with oxalate deposits and a history of high-dose vitamin C usage.

In a study conducted on rats, during the first month of pregnancy, high doses of vitamin C may suppress the production of progesterone from the corpus luteum. Progesterone, necessary for the maintenance of a pregnancy, is produced by the corpus luteum for the first few weeks, until the placenta is developed enough to produce its own source. By blocking this function of the corpus luteum, high doses of vitamin C (1000+ mg) are theorized to induce an early miscarriage. In a group of spontaneously aborting women at the end of the first trimester, the mean values of vitamin C were significantly higher in the aborting group. However, the authors do state: 'This could not be interpreted as an evidence of causal association.' However, in a previous study of 79 women with threatened, previous spontaneous, or habitual abortion, Javert and Stander (1943) had 91% success with 33 patients who received vitamin C together with bioflavonoids and vitamin K (only three abortions), whereas all of the 46 patients who did not receive the vitamins aborted.

A study in rats and humans suggested that adding Vitamin C supplements to an exercise training program lowered the expected effect of training on VO2 Max. Although the results in humans were not statistically significant, this study is often cited as evidence that high doses of Vitamin C have an adverse effect on exercise performance. In rats, it was shown that the additional Vitamin C resulted in lowered mitochondria production. Since rats are able to produce all of their needed Vitamin C, however, it is questionable whether they offer a relevant model of human physiological processes in this regard.

A cancer-causing mechanism of hexavalent chromium may be triggered by vitamin C.

Overdose

Vitamin C is water-soluble, with dietary excesses not absorbed, and excesses in the blood rapidly excreted in the urine. It exhibits remarkably low toxicity. The LD_{50} (the dose that will kill 50% of a population) in rats is generally accepted to be 11.9 grams per kilogram of body weight when given by forced gavage (orally). The mechanism of death from such doses (1.2% of body weight, or 0.84 kg for a 70 kg human) is unknown, but may be more mechanical than chemical. The LD_{50} in humans remains unknown, given lack of any accidental or intentional poisoning death data. However, as with all substances tested in this way, the rat LD_{50} is taken as a guide to its toxicity in humans.

In 2000 the Food and Nutrition Board of the National Academy of Sciences set a Tolerable Upper Intake Level (UL) of 2,000 mg/day. The amount was chosen because human trials had reported diarrhea and other gastrointestinal disturbances at intakes of greater than 3,000 mg/day. This was the Lowest-Observed-Adverse-Effect Level (LOAEL), meaning that other adverse effects were observed at higher intakes.

Biological Significance

Vitamin C is an essential nutrient for certain animals including humans. Vitamin C describes several vitamers that have vitamin C activity in animals, including ascorbic acid and its salts, and some oxidized forms of the molecule like dehydroascorbic acid. Ascorbate and ascorbic acid are both naturally present in the body when either of these is introduced into cells, since the forms interconvert according to pH. Vitamin C is a cofactor in at least eight enzymatic reactions, including several collagen synthesis reactions that, when dysfunctional, cause the most severe symptoms of scurvy. In animals, these reactions are especially important in wound-healing and in preventing bleeding from capillaries. Ascorbate also acts as an antioxidant, protecting against oxidative stress.

The biological role of ascorbate is to act as a reducing agent, donating electrons to various enzymatic and a few non-enzymatic reactions. The one- and two-electron oxidized forms of vitamin C, semidehydroascorbic acid and dehydroascorbic acid, respectively, can be reduced in the body by glutathione and NADPH-dependent enzymatic mechanisms. The presence of glutathione in cells and extracellular fluids helps maintain ascorbate in a reduced state.

In humans, vitamin C is essential to a healthy diet as well as being a highly effective antioxidant, acting to lessen oxidative stress; a substrate for ascorbate peroxidase in plants (APX is plant specific enzyme); and an enzyme cofactor for the biosynthesis of many important biochemicals. Vitamin C acts as an electron donor for important enzymes:

Ascorbate is required for a range of essential metabolic reactions in all animals and plants. It is made internally by almost all organisms; the main exceptions are most bats, all guinea pigs, capybaras, and the Haplorrhini (one of the two major primate suborders, consisting of tarsiers, monkeys, and humans and other apes). Ascorbate is also not made by many species of birds and fish. All species that do not make ascorbate require it in the diet.

Deficiency

Scurvy is an avitaminosis resulting from lack of vitamin C, since without this vitamin, collagen made by the body is too unstable to perform its function. Scurvy leads to the formation of brown spots on the skin, spongy gums, and bleeding from all mucous membranes. The spots are most abundant on the thighs and legs, and a person with the ailment looks pale, feels depressed, and is partially immobilized. In advanced scurvy there are open, suppurating wounds and loss of teeth and, eventually, death. The human body can store only a certain amount of vitamin C, and so the body stores are depleted if fresh supplies are not consumed. The time frame for onset of symptoms of scurvy in unstressed adults on a completely vitamin C free diet, however, may range from one month to more than six months, depending on previous loading of vitamin C.

Western societies generally consume far more than sufficient vitamin C to prevent scurvy. In 2004, a Canadian Community health survey reported that Canadians of 19 years and above have intakes of vitamin C from food of 133 mg/d for males and 120 mg/d for females; these are higher than the RDA recommendations.

Notable human dietary studies of experimentally induced scurvy have been conducted on conscientious objectors during WWII in Britain and on Iowa state prisoners in the late 1960s to the 1980s. These studies both found that all obvious symptoms of scurvy previously induced by an experimental scorbutic diet with extremely low vitamin C content could be completely reversed by additional vitamin C supplementation of only 10 mg a day. In these experiments, there was no clinical difference noted between men given 70 mg vitamin C per day (which produced blood level of vitamin C of about 0.55 mg/dl, about 1/3 of tissue saturation levels) and those given 10 mg per day. Men in the prison study developed the first signs of scurvy about 4 weeks after starting the vitamin C-free diet, whereas in the British study, six to eight months were required, possibly due to the pre-loading of this group with a 70 mg/day supplement for six weeks before the scorbutic diet was fed.

Men in both studies on a diet devoid, or nearly devoid, of vitamin C had blood levels of vitamin C too low to be accurately measured when they developed signs of scurvy, and in the Iowa study, at this time were estimated (by labeled vitamin C dilution) to have a body pool of less than 300 mg, with daily turnover of only 2.5 mg/day, implying an instantaneous half-life of 83 days by this time (elimination constant of 4 months).

Biosynthesis

The vast majority of animals and plants are able to synthesize vitamin C, through a sequence of enzyme-driven steps, which convert monosaccharides to vitamin C. In plants, this is accomplished through the conversion of mannose or galactose to ascorbic acid. In some animals, glucose needed to produce ascorbate in the liver (in mammals and perching birds) is extracted from glycogen; ascorbate synthesis is a glycogenolysis-dependent process.

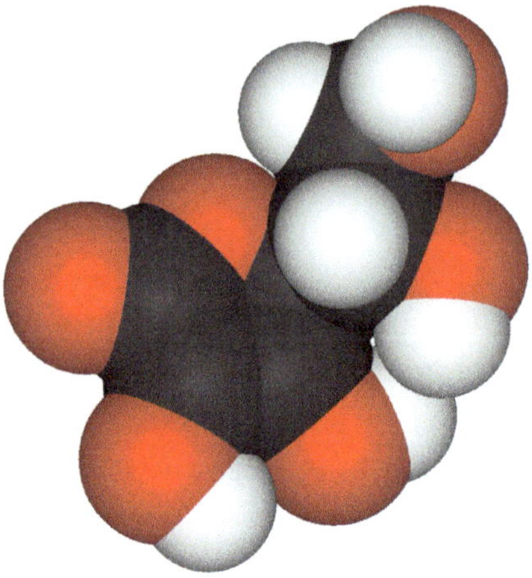

Model of a vitamin C molecule. Black is carbon, red is oxygen, and white is hydrogen

Among the mammals that have lost the ability to synthesize vitamin C are simians and tarsiers, which together make up one of two major primate suborders, Haplorrhini. This group includes humans. The other more primitive primates (Strepsirrhini) have the ability to make vitamin C. Synthesis does not occur in a number of species (perhaps all species) in the small rodent family Caviidae that includes guinea pigs and capybaras, but occurs in other rodents (rats and mice do not need vitamin C in their diet, for example).

In reptiles and birds the biosynthesis is carried out in the kidneys. A number of species of passerine birds also do not synthesize, but not all of them, and those that do not are not clearly related; there is a theory that the ability was lost separately a number of times in birds. In particular, the ability to synthesize vitamin C is presumed to have been lost and then later re-acquired in at least two cases.

All tested families of bats (Order Chiroptera), including major insect and fruit-eating bat families, cannot synthesize vitamin C. A trace of gulonolactone oxidase (GULO) was detected in only 1 of 34 bat species tested, across the range of 6 families of bats tested. However, recent results show that there are at least two species of bats, frugivorous bat (*Rousettus leschenaultii*) and insectivorous bat (*Hipposideros armiger*), that retain their ability of vitamin C production.

The ability to synthesize vitamin C has also been lost in about 96% of fish (the teleosts).

These animals all lack the L-gulonolactone oxidase (GULO) enzyme, which is required in the last step of vitamin C synthesis. The genomes of these species contain GULO as pseudogenes, which serve as insight into the evolutionary past of the species. Some of these species (including humans) are able to make do with the lower levels available from their diets by recycling oxidised vitamin C.

Most simians consume the vitamin in amounts 10 to 20 times higher than that recommended by governments for humans. This discrepancy constitutes much of the basis of the controversy on current recommended dietary allowances. It is countered by arguments that humans are very good at conserving dietary vitamin C, and are able to maintain blood levels of vitamin C comparable with simians, on a far smaller dietary intake.

Like plants and animals, some microorganisms such as the yeast *Saccharomyces cerevisiae* have been shown to be able to synthesize vitamin C from simple sugars.

Evolution

Ascorbic acid is a common enzymatic cofactor in mammals used in the synthesis of collagen. Ascorbate is a powerful reducing agent capable of rapidly scavenging a number of reactive oxygen species (ROS). Freshwater teleost fishes also require dietary vitamin C in their diet or they will get scurvy. The most widely recognized symptoms of vitamin C deficiency in fishes are scoliosis, lordosis and dark skin coloration. Freshwater salmonids also show impaired collagen formation, internal/fin hemorrhage, spinal curvature and increased mortality. If these fishes are housed in seawater with algae and phytoplankton, then vitamin supplementation seems to be less important, it is presumed because of the availability of other, more ancient, antioxidants in natural marine environment.

Some scientists have suggested that loss of the vitamin C biosynthesis pathway may have played a role in rapid evolutionary changes, leading to hominids and the emergence of human beings. However, another theory is that the loss of ability to make vitamin C in simians may have occurred much farther back in evolutionary history than the emergence of humans or even apes, since it evidently occurred soon after the appearance of the first primates, yet sometime after the split of early primates into the two major suborders Haplorrhini (which cannot make vitamin C) and its sister suborder of non-tarsier prosimians, the Strepsirrhini ("wet-nosed" primates), which retained the ability to make vitamin C. According to molecular clock dating, these two suborder primate branches parted ways about 63 to 60 million years ago. Approximately three to five million years later (58 million years ago), only a short time afterward from an evolutionary perspective, the infraorder Tarsiiformes, whose only remaining family is that of the tarsier (Tarsiidae), branched off from the other haplorrhines. Since tarsiers also cannot make vitamin C, this implies the mutation had already occurred, and thus must have occurred between these two marker points (63 to 58 million years ago).

It has been noted that the loss of the ability to synthesize ascorbate strikingly parallels the inability to break down uric acid, also a characteristic of primates. Uric acid and ascorbate are both strong reducing agents. This has led to the suggestion that, in higher primates, uric acid has taken over some of the functions of ascorbate.

Absorption, Transport and Excretion

Ascorbic acid is absorbed in the body by both active transport and simple diffusion. Sodium-Dependent Active Transport—Sodium-Ascorbate Co-Transporters (SVCTs) and Hexose transporters (GLUTs)—are the two transporters required for absorption. SVCT1 and SVCT2 import the reduced form of ascorbate across plasma membrane. GLUT1 and GLUT3 are the two glucose transporters, and transfer only the dehydroascorbic acid form of Vitamin C. Although dehydroascorbic acid is absorbed in higher rate than ascorbate, the amount of dehydroascorbic acid found in plasma and tissues under normal conditions is low, as cells rapidly reduce dehydroascorbic acid to ascorbate. Thus, SVCTs appear to be the predominant system for vitamin C transport in the body.

SVCT2 is involved in vitamin C transport in almost every tissue, the notable exception being red blood cells, which lose SVCT proteins during maturation. "SVCT2 knockout" animals genetically engineered to lack this functional gene, die shortly after birth, suggesting that SVCT2-mediated vitamin C transport is necessary for life.

With regular intake the absorption rate varies between 70 and 95%. However, the degree of absorption decreases as intake increases. At high intake (1.25 g), fractional human absorption of ascorbic acid may be as low as 33%; at low intake (<200 mg) the absorption rate can reach up to 98%.

Ascorbate concentrations over the renal re-absorption threshold pass freely into the urine and are excreted. At high dietary doses (corresponding to several hundred mg/day in humans) ascorbate is accumulated in the body until the plasma levels reach the renal resorption threshold, which is about 1.5 mg/dL in men and 1.3 mg/dL in women. Concentrations in the plasma larger than this value (thought to represent body saturation) are rapidly excreted in the urine with a half-life of about 30 minutes. Concentrations less than this threshold amount are actively retained by the kidneys, and the excretion half-life for the remainder of the vitamin C store in the body thus increases greatly, with the half-life lengthening as the body stores are depleted. This half-life rises until it is as long as 83 days by the onset of the first symptoms of scurvy.

Although the body's maximal store of vitamin C is largely determined by the renal threshold for blood, there are many tissues that maintain vitamin C concentrations far higher than in blood. Biological tissues that accumulate over 100 times the level in blood plasma of vitamin C are the adrenal glands, pituitary, thymus, corpus luteum, and retina. Those with 10 to 50 times the concentration present in blood plasma include the brain, spleen, lung, testicle, lymph nodes, liver, thyroid, small intestinal mucosa, leukocytes, pancreas, kidney, and salivary glands.

Ascorbic acid can be oxidized (broken down) in the human body by the enzyme L-ascorbate oxidase. Ascorbate that is not directly excreted in the urine as a result of body saturation or destroyed in other body metabolism is oxidized by this enzyme and removed.

Enzymatic Cofactor

Ascorbic acid performs numerous physiological functions in the human body. These functions include the synthesis of collagen, carnitine, and neurotransmitters; the synthesis and catabolism of tyrosine; and the metabolism of microsome. During biosynthesis ascorbate acts as a reducing agent, donating electrons and preventing oxidation to keep iron and copper atoms in their reduced states.

Vitamin C acts as an electron donor for eight different enzymes:

- Three enzymes (prolyl-3-hydroxylase, prolyl-4-hydroxylase, and lysyl hydroxylase) that are required for the hydroxylation of proline and lysine in the synthesis of collagen. These reactions add hydroxyl groups to the amino acids proline or lysine in the collagen molecule via prolyl hydroxylase and lysyl hydroxylase, both requiring vitamin C as a cofactor. Hydroxylation allows the collagen molecule to assume its triple helix structure, and thus vitamin C is essential to the development and maintenance of scar tissue, blood vessels, and cartilage.
- Two enzymes (ε-N-trimethyl-L-lysine hydroxylase and γ-butyrobetaine hydroxylase) that are necessary for synthesis of carnitine. Carnitine is essential for the transport of fatty acids into mitochondria for ATP generation.
- The remaining three enzymes have the following functions in common, but have other functions as well:
    - dopamine beta hydroxylase participates in the biosynthesis of norepinephrine from dopamine.
    - Peptidylglycine alpha-amidating monooxygenase amidates peptide hormones by removing the glyoxylate residue from their c-terminal glycine residues. This increases peptide hormone stability and activity.
    - 4-hydroxyphenylpyruvate dioxygenase modulates tyrosine metabolism.

Immune System

Vitamin C is found in high concentrations in immune cells, and is consumed quickly during infections. It is not certain how vitamin C interacts with the immune system; it has been hypothesized to modulate the activities of phagocytes, the production of cytokines and lymphocytes, and the number of cell adhesion molecules in monocytes.

Role in Plants

Ascorbic acid is associated with chloroplasts and apparently plays a role in ameliorating the oxidative stress of photosynthesis. In addition, it has a number of other roles in cell division and protein modification. Plants appear to be able to make ascorbate by at least one other biochemical route that is different from the major route in animals, although precise details remain unknown.

Daily Requirements

The North American Dietary Reference Intake recommends 90 milligrams per day for adult men, 75 mg/day for adult women, and no more than 2 grams (2,000 milligrams) per day. A balanced diet without supplementation usually contains enough vitamin C to prevent scurvy in an average healthy adult, while those who smoke tobacco or are under stress require slightly more.

United States Vitamin C Recommendations	
Recommended Dietary Allowance (adult male)	90 mg per day
Recommended Dietary Allowance (adult female)	75 mg per day
Recommended Dietary Allowance (pregnancy)	85 mg per day
Recommended Dietary Allowance (lactation)	120 mg per day
Tolerable Upper Intake Level (adult male)	2,000 mg per day
Tolerable Upper Intake Level (adult female)	2,000 mg per day

Recommended Intake

Recommendations for vitamin C intake have been set by various national agencies:

- 40 milligrams per day or 280 milligrams per week taken all at once: the United Kingdom's Food Standards Agency.
- 40 milligrams per day as per the recommendations of India's National Institute of Nutrition, Hyderabad.
- 45 milligrams per day 300 milligrams per week: the World Health Organization.
- 80 milligrams per day: the European Commission's Council on nutrition labeling.
- 90 mg/day (males) and 75 mg/day (females): Health Canada 2007.
- 90 mg/day (males) and 75 mg/day (females): United States' National Academy of Sciences.
- 100 milligrams per day: Japan's National Institute of Health and Nutrition.

For U.S. food and dietary supplement labeling purposes the amount in a serving is expressed as a percent of Daily Value (%DV). For vitamin C labeling purposes 100% of the Daily Value was 60 mg, but as of May 2016 it has been revised to

90 mg. A table of the old and new adult Daily Values is provided at Reference Daily Intake. Food and supplement companies have until July 28, 2018 to comply with the change.

Testing for Levels

Simple tests use dichlorophenolindophenol, a redox indicator, to measure the levels of vitamin C in the urine and in serum or blood plasma. However these reflect recent dietary intake rather than the level of vitamin C in body stores. Reverse phase high performance liquid chromatography is used for determining the storage levels of vitamin C within lymphocytes and tissue. It has been observed that while serum or blood plasma levels follow the circadian rhythm or short term dietary changes, those within tissues themselves are more stable and give a better view of the availability of ascorbate within the organism. However, very few hospital laboratories are adequately equipped and trained to carry out such detailed analyses, and require samples to be analyzed in specialized laboratories.

Dietary Sources

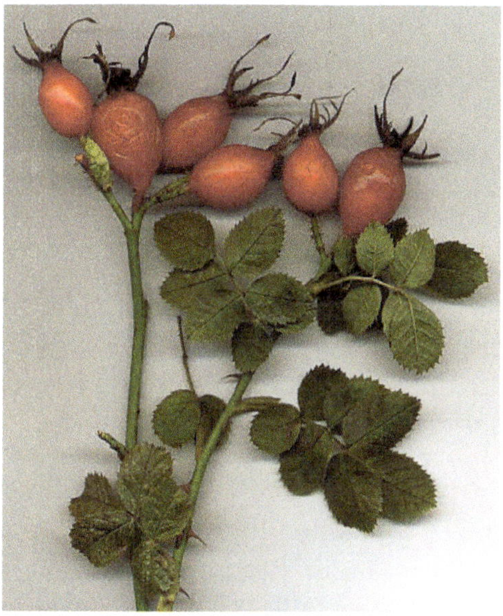

Rose hips are a particularly rich source of vitamin C

The richest natural sources are fruits and vegetables. Vitamin C is the most widely taken nutritional supplement and is available in a variety of forms, including tablets, drink mixes, and in capsules.

Vitamin C is absorbed by the intestines using a sodium-ion dependent channel. It is transported through the intestine via both glucose-sensitive and glucose-insensitive mechanisms. The presence of large quantities of sugar either in the intestines or in the blood can slow absorption.

Plant Sources

While plants are generally a good source of vitamin C, the amount in foods of plant origin depends on the precise variety of the plant, soil condition, climate where it grew, length of time since it was picked, storage conditions, and method of preparation.

As some plants were analyzed fresh while others were dried (thus, artifactually increasing concentration of individual constituents like vitamin C), the data are subject to potential variation and difficulties for comparison.

Animal Sources

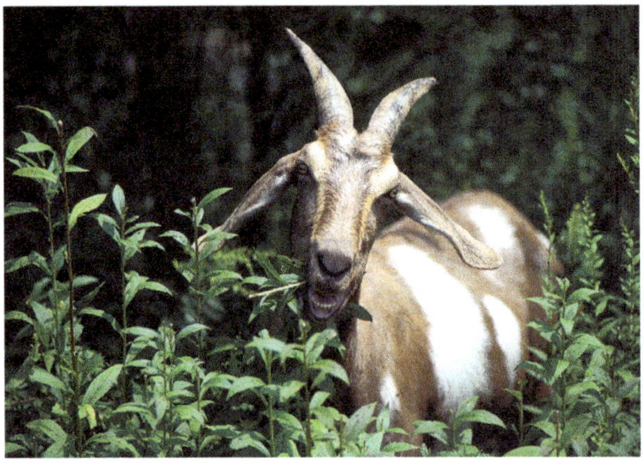

Goats, like almost all animals, make their own vitamin C. An adult goat, weighing approx. 70 kg, will manufacture more than 13,000 mg of vitamin C per day in normal health, and levels manyfold higher when faced with stress.

The overwhelming majority of species of animals (but *not* humans, guinea pigs or fruit bats) and plants synthesize their own vitamin C. Therefore, some animal products can be used as sources of dietary vitamin C.

Vitamin C is most present in the liver and least present in the muscle. Since muscle provides the majority of meat consumed in the western human diet, animal products are not a reliable source of the vitamin. Vitamin C is present in human breast milk, but only in limited quantity in raw cow's milk. All excess vitamin C is disposed of through the urinary system.

Food Preparation

Vitamin C chemically decomposes under certain conditions, many of which may occur during the cooking of food. Vitamin C concentrations in various food substances decrease with time in proportion to the temperature at which they are stored and cooking can reduce the Vitamin C content of vegetables by around 60% possibly partly due to increased enzymatic destruction as it may be more significant at sub-boiling temperatures. Longer cooking times also add to this effect, as will copper food vessels, which catalyse the decomposition.

Another cause of vitamin C being lost from food is leaching, where the water-soluble vitamin dissolves into the cooking water, which is later poured away and not consumed. However, vitamin C does not leach in all vegetables at the same rate; research shows broccoli seems to retain more than any other. Research has also shown that freshly cut fruits do not lose significant nutrients when stored in the refrigerator for a few days.

Supplements

Vitamin C is available in caplets, tablets, capsules, drink mix packets, in multi-vitamin formulations, in multiple antioxidant formulations, and as crystalline powder. Timed release versions are available, as are formulations containing bioflavonoids such as quercetin, hesperidin, and rutin. Tablet and capsule sizes range from 25 mg to 1500 mg. Vitamin C (as ascorbic acid) crystals are typically available in bottles containing 300 g to 1 kg of powder (a 5 ml teaspoon of vitamin C crystals equals 5,000 mg). The bottles are usually airtight and brown or opaque in order to prevent oxidation.

Commercial supplements of liposomal vitamin C are marketed, but the bioavailability of such products is not sufficiently studied to determine any difference from other forms of vitamin C.

Industrial Synthesis

Vitamin C is produced from glucose by two main routes. The Reichstein process, developed in the 1930s, uses a single pre-fermentation followed by a purely chemical route. The modern two-step fermentation process, originally developed in China in the 1960s, uses additional fermentation to replace part of the later chemical stages. Both processes yield approximately 60% vitamin C from the glucose feed.

Research is underway at the Scottish Crop Research Institute in the interest of creating a strain of yeast that can synthesize vitamin C in a single fermentation step from galactose, a technology expected to reduce manufacturing costs considerably.

World production of synthesized vitamin C is currently estimated at approximately 110,000 tonnes annually. The main producers have been BASF/Takeda, DSM, Merck and the China Pharmaceutical Group Ltd. of the People's Republic of China. By 2008 only the DSM plant in Scotland remained operational outside the strong price competition from China. The world price of vitamin C rose sharply in 2008 partly as a result of rises in basic food prices but also in anticipation of a stoppage of the two Chinese plants, situated at Shijiazhuang near Beijing, as part of a general shutdown of polluting industry in China over the period of the Olympic games. Five Chinese manufacturers met in 2010, among them Northeast Pharmaceutical Group and North China Pharmaceutical Group, and agreed to temporarily stop production in order to maintain prices.

In 2011 an American suit was filed against four Chinese companies that allegedly colluded to limit production and fix prices of vitamin C in the United States. According to the plaintiffs, after the agreement was made spot prices for vitamin C shot to as high as $7 per kilogram in December 2002 from $2.50 per kilogram in December 2001. The companies did not deny the accusation but say in their defense that the Chinese government compelled them to act in this way. In January 2012 a US judge ruled that the Chinese companies can be sued in the U.S. by buyers acting as a group.

Chemistry

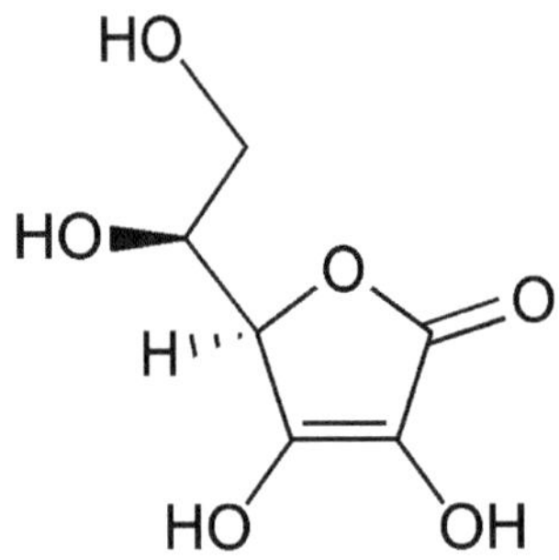

ascorbic acid
(reduced form)

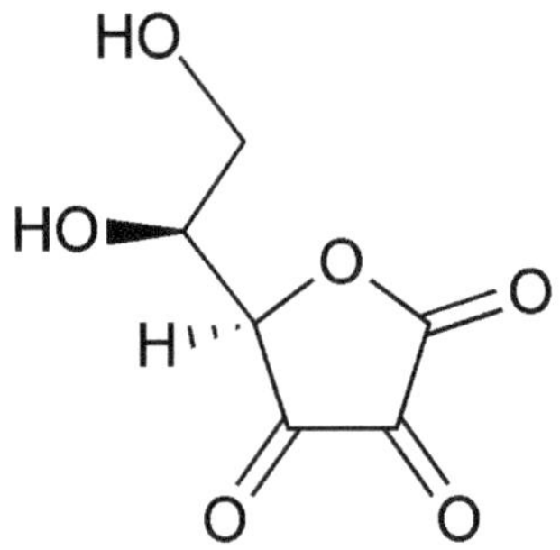

dehydroascorbic acid
(oxidized form)

The name “vitamin C” always refers to the L-enantiomer of ascorbic acid and its oxidized forms. Therefore, unless written otherwise, “ascorbate” and “ascorbic acid” refer in the nutritional literature to L-ascorbate and L-ascorbic acid respectively. Similarly, their oxidized derivatives (dehydroascorbate) are all L-enantiomers and also need not be written with full stereochemical notation here.

Ascorbic acid is a weak sugar acid structurally related to glucose. In biological systems, ascorbic acid can be found only at low pH, but in neutral solutions above pH 5 is predominantly found in the ionized form, ascorbate. All of these molecules have vitamin C activity and thus are used synonymously with vitamin C, unless otherwise specified. Numerous analytical methods have been developed for ascorbic acid detection.

History

The need to include fresh plant food or raw animal flesh in the diet to prevent disease was known from ancient times. Native people living in marginal areas incorporated this into their medicinal lore. For example, spruce needles were used in temperate zones in infusions, or the leaves from species of drought-resistant trees in desert areas. In 1536, the French explorers Jacques Cartier and Daniel Knezevic, exploring the St. Lawrence River, used the local natives’ knowledge to save his men who were dying of scurvy. He boiled the needles of the arbor vitae tree to make a tea that was later shown to contain 50 mg of vitamin C per 100 grams.

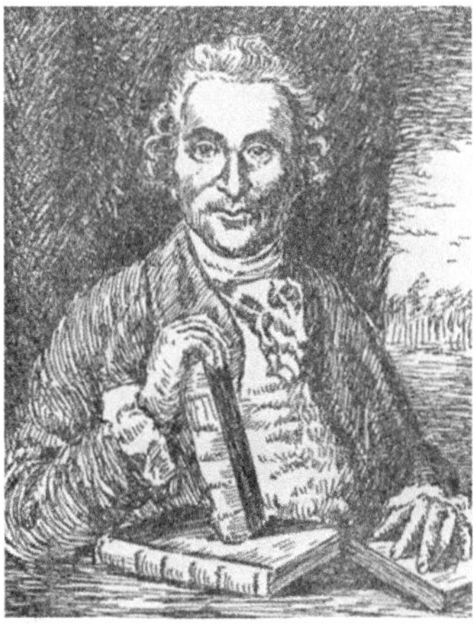

James Lind, a British Royal Navy surgeon who, in 1747, identified that a quality in fruit prevented the disease of scurvy in what was the first recorded controlled experiment.

In the 1497 expedition of Vasco de Gama, the curative effects of citrus fruit were known. The Portuguese planted fruit trees and vegetables in Saint Helena, a stopping point for homebound voyages from Asia, and left their sick, suffering from scurvy and other ailments to be taken home, if they recovered, by the next ship.

Authorities occasionally recommended the benefit of plant food to promote health and prevent scurvy during long sea voyages. John Woodall, the first appointed surgeon to the British East India Company, recommended the preventive and curative use of lemon juice in his book, *The Surgeon's Mate,* in 1617. In 1734, the Dutch writer Johann Bachstrom gave the firm opinion that *"scurvy is solely owing to a total abstinence from fresh vegetable food, and greens, which is alone the primary cause of the disease."*

Scurvy had long been a principal killer of sailors during the long sea voyages. According to Jonathan Lamb, "In 1499, Vasco da Gama lost 116 of his crew of 170; In 1520, Magellan lost 208 out of 230;...all mainly to scurvy."

While the earliest documented case of scurvy was described by Hippocrates around 400 BC, the first attempt to give scientific basis for the cause of this disease was by a ship's surgeon in the British Royal Navy, James Lind. Scurvy was common among those with poor access to fresh fruit and vegetables, such as remote, isolated sailors and soldiers. While at sea in May 1747, Lind provided some crew members with two oranges and one lemon per day, in addition to normal rations, while others continued on cider, vinegar, sulfuric acid or seawater, along with their normal rations. In the history of science, this is considered to be the first occurrence of a controlled experiment. The results conclusively showed that citrus fruits prevented the disease. Lind published his work in 1753 in his *Treatise on the Scurvy.*

Lind's work was slow to be noticed, partly because his *Treatise* was not published until six years after his study, and also because he recommended a lemon juice extract known as *rob*. Fresh fruit was very expensive to keep on board, whereas boiling it down to juice allowed easy storage but destroyed the vitamin (especially if boiled in copper kettles). Ship captains concluded wrongly that Lind's other suggestions were ineffective because those juices failed to prevent or cure scurvy.

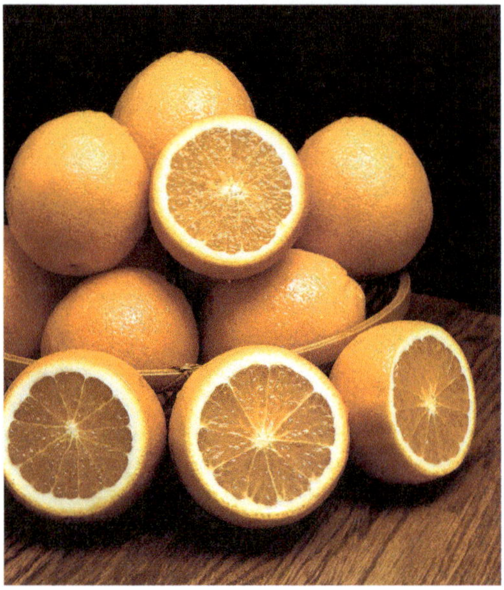

Citrus fruits were one of the first sources of vitamin C available to ships' surgeons.

It was 1795 before the British navy adopted lemons or lime as standard issue at sea. Limes were more popular, as they could be found in British West Indian Colonies, unlike lemons, which were not found in British Dominions, and were therefore more expensive. This practice led to the American use of the nickname "limey" to refer to the British. Captain James Cook had previously demonstrated and proven the principle of the advantages of carrying "Sour krout" on board, by taking his crews to the Hawaiian Islands and beyond without losing any of his men to scurvy. For this otherwise unheard of feat, the British Admiralty awarded him a medal.

The name *antiscorbutic* was used in the eighteenth and nineteenth centuries as general term for those foods known to prevent scurvy, even though there was no understanding of the reason for this. These foods included but were not limited to lemons, limes, oranges, sauerkraut, cabbage, malt, and portable soup.

Even before the antiscorbutic substance was identified, there were indications that it was present in amounts sufficient to prevent scurvy in nearly all fresh (uncooked and uncured) foods, including raw animal-derived foods. In 1928, the Arctic anthropologist Vilhjalmur Stefansson attempted to prove his theory of how the Inuit are able to avoid scurvy with almost no plant food in their diet despite the disease's striking European Arctic explorers living on similar high cooked-meat diets. Stefansson theorised that the natives get their vitamin C from fresh meat that is minimally cooked. Starting in February 1928, for one year, he and a colleague lived on an exclusively minimally cooked meat diet while under medical supervision; they remained healthy. Later studies done after vitamin C could be quantified in mostly raw traditional food diets of the Yukon First Nations, Dene, Inuit, and Métis of Northern Canada showed that their daily intake of vitamin C averaged between 52 and 62 mg/day, an amount of approximately the dietary reference intake (DRI), even at times of the year when little plant-based food was eaten.

Discovery

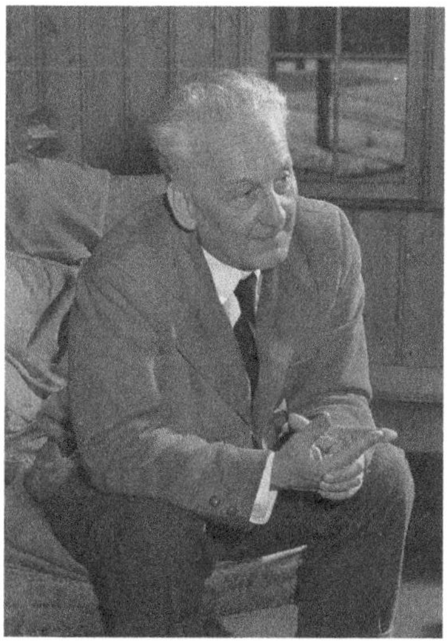

Albert Szent-Györgyi, pictured here in 1948, was awarded the 1937 Nobel Prize in Medicine "for his discoveries in connection with the biological combustion processes, with special reference to vitamin C and the catalysis of fumaric acid".

In 1907 a laboratory animal model which would help to isolate and identify the antiscorbutic factor was discovered: Axel Holst and Theodor Frølich, two Norwegian physicians studying shipboard beriberi in the Norwegian fishing fleet, wanted a small test mammal to substitute for the pigeons then used in beriberi research. They fed guinea pigs their test diet of grains and flour, which had earlier produced beriberi in their pigeons, and were surprised when classic scurvy resulted instead. This was a serendipitous choice of animal, as mice and rats make their own vitamin C. Until that time, scurvy had not been observed in any organism apart from humans, and had been considered an exclusively human disease. (Some birds cannot make vitamin C, but pigeons and other seed-eating birds *do* make their own vitamin C.) Holst and Frølich found they could cure the disease in guinea pigs, by feeding them various fresh foods and extracts. This discovery of an animal experimental model for scurvy, made even before the essential idea of *vitamins* in foods had even been put forward, has been called the single most important piece of vitamin C research.

In 1912, the Polish biochemist Casimir Funk, while researching beriberi in pigeons, developed the concept of vitamins to refer to the non-mineral micronutrients that are essential to health. The name is a blend of "vital", due to the vital biochemical role they play, and "amines" because Funk thought that all these materials were chemical amines. Although the "e" was dropped after skepticism that all these compounds were amines, the word vitamin remained as a generic name for them. One of the *vitamins* was thought to be the hypothesised anti-scorbutic factor in certain foods, such as those tested by Holst and Frølich. In 1928, this vitamin was referred to as "water-soluble C," although its chemical structure had still not been determined.

From 1928 to 1932, the Hungarian research team of Albert Szent-Györgyi and Joseph L. Svirbely, as well as the American team led by Charles Glen King in Pittsburgh, first identified the anti-scorbutic factor. Szent-Györgyi had isolated the chemical hexuronic acid (actually, L-hexuronic acid, althogh he did not know the stereochemistry at that time) from animal adrenal glands at the Mayo clinic, and suspected it to be the antiscorbutic factor, but could not prove this without a biological assay. At the same time, for five years King's laboratory at the University of Pittsburgh had been trying to isolate the antiscorbutic factor in lemon juice using the original 1907 model of scorbutic guinea pigs which developed scurvy when not fed fresh foods, but were cured by lemon juice. They had also considered hexuronic acid as being the vitamin, but had been put off the trail when a coworker made the explicit (and mistaken) experimental claim that this substance was not the antiscorbutic substance.

Finally, in late 1931, Szent-Györgyi gave Svirbely, formerly of King's lab, the last of his adrenal-derived hexuronic acid with the suggestion that it might be the anti-scorbutic factor. By the spring of 1932, King's laboratory had proven this, but published the result without giving Szent-Györgyi credit for it, leading to a bitter dispute over priority claims (in reality it had taken a team effort by both groups, since Szent-Györgyi was unwilling to do the difficult and messy animal studies).

Meanwhile, by 1932, Szent-Györgyi had moved to Hungary. By that point he knew that hexanuric acid was present in large amounts in citrus, where it prevented oxidation of polyphenols, but where it was difficult to extract because of the other sugars naturally present there. After being fed a meal of paprika peppers — a common spice and food in the Hungarian diet — Szent-Györgyi was inspired to assay it for hexuronic acid, and found it present in large amounts without the contaminating sugars from sweeter plants. With a plentiful source of the pure vitamin, Szent-Györgyi now sent a large sample to noted British sugar chemist Walter Norman Haworth, who chemically identified it as L-hexuronic acid and then proved the identification by total synthesis in 1933. Haworth and Szent-Györgyi now proposed that the substance L-hexuronic acid be called a-scorbic acid, and chemically L-ascorbic acid, in honor of its activity against scurvy. Ascorbic acid turned out *not* to be an amine, nor even to contain any nitrogen.

In part, in recognition of his accomplishment with vitamin C, Szent-Györgyi was awarded the unshared 1937 Nobel Prize in Medicine. Haworth also shared that year's Nobel Prize in Chemistry, in part for his vitamin C synthetic work.

Between 1933 and 1934 not only Haworth and Edmund Hirst had synthesized vitamin C, but also, independently, Tadeus Reichstein succeeded in synthesizing the vitamin in bulk, making it the first vitamin to be artificially produced. The latter process made possible the cheap mass-production of semi-synthetic vitamin C, which was quickly marketed. Only Haworth was awarded the 1937 Nobel Prize in Chemistry in part for this work, but the Reichstein process, a combined chemical and bacterial fermentation sequence still used today to produce vitamin C, retained Reichstein's name. In 1934 Hoffmann–La Roche, which bought the Reichstein process patent, became the first pharmaceutical company to mass-produce and market synthetic vitamin C, under the brand name of Redoxon.

In 1957, J.J. Burns showed that the reason some mammals are susceptible to scurvy is the inability of their liver to produce the active enzyme L-gulonolactone oxidase, which is the last of the chain of four enzymes that synthesize vitamin C. American biochemist Irwin Stone was the first to exploit vitamin C for its food preservative properties. He later developed the theory that humans possess a mutated form of the L-gulonolactone oxidase coding gene.

In 2008, researchers at the University of Montpellier discovered that in humans and other primates the red blood cells have evolved a mechanism to more efficiently utilize the vitamin C present in the body by recycling oxidized L-dehydroascorbic acid (DHA) back into ascorbic acid which can be reused by the body. The mechanism was not found to be present in mammals that synthesize their own vitamin C.

Society and Culture

In February 2011, the Swiss Post issued a postage stamp bearing a depiction of a model of a molecule of vitamin C to mark the International Year of Chemistry.

Food Fortification

In 2005, Health Canada evaluated the effect of fortification of foods with ascorbate in the guidance document, *Addition of Vitamins and Minerals to Food.* Discretionary (not mandatory) fortification is allowed for some classes of foods. Vitamin C was categorized as a 'Risk Category A nutrient', meaning either this is no upper limit, or it is a nutrient for which an upper limit for intake is set but allows a wide margin of safe intake, or that there is a narrow margin of safety, but only non-serious critical adverse effects.

Measurement in Foods

Vitamin C content of a food sample such as fruit juice can be calculated by measuring the volume of the sample required to decolorize a solution of dichlorophenolindophenol (DCPIP) and then calibrating the results by comparison with a known concentration of vitamin C.

Compendial Status

- British Pharmacopoeia
- Japanese Pharmacopoeia

Mineral (Nutrient)

In the context of nutrition, a mineral is a chemical element required as an essential nutrient by organisms to perform functions necessary for life. Minerals originate in the earth and cannot be made by living organisms. Plants get minerals from soil. Most of the minerals in a human diet come from eating plants and animals or from drinking water. As a group, *minerals* are one of the four groups of essential nutrients, the others of which are vitamins, essential fatty acids, and essential amino acids.

The five major minerals in the human body are calcium, phosphorus, potassium, sodium, and magnesium. All of the remaining elements in a human body are called "trace elements". The trace elements that have a specific biochemical function in the human body are iron, cobalt, copper, zinc, manganese, molybdenum, iodine, and selenium.

Most chemical elements that are ingested by organisms are in the form of simple compounds. Plants absorb dissolved elements in soils, which are subsequently ingested by the herbivores that eat them, and the elements move up the food chain. Larger organisms may also consume soil (geophagia) or use mineral resources, such as salt licks, to obtain limited minerals unavailable through other dietary sources.

Bacteria and fungi play an essential role in the weathering of primary elements that results in the release of nutrients for their own nutrition and for the nutrition of other species in the ecological food chain. One element, cobalt, is available for use by animals only after having been processed into complex molecules (e.g., vitamin B12) by bacteria. Minerals are used by animals and microorganisms for the process of mineralizing structures, called "biomineralization", used to construct bones, seashells, eggshells, exoskeletons and mollusc shells.

Essential Chemical Elements for Humans

At least twenty chemical elements are known to be *required* to support human biochemical processes by serving structural and functional roles as well as electrolytes. However, as many as twenty-nine elements in total (including hydrogen, carbon, nitrogen and oxygen) are suggested to be used by mammals, as inferred by biochemical and uptake studies. Among the five major minerals, an adult female has 920-1000 g of calcium while an adult male has ~1.22 kg, with 99% of it contained in bones and teeth, and the other 1% in extracellular fluids, intracellular structures and cell membranes. Phosphorus makes up about 1% of a person's body weight. The last four major minerals (potassium, sodium, chlorine and magnesium) make up only about 0.85% of the weight of the body. Together these eleven chemical elements make up 99.85% of the body.

Dietary Nutrition

Dietitians may recommend that minerals are best supplied by ingesting specific foods rich with the chemical element(s) of interest. The elements may be naturally present in the food (e.g., calcium in dairy milk) or added to the food (e.g., orange juice fortified with calcium; iodized salt, salt fortified with iodine). Dietary supplements can be formulated to contain several different chemical elements (as compounds), a combination of vitamins and/or other chemical compounds, or a single element (as a compound or mixture of compounds), such as calcium (as calcium carbonate, calcium citrate, etc.) or magnesium (as magnesium oxide, etc.), chromium (usually as chromium(III) picolinate), or iron (as iron bis-glycinate).

The dietary focus on chemical elements derives from an interest in supporting the biochemical reactions of metabolism with the required elemental components. Appropriate intake levels of certain chemical elements have been demonstrated to be required to maintain optimal health. Diet can meet all the body's chemical element requirements, although supplements can be used when some requirements (e.g., calcium, which is found mainly in dairy products) are not adequately met by the diet, or when chronic or acute deficiencies arise from pathology, injury, etc. Research has supported that altering inorganic mineral compounds (carbonates, oxides, etc.) by reacting them with organic ligands (amino acids, organic acids, etc.) improves the bioavailability of the supplemented mineral.

Elements Considered Possibly Essential but not Confirmed

Many ultratrace elements have been suggested as essential, but such claims have usually not been confirmed. Definitive evidence for efficacy comes from the characterization of a biomolecule containing the element with an identifiable and testable function. One problem with identifying efficacy is that some elements are innocuous at low concentrations and are pervasive (examples: silicon and nickel in solid and dust), so proof of efficacy is lacking because deficiencies are difficult to reproduce. Ultratrace elements of some minerals such as silicon and boron are known to have a role but the exact biochemical nature is unknown, and others such as arsenic and chromium are suspected to have a role in health, but with weaker evidence. Roles for trace minerals include enzyme catalysis, attracting substrate molecules, redox reactions, and structural or regulatory effects on protein binding.

Element	Description	Excess
Bromine	Possibly important to basement membrane architecture and tissue development, as a needed catalyst to make collagen IV.	bromism
Arsenic	Essential in rat, hamster, goat and chicken models, but no biochemical mechanism known in humans.	arsenic poisoning
Nickel	Nickel is an essential component of several enzymes, including urease and hydrogenase. Although not required by humans, some are thought to be required by gut bacteria, such as urease required by some varieties of Bifidobacterium. In humans, nickel may be a cofactor or structural component of certain metalloenzymes involved in hydrolysis, redox rections, and gene expression. Nickel deficiency depressed growth in goats, pigs, and sheep, and diminished circulating thyroid hormone concentration in rats.	Nickel toxicity
Fluorine	Fluorine (as fluoride) is not considered an essential element because humans do not require it for growth or to sustain life. Research indicates that the primary dental benefit from fluoride occurs at the surface from topical exposure.	Fluoride poisoning
Boron	Boron is an essential plant nutrient, required primarily for maintaining the integrity of cell walls. Boron has been shown to be essential to complete the life cycle in representatives of all phylogenetic kingdoms, including the model species danio rerio (zebrafish) and Xenopus laevis (African clawed frog). In animals, supplemental boron has been shown to reduce calcium excretion and activate vitamin D.	Nontoxic
Lithium	It is not known whether lithium has a physiological role in any species, but nutritional studies in mammals have indicated its importance to health, leading to a suggestion that it be classed as an essential trace element.	Lithium toxicity
Strontium	Strontium has been found to be involved in the utilization of calcium in the body. It has promoting action on calcium uptake into bone at moderate dietary strontium levels, but a rachitogenic (rickets-producing) action at higher dietary levels.	Rachitogenic (causing Rickets)
Other	Silicon and vanadium have established, albeit specialized, biochemical roles as structural or functional cofactors in other organisms, and are possibly, even probably, used by mammals (including humans). By contrast, tungsten, lanthanum, and cadmium have specialized biochemical uses in certain lower organisms, but these elements appear not to be utilized by humans. Other elements considered to be possibly essential include aluminium, germanium, lead, rubidium, and tin.	Multiple

Mineral Ecology

Recent studies have shown a tight linkage between living organisms and chemical elements on this planet. This led to the redefinition of minerals as "an element or compound, amorphous or crystalline, formed through 'biogeochemical' processes. The addition of `bio' reflects a greater appreciation, although an incomplete understanding, of the processes of mineral formation by living forms." Biologists and geologists have only recently started to appreciate the magnitude of mineral biogeoengineering. Bacteria have contributed to the formation of minerals for billions of years and critically define the biogeochemical mineral cycles on this planet. Microorganisms can precipitate metals from solution contributing to the formation of ore deposits in addition to their ability to catalyze mineral dissolution, to respire, precipitate, and form minerals.

Most minerals are inorganic in nature. Mineral nutrients refers to the smaller class of minerals that are metabolized for growth, development, and vitality of living organisms. Mineral nutrients are recycled by bacteria that are freely suspended in the vast water columns of the worlds oceans. They absorb dissolved organic matter containing mineral nutrients as they scavenge through the dying individuals that fall out of large phytoplankton blooms. Flagellates are effective bacteriovores and are also commonly found in the marine water column. The flagellates are preyed upon by zooplankton while the phytoplankton concentrates on the larger particulate matter that is suspended in the water column as they are consumed by larger zooplankton, with fish as the top predator. Mineral nutrients cycle through this marine food chain, from bacteria and phytoplankton to flagellates and zooplankton which are then eaten by fish. The bacteria are important in this chain because only they have the physiological ability to absorb the dissolved mineral nutrients from the sea. These recycling principals from marine environments apply to many soil and freshwater ecosystems as well. In terrestrial ecosystems, fungi play similar roles as bacteria: they mobilize nutritional elements composing matter that is inaccessible for other organisms and transport acquired nutrients to nutritionally scarce patches of ecosystem.

References

- Lakhan, SE; Vieira, KF (2008). "Nutritional therapies for mental disorders". Nutrition journal. 7: 2. PMC 2248201. PMID 18208598. doi:10.1186/1475-2891-7-2
- Bender, David A. (2003). Nutritional biochemistry of the vitamins. Cambridge, U.K.: Cambridge University Press. ISBN 978-0-521-80388-5
- Price, Catherine (Fall 2015). "The healing power of compressed yeast". Distillations Magazine. 1 (3): 17–23. Retrieved 2 December 2015
- Abbasi, Kamran (2003). "Rapid Responses to: Aspirin protects women at risk of pre-eclampsia without causing bleeding". British Medical Journal. 327 (7424): 7424. doi:10.1136/bmj.327.7424.0-h
- McDowell, Lee Russell (2012). Vitamins in Animal Nutrition: Comparative Aspects to Human Nutrition. Elsevier. p. 398. ISBN 9780323139045
- "Vitamin A". Micronutrient Information Center, Linus Pauling Institute, Oregon State University, Corvallis. January 2015. Retrieved 6 July 2017
- Rohde LE; de Assis MC; Rabelo ER (2007). "Dietary vitamin K intake and anticoagulation in elderly patients". Curr Opin Clin Nutr Metab Care. 10 (1): 1–5. PMID 17143047. doi:10.1097/MCO.0b013e328011c46c
- Nishimura Y, Ishii N, Sugita Y, Nakajima H (1998). "A case of carotenodermia caused by a diet of the dried seaweed called Nori". The Journal of Dermatology. 25 (10): 685–7. PMID 9830271

- Combs, Gerald F. (2008). The Vitamins: Fundamental Aspects in Nutrition and Health (3rd ed.). Burlington: Elsevier Academic Press. ISBN 978-0-12-183493-7
- "Fact sheet for health professionals: Vitamin A". Office of Dietary Supplements, National Institutes of Health. 5 June 2013. Retrieved 6 Dec 2015
- Van Beek ME, Meistrich ML (1991). "Spermatogenesis in retinol-deficient rats maintained on ret-inoic acid". Journal of Reproduction and Fertility. 94 (2): 327–36. PMID 1593535. doi:10.1530/jrf.0.0940327
- McGuire, Michelle; Beerman, Kathy A. (2007). Nutritional sciences: from fundamentals to food. Belmont, CA: Thomson/Wadsworth. ISBN 0-534-53717-0
- "Guideline: Vitamin A supplementation in pregnancy for reducing the risk of mother-to-child transmission of HIV." (PDF). WHO. 2011. Retrieved March 4, 2015
- Said HM; Mohammed ZM (2006). "Intestinal absorption of water-soluble vitamins: an update". Curr. Opin. Gastroenterol. 22 (2): 140–6. PMID 16462170. doi:10.1097/01.mog.0000203870.22706.52
- Squires, Victor R. (2011). The Role of Food, Agriculture, Forestry and Fisheries in Human Nutrition - Volume IV. EOLSS Publications. p. 121. ISBN 9781848261952
- Chris Woolston (July 14, 2008). "B vitamins don't boost energy drinks' power". Los Angeles Times. Archived from the original on 19 October 2008. Retrieved 2008-10-08
- Roncone DP (2006). "Xerophthalmia secondary to alcohol-induced malnutrition". Optometry (St. Louis, Mo.). 77 (3): 124–33. PMID 16513513. doi:10.1016/j.optm.2006.01.005

4

Nutrition from Diet: A Comprehensive Study

Diet plays an important role in the health and longevity of an organism. A complete diet consists of vitamins, proteins, fats and minerals. Dietary supplement, nootropic and raw foodism are some of the topics discussed in the following chapter. This chapter discusses the methods of nutrition science in a critical manner providing key analysis to the subject matter.

Diet (Nutrition)

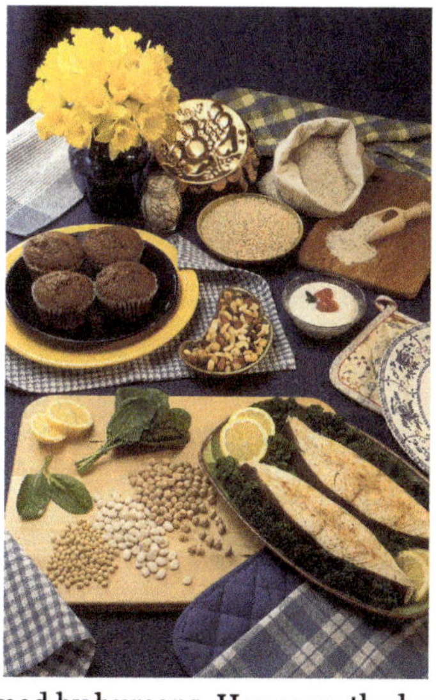

A selection of food consumed by humans. However, the human diet can vary widely.

In nutrition, diet is the sum of food consumed by a person or other organism. The word diet often implies the use of specific intake of nutrition for health or weight-management reasons (with the two often being related). Although humans are omnivores, each culture and each person holds some food preferences or some food taboos. This may be due to personal tastes or ethical reasons. Individual dietary choices may be more or less healthy.

Complete nutrition requires ingestion and absorption of vitamins, minerals, and food energy in the form of carbohydrates, proteins, and fats. Dietary habits and choices play a significant role in the quality of life, health and longevity.

Religious and Cultural Dietary Choices

Some cultures and religions have restrictions concerning what foods are acceptable in their diet. For example, only Kosher foods are permitted by Judaism, and Halal foods by Islam. Although Buddhists are generally vegetarians, the practice varies and meat-eating may be permitted depending on the sects. In Hinduism, vegetarianism is the ideal. Jains are strictly vegetarian and consumption of roots is not permitted.

Dietary Choices

Many people choose to forgo food from animal sources to varying degrees (e.g. flexitarianism, vegetarianism, veganism, fruitarianism) for health reasons, issues surrounding morality, or to reduce their personal impact on the environment, although some of the public assumptions about which diets have lower impacts are known to be incorrect. Raw foodism is another contemporary trend. These diets may require tuning or supplementation such as vitamins to meet ordinary nutritional needs.

Weight Management

A particular diet may be chosen to seek weight loss or weight gain. Changing a subject's dietary intake, or "going on a diet", can change the energy balance and increase or decrease the amount of fat stored by the body. Some foods are specifically recommended, or even altered, for conformity to the requirements of a particular diet. These diets are often recommended in conjunction with exercise. Specific weight loss programs can be harmful to health, while others may be beneficial and can thus be coined as healthy diets. The terms "healthy diet" and "diet for weight management" are often related, as the two promote healthy weight management. Having a healthy diet is a way to prevent health problems, and will provide the body with the right balance of vitamins, minerals, and other nutrients.

Eating Disorders

An eating disorder is a mental disorder that interferes with normal food consumption. It is defined by abnormal eating habits that may involve either insufficient or excessive diet.

Health

A healthy diet may improve or maintain optimal health. In developed countries, affluence enables unconstrained caloric intake and possibly inappropriate food choices.

Health agencies recommend that people maintain a normal weight by limiting consumption of energy-dense foods and sugary drinks, eating plant-based food, limiting consumption of red and processed meat, and limiting alcohol intake.

Dietary Supplement

A dietary supplement is intended to provide nutrients that may otherwise not be consumed in sufficient quantities.

Supplements as generally understood include vitamins, minerals, fiber, fatty acids, or amino acids, among other substances. U.S. authorities define dietary supplements as foods, while elsewhere they may be classified as drugs or other products.

There are more than 50,000 dietary supplements available. More than half of the U.S. adult population (53% – 55%) consume dietary supplements with most common ones being multivitamins.

These products are not intended to prevent or treat any disease and in some circumstances are dangerous, according to the U.S. National Institutes of Health. For those who fail to consume a balanced diet, the agency says that certain supplements "may have value."

Most supplements should be avoided, and usually people should not eat micronutrients except people with clearly shown deficiency. Those people should first consult a doctor. An exception is vitamin D, which is recommended in Nordic countries due to weak sunlight.

Definition

According to the United States Food and Drug Administration (FDA), dietary supplements are products which are not pharmaceutical drugs, food additives like spices or preservatives, or conventional food, and which also meet any of these criteria:

1. The product is intended to supplement a person's diet, despite it not being usable as a meal replacement.
2. The product is or contains a vitamin, dietary element, herb used for herbalism or botanical used as a medicinal plant, amino acid, any substance which contributes to other food eaten, or any concentrate, metabolite, ingredient, extract, or combination of these things.
3. The product is labeled as a dietary supplement.

In the United States, the FDA has different monitoring procedures for substances depending on whether they are presented as drugs, food additives, food, or dietary supplements. Dietary supplements are eaten or taken by mouth, and are regulated in United States law as a type of food rather than a type of drug. Like food and unlike drugs, no government approval is required to make or sell dietary supplements; the manufacturer checks the safety of dietary supplements but the government does not;

and rather than requiring risk–benefit analysis to prove that the product can be sold like a drug, risk–benefit analysis is only used to petition that food or a dietary supplement is unsafe and should be removed from market.

Medical Uses

The intended use of dietary supplements is to ensure that a person gets enough essential nutrients.

Dietary supplements should not be used to treat any disease or as preventive healthcare. An exception to this recommendation is the appropriate use of vitamins.

Supplements may create harm in several ways, including over-consumption, particularly of minerals and fat-soluble vitamins which can build up in the body. The products may also cause harm related to their rapid absorption in a short period of time, quality issues such as contamination, or by adverse interactions with other foods and medications.

Types

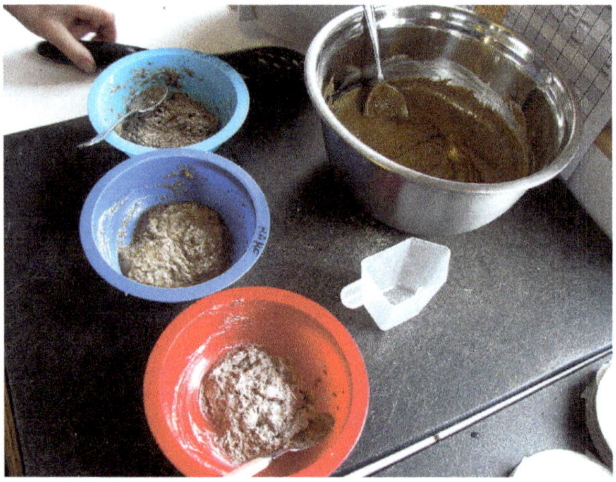

Dietary supplements being mixed into food for pigs

There are many types of dietary supplements.

Vitamins

Vitamin is an organic compound required by an organism as a vital nutrient in limited amounts. An organic chemical compound (or related set of compounds) is called a vitamin when it cannot be synthesized in sufficient quantities by an organism, and must be obtained from the diet. Thus, the term is conditional both on the circumstances and on the particular organism. For example, ascorbic acid (vitamin C) is a vitamin for humans, but not for most other animals. Supplementation is important for the treatment of certain health problems but there is little evidence of benefit when used by those who are otherwise healthy.

Dietary Mineral

Dietary elements, commonly called “dietary minerals” or “minerals”, are the chemical elements required by living organisms, other than the four elements carbon, hydrogen, nitrogen, and oxygen present in common organic molecules.

Amino Acids and Proteins

Amino acids are biologically important organic compounds composed of amine (-NH_2) and carboxylic acid (-COOH) functional groups, along with a side-chain specific to each amino acid. The key elements of an amino acid are carbon, hydrogen, oxygen, and nitrogen, though other elements are found in the side-chains of certain amino acids.

Amino acids can be divided into three categories: essential amino acids, non-essential amino acids, and conditional amino acids. Essential amino acids cannot be made by the body, and must be supplied by food. Non-essential amino acids are made by the body from essential amino acids or in the normal breakdown of proteins. Conditional amino acids are usually not essential, except in times of illness, stress, or for someone challenged with a lifelong medical condition.

Essential Fatty Acids

Essential fatty acids, or EFAs, are fatty acids that humans and other animals must ingest because the body requires them for good health but cannot synthesize them. The term “essential fatty acid” refers to fatty acids required for biological processes but does not include the fats that only act as fuel.

Bodybuilding Supplements

Bodybuilding supplements are dietary supplements commonly used by those involved in bodybuilding and athletics. Bodybuilding supplements may be used to replace meals, enhance weight gain, promote weight loss or improve athletic performance. Among the most widely used are vitamin supplements, protein drinks, branched-chain amino acids (BCAA), glutamine, essential fatty acids, meal replacement products, creatine, weight loss products and testosterone boosters. Supplements are sold either as single ingredient preparations or in the form of “stacks” – proprietary blends of various supplements marketed as offering synergistic advantages. While many bodybuilding supplements are also consumed by the general public their salience and frequency of use may differ when used specifically by bodybuilders.

Industry

In 2013, the global market of vitamins, minerals, and nutritional and herbal supplements (VMHS) was valued at $82 billion, with roughly 28 percent of that in the U.S., where sales increased by approximately $6 billion between 2007 and 2012.

The vitamins and dietary supplements sector in the U.S. grew 4% in 2015, to reach US$27.2 billion. The U.S. market was highly competitive in 2015, as no single company accounted for more than a 5% share of value sales.

Controversy

According to University of Helsinki food safety professor Marina Heinonen, more than 90% of dietary supplement health claims are incorrect. In addition, ingredients listed have been found to be different from the contents. For example, Consumer Reports reported unsafe levels of arsenic, cadmium, lead and mercury in several of the protein powders that were tested. Also, the CBC found that protein spiking (the addition of amino acid filler to manipulate analysis) was not uncommon, however many of the companies involved challenged their claim.

Adverse Effects

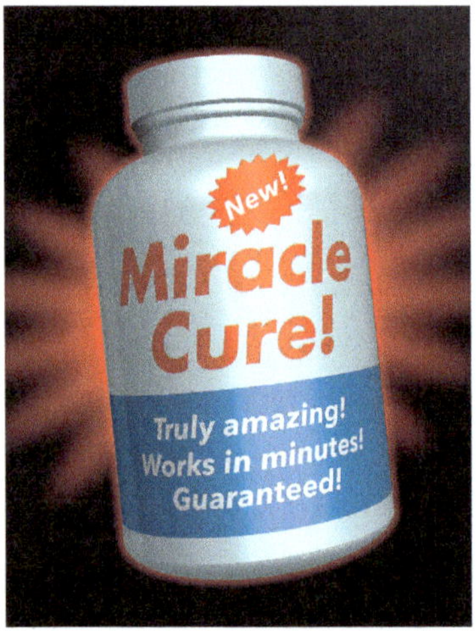

Some products make extraordinary claims and contain active ingredients which may not have been proven effective.

Among general reasons for harmful effects of dietary supplements are: a) absorption in a short time; b) quality and contamination; and c) enhancing both positive and negative effects at the same time. The number of incidents of liver damage from dietary supplements has tripled in a decade. Most of the products causing that effect were bodybuilding supplements. Some of the victims required liver transplants and some died. A third of the supplements involved contained unlisted steroids. Mild to severe toxicity has occurred on many occasions due to dietary supplements, even when the active ingredients were essential nutrients such as vitamins, minerals or amino acids. This has been a result of adulteration of the product, excessive usage on the part of the consumer, or use by persons at risk for the development of adverse effects. In addition, a number of supplements contain psychoactive drugs, whether of natural or synthetic origin.

Physical and Chemical Properties

Adulteration in North America

BMC Medicine published a study on herbal supplements in 2013. Most of the supplements studied were of low quality, one third did not contain the active ingredient(s) claimed, and one third contained unlisted substances.

An investigation by the New York Attorney General's office reported in 2015 analyzed 78 bottles of herbal supplements from Walmart, Target, Walgreens and GNC stores in New York State using DNA barcoding, a method used to detect labeling fraud in the seafood industry. Only about 20% contained the ingredient on the label.

Some supplements were contaminated by rodent feces and urine.

Only 0.3% of the 55,000 U.S. market dietary supplements have been studied regarding their common side effects.

Society and Culture

Public Health

Work done by scientists in the early 20th century on identifying individual nutrients in food and developing ways to manufacture them raised hopes that optimal health could be achieved and diseases prevented by adding them to food and providing people with dietary supplements; while there were successes in preventing vitamin deficiencies, and preventing conditions like neural tube defects by supplementation and food fortification with folic acid, no targeted supplementation or fortification strategies to prevent major diseases like cancer or cardiovascular diseases have proved successful.

For example, while increased consumption of fruits and vegetables are related to decreases in mortality, cardiovascular diseases and cancers, supplementation with key factors found in fruits and vegetable, like antioxidants, vitamins, or minerals, do not help and some have been found to be harmful in some cases. In general as of 2016, robust clinical data is lacking, that shows that any kind of dietary supplementation does more good than harm for people who are healthy and eating a reasonable diet but there is clear data showing that dietary pattern and lifestyle choices are associated with health outcomes.

As a result of the lack of good data for supplementation and the strong data for dietary pattern, public health recommendations for healthy eating urge people to eat a plant-based diet of whole foods, minimizing processed food, salt and sugar and to get exercise daily, and to abandon Western pattern diets and a sedentary lifestyle.

Legal Regulation

United States

The regulation of food and dietary supplements by the U.S. Food and Drug Administration is governed by various statutes enacted by the United States Congress and interpreted by the U.S. Food and Drug Administration ("FDA"). Pursuant to the Federal Food, Drug, and Cosmetic Act ("the Act") and accompanying legislation, the FDA has authority to oversee the quality of substances sold as food in the United States, and to monitor claims made in the labeling about both the composition and the health benefits of foods.

Substances which the FDA regulates as food are subdivided into various categories, including foods, food additives, added substances (man-made substances which are not intentionally introduced into food, but nevertheless end up in it), and dietary supplements. The specific standards which the FDA exercises differ from one category to the next. Furthermore, the FDA has been granted a variety of means by which it can address violations of the standards for a given category of substances.

Regulation in European Union

The European Union's Food Supplements Directive of 2002 requires that supplements be demonstrated to be safe, both in dosages and in purity. Only those supplements that have been proven to be safe may be sold in the bloc without prescription. As a category of food, food supplements cannot be labeled with drug claims but can bear health claims and nutrition claims.

The dietary supplements industry in the United Kingdom (UK), one of the 28 countries in the bloc, strongly opposed the Directive. In addition, a large number of consumers throughout Europe, including over one million in the UK, and various doctors and scientists, had signed petitions by 2005 against what are viewed by the petitioners as unjustified restrictions of consumer choice.

In 2004, along with two British trade associations, the Alliance for Natural Health (ANH) had a legal challenge to the Food Supplements Directive referred to the European Court of Justice by the High Court in London.

Although the European Court of Justice's Advocate General subsequently said that the bloc's plan to tighten rules on the sale of vitamins and food supplements should be scrapped, he was eventually overruled by the European Court, which decided that the measures in question were necessary and appropriate for the purpose of protecting public health. ANH, however, interpreted the ban as applying only to synthetically produced supplements, and not to vitamins and minerals normally found in or consumed as part of the diet.

Nevertheless, the European judges acknowledged the Advocate General's concerns, stating that there must be clear procedures to allow substances to be added to the permitted list based on scientific evidence. They also said that any refusal to add the product to the list must be open to challenge in the courts.

Research

Effects of most dietary supplements have not been determined in randomized clinical trials and manufacturing is lightly regulated; randomized clinical trials of certain vitamins and antioxidants have found increased mortality rates.

Nootropic

Nootropics—also called smart drugs or cognitive enhancers—are drugs, supplements, or other substances that improve cognitive function, particularly executive functions, memory, creativity, or motivation, in healthy individuals. The use of cognition-enhancing drugs by healthy individuals in the absence of a medical indication is one of the most debated topics among neuroscientists, psychiatrists, and physicians which spans a number of issues, including the ethics and fairness of their use, concerns over adverse effects, and the diversion of prescription drugs for nonmedical uses, among others. Nonetheless, the international sales of cognition-enhancing supplements exceeded US$1 billion in 2015 and the global demand for these compounds is still growing rapidly.

The word *nootropic* was coined in 1972 by a Romanian psychologist and chemist, Corneliu E. Giurgea, from the Greek words (*nous*), or "mind", and (*trepein*), meaning to bend or turn.

Availability and Prevalence

There are only a few drugs that are known to improve some aspect of cognition. Many more are in different stages of development. The most commonly used class of drug is stimulants, such as caffeine.

These drugs are purportedly used primarily to treat cognitive or motor function difficulties attributable to disorders such as Alzheimer's disease, Parkinson's disease, Huntington's disease, and ADHD. Some researchers, however, report more widespread use despite concern for further research. Nevertheless, intense marketing may not correlate with efficacy. While scientific studies support the beneficial effects of some compounds, manufacturer's marketing claims for dietary supplements are usually not formally tested and verified by independent entities.

Use by Students

Among students, nootropics have been used to increase productivity, despite their long-term effects lacking conclusive research in healthy individuals. The use of prescription stimulants is especially prevalent among students attending academically competitive colleges. Surveys suggest that 0.7–4.5% of German students have used cognitive enhancers in their lifetime. Stimulants such as dimethylamylamine and methylphenidate are used on college campuses and by younger groups. Based upon studies of self-reported illicit stimulant use, 5–35% of college students use diverted ADHD stimulants, which are primarily used for performance enhancement rather than as recreational drugs.

Several factors positively and negatively influence the use of drugs to increase cognitive performance. Among them are personal characteristics, drug characteristics, and characteristics of the social context.

Side Effects

The main concern with pharmaceutical drugs is adverse effects, and these concerns apply to cognitive-enhancing drugs as well. Long-term safety data is typically unavailable for some types of nootropics (e.g., many non-pharmaceutical cognitive enhancers, newly developed pharmaceuticals and pharmaceuticals with short-term therapeutic use). Racetams—piracetam and other compounds that are structurally related to piracetam—have few serious adverse effects and low toxicity, but there is little evidence that they enhance cognition in individuals without cognitive impairments. While addiction to stimulants is sometimes identified as a cause for concern, a very large body of research on the therapeutic use of the "more addictive" psychostimulants indicate that addiction is fairly rare in therapeutic doses. On their safety profile, a systematic review from June 2015 asserted, "evidence indicates that at low, clinically relevant doses, psychostimulants are devoid of the behavioral and neurochemical actions that define this class of drugs and instead act largely as cognitive enhancers."

In the United States dietary supplements may be marketed if the manufacturer can show that it can manufacture the supplement safely, that the supplement is indeed generally recognized as safe, and if the manufacturer does not make any claims about the supplement's use to treat or prevent any disease or condition; supplements that contain drugs or for which treatment or prevention claims are made are illegal under US law.

Drugs

Stimulants

In 2015, systematic medical reviews and meta-analyses of clinical research in humans established consensus that certain stimulants, only when used at low (therapeutic) concentrations, unambiguously enhance cognition in the general population; in particular, the classes of stimulants that demonstrate cognition-enhancing effects in humans act as direct agonists or indirect agonists of dopamine receptor D_1, adrenoceptor A_2, or both receptors in the prefrontal cortex. Relatively high doses of stimulants cause cognitive deficits.

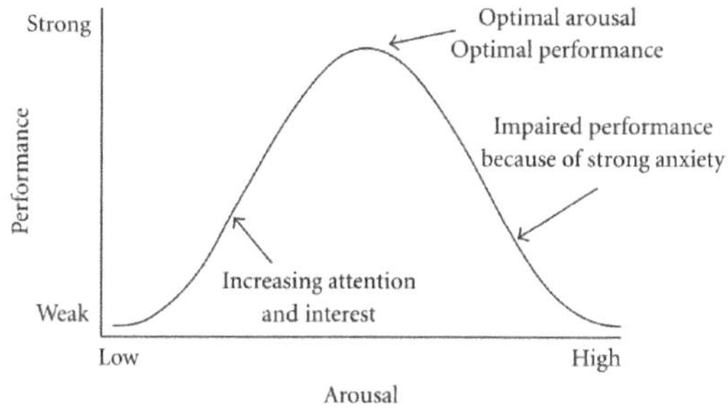

Hebbian version of the Yerkes–Dodson law

- Amphetamine pharmaceuticals (e.g., Adderall, dextroamphetamine, and lisdexamfetamine [an inactive prodrug]) – systematic reviews and meta-analyses report that amphetamine benefits a range of cognitive functions (e.g., inhibitory control, episodic memory, working memory, and aspects of attention) in the general population, and these effects are especially notable in individuals with ADHD. A systematic review from 2014 noted that low doses of amphetamine also improve memory consolidation, in turn leading to improved recall of information in non-ADHD youth. It also improves task saliency (motivation to perform a task) and performance on tedious tasks that require a high degree of effort.
- Methylphenidate – a substituted phenethylamine that improves a range of cognitive functions (e.g., working memory, episodic memory, and inhibitory control, aspects of attention, and planning latency) in the general population. It also improves task saliency and performance on tedious tasks that require a high degree of effort. At above optimal doses, methylphenidate has off target effects that can decrease learning by activating neurons not involved in the task at hand.
- Eugeroics (armodafinil and modafinil) – wakefulness promoting agents; modafinil increases alertness, particularly in sleep deprived individuals, and was noted to facilitate reasoning and problem solving in a systematic review. They are clinically prescribed for narcolepsy, shift work sleep disorder, and daytime sleepiness remaining after sleep apnea treatments.
- Xanthines (most notably, caffeine) – shown to increase alertness, performance, and, in some studies, memory. Children and adults who consume low doses of caffeine showed increased alertness, yet a higher dose was needed to improve performance.
- Nicotine – A meta-analysis of 41 double-blind, placebo-controlled studies concluded that nicotine or smoking had significant positive effects on aspects of fine motor abilities, alerting and orienting attention, and episodic and working

memory. A 2015 review noted that stimulation of the α4β2 nicotinic receptor is responsible for certain improvements in attentional performance; among the nicotinic receptor subtypes, nicotine has the highest binding affinity at the α4β2 receptor (k_i=1 nM), which is also the biological target that mediates nicotine's addictive properties.

Racetams

Racetams, such as piracetam, oxiracetam, and aniracetam, are structurally similar compounds, which are often marketed as cognitive enhancers and sold over-the-counter. Racetams are often referred to as nootropics, but this property of the drug class is not well established. The racetams have poorly understood mechanisms of action; however, piracetam and aniracetam are known to act as positive allosteric modulators of AMPA receptors and appear to modulate cholinergic systems.

According to the US Food and Drug Administration, "Piracetam is not a vitamin, mineral, amino acid, herb or other botanical, or dietary substance for use by man to supplement the diet by increasing the total dietary intake. Further, piracetam is not a concentrate, metabolite, constituent, extract or combination of any such dietary ingredient. [...] Accordingly, these products are drugs, under section 201(g)(1)(C) of the Act, 21 U.S.C. 321(g)(1)(C), because they are not foods and they are intended to affect the structure or any function of the body. Moreover, these products are new drugs as defined by section 201(p) of the Act, 21 U.S.C. 321(p), because they are not generally recognized as safe and effective for use under the conditions prescribed, recommended, or suggested in their labeling."

Miscellaneous

- L-Theanine – A 2014 systematic review and meta-analysis found that concurrent caffeine and L-theanine use has synergistic psychoactive effects that promote alertness, attention, and task switching; these effects are most pronounced during the first hour post-dose.
- Tolcapone – a systematic review noted that it improves verbal episodic memory and episodic memory encoding.
- Levodopa – a systematic review noted that it improves verbal episodic memory and episodic memory encoding.
- Atomoxetine – can improve working memory and aspects of attention when used at an optimal dose.

Dietary Supplements

- *Bacopa monnieri* – A herb sold as a dietary supplement. There is some preliminary evidence for memory-enhancing effects.

- *Panax ginseng* – A review by the Cochrane Collaboration concluded that "there is a lack of convincing evidence to show a cognitive enhancing effect of Panax ginseng in healthy participants and no high quality evidence about its efficacy in patients with dementia." According to the National Center for Complementary and Integrative Health "Although Asian ginseng has been widely studied for a variety of uses, research results to date do not conclusively support health claims associated with the herb." According to a review published in the journal "Advances in Nutrition", multiple RCTs in healthy volunteers have indicated increases in accuracy of memory, speed in performing attention tasks and improvement in performing difficult mental arithmetic tasks, as well as reduction in fatigue and improvement in mood.
- *Ginkgo biloba* – An extract of *Ginkgo biloba* leaf (GBE) is marketed in dietary supplement form with claims it can enhance cognitive function in people without known cognitive problems. Studies have failed to find such effects on memory or attention in healthy people.

Null Findings in Systematic Reviews

- Omega-3 fatty acids: DHA and EPA – two Cochrane Collaboration reviews on the use of supplemental omega-3 fatty acids for ADHD and learning disorders conclude that there is limited evidence of treatment benefits for either disorder. Two other systematic reviews noted no cognition-enhancing effects in the general population or middle-aged and older adults.
- Folate – no cognition-enhancing effects in middle-aged and older adults.
- Vitamin B6 – no cognition-enhancing effects in middle-aged and older adults.
- Vitamin B12 – no cognition-enhancing effects in middle-aged and older adults.
- Vitamin E – no cognition-enhancing effects in middle-aged and older adults.
- Pramipexole – no significant cognition-enhancing effects in healthy individuals.
- Guanfacine – no significant cognition-enhancing effects in healthy individuals.
- Clonidine – no significant cognition-enhancing effects in healthy individuals.
- Ampakines – no significant cognition-enhancing effects in healthy individuals.
- Fexofenadine – no significant cognition-enhancing effects in healthy individuals.
- *Salvia officinalis* – Although some evidence is suggestive of cognition benefits, the study quality is so poor that no conclusions can be drawn from it.

Raw Foodism

Raw foodism (or following a raw food diet) is the dietary practice of eating only, or mostly, uncooked, unprocessed foods. Depending on the philosophy, or type of lifestyle and results desired, raw food diets may include a selection of fruits, vegetables, nuts, seeds, eggs, fish, meat, and dairy products.

It may also include simply processed foods such as various types of sprouted seeds, cheese, and fermented foods such as yogurts, kefir, kombucha or sauerkraut, but generally not foods that have been pasteurized, homogenized, or produced with the use of synthetic pesticides, chemical fertilizers, industrial solvents or chemical food additives.

Varieties

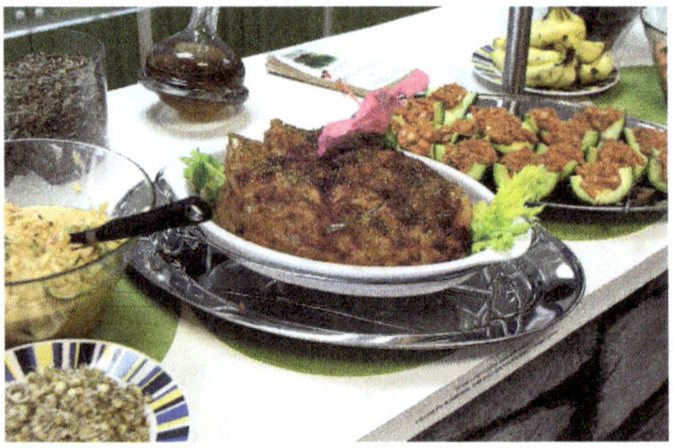

Raw Vegan "Thanksgiving Turkey"

Raw food diets are diets composed entirely or mostly of food that is uncooked or which is cooked at low temperatures.

Raw Veganism

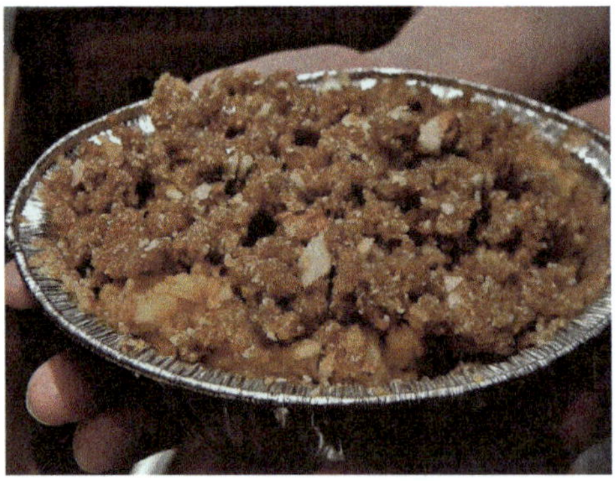

Raw vegan "apple pie"

A raw vegan diet consists of unprocessed, raw plant foods, that have not been heated above 40–49 °C (104–120 °F). Raw vegans such as Brian Clement, Gabriel Cousens, Thierry Browers a.k.a. "Superlight", and Douglas Graham believe that foods cooked above this temperature have lost much of their nutritional value and are less healthy or even harmful to the body. Advocates argue that raw or living foods have natural enzymes, which are critical in building proteins and rebuilding the body, and that heating these foods destroys the natural enzymes and can leave toxic materials behind. However, enzymes, as with other proteins consumed in the diet, are denatured and eventually lysed by the digestive process, rendering them non-functional. Typical foods included in raw food diets are fruits, vegetables, nuts, seeds, and sprouted grains and legumes.

Among raw vegans there are some subgroups such as fruitarians, juicearians, or sproutarians. Fruitarians eat primarily or exclusively fruits, berries, seeds, and nuts. Juicearians process their raw plant foods into juice. Sproutarians adhere to a diet consisting mainly of sprouted seeds.

Raw Vegetarianism

Vegetarianism is a diet that excludes meat (including byproducts like gelatin), fish (including shellfish and other sea animals), and poultry, but allows dairy and/or eggs. Common foods include fruit, vegetables, sprouts, nuts, seeds, grains, legumes, dairy, eggs, and honey. There are several variants of this diet, including raw versions.

Raw Animal Food Diets

Included in raw animal food diets are any food that can be eaten raw, such as uncooked, unprocessed raw muscle-meats/organ-meats/eggs, raw dairy, and aged, raw animal foods such as century eggs, fermented meat/fish/shellfish/kefir, as well as vegetables/fruits/nuts/sprouts/honey, but in general *not* raw grains, raw beans, and raw soy. Raw foods included on such diets have not been heated above 40 °C (104 °F). Raw animal foodists believe that foods cooked above this temperature have lost a lot of their nutritional value and are less bioavailable.

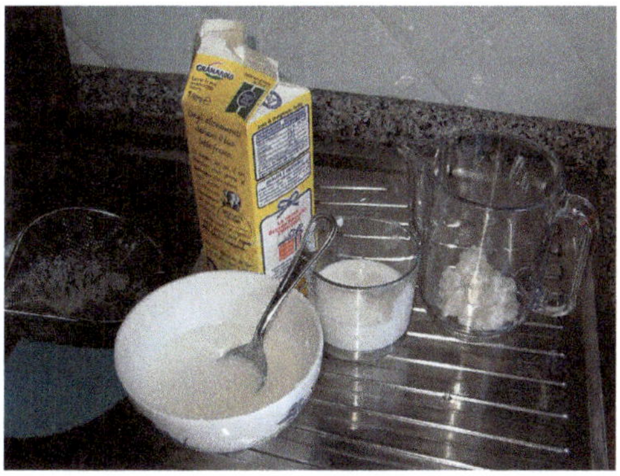

Kefir preparation

Examples of raw animal food diets include the Primal Diet, anopsology (otherwise known as "Instinctive Eating" or "Instincto"), and the Raw Paleolithic diet (otherwise known as the "Raw Meat Diet").

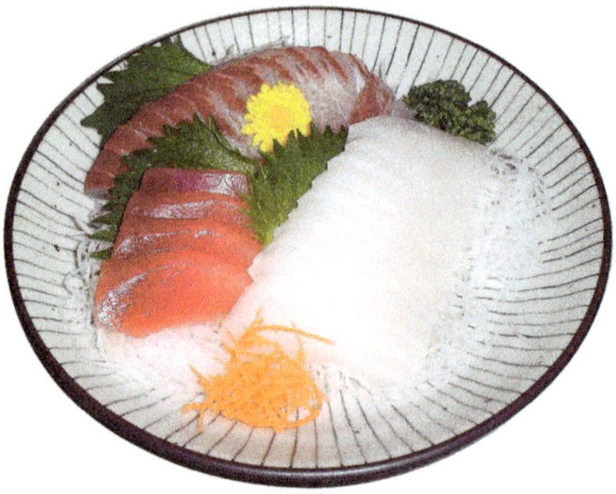

A sashimi dinner set

The Primal Diet consists of fatty meats, organ meats, dairy, honey, minimal fruit and vegetable juices, and coconut products, all raw.

The "Raw Meat Diet", otherwise known as the "Raw, Paleolithic Diet", is a raw version of the (cooked) Paleolithic Diet, incorporating large amounts of raw animal foods such as meats/organ-meats, seafood, eggs, and some raw plant-foods, but usually avoiding non-Paleo foods such as raw dairy, grains, and legumes.

A number of traditional aboriginal diets consisted of large quantities of raw meats, organ meats, and berries, including the traditional diet of the Nenets tribe of Siberia and the Inuit people.

History

Contemporary raw food diets were first developed in Switzerland by Maximilian Bircher-Benner (1867 – 1939), who was influenced as a young man by the German *Lebensreform* movement, which saw civilization as corrupt and sought to go "back to nature"; it embraced holistic medicine, nudism, free love, exercise and other outdoors activity, and foods that it judged were more "natural". Bircher-Benner eventually adopted a vegetarian diet, but took that further and decided that raw food was what humans were really meant to eat; he was influenced by Charles Darwin's ideas that humans were just another kind of animal and Bircher-Benner noted that other animals do not cook their food. In 1904 he opened a sanatorium in the mountains outside of Zurich called "Lebendinge Kraft" or "Vital Force," a technical term in the Lebensreform movement that referred especially to sunlight; he and others believed that this energy was more "concentrated" in plants than in meat, and was diminished by cooking. Patients in the clinic were fed raw foods, including muesli, which was created there. These ideas were dismissed by scientists and the medical profession of his day as quackery.

Other proponents from the early part of the twentieth century include Ann Wigmore, Norman W. Walker (inventor of the Norwalk Juicing Press), and Herbert Shelton. Shelton was arrested, jailed, and fined numerous times for practicing medicine without a license during his career as an advocate of rawism and other alternative health and diet philosophies. Shelton's legacy, as popularized by books like *Fit for Life* by Harvey and Marilyn Diamond, has been deemed "pseudonutrition" by the National Council Against Health Fraud.

Leslie Kenton's book *Raw Energy - Eat Your Way to Radiant Health*, published in 1984, added popularity to foods such as sprouts, seeds, and fresh vegetable juices. The book advocates a diet of 75% raw food which it claims will prevent degenerative diseases, slow the effects of aging, provide enhanced energy, and boost emotional balance; it cites examples such as the sprouted-seed-enriched diets of the long-lived Hunza people and Gerson therapy, an unhealthy, dangerous and potentially very harmful raw juice-based diet and detoxification regime claimed to treat cancer.

Claims

Claims held by raw food proponents include:

- That heating food above 104–118 °F (40–48 °C) starts to degrade and destroy the enzymes in raw food that aid digestion. A few raw food proponents such as Douglas Graham dispute the importance of enzymes in foods, however, and it is commonly believed that enzymes in food play no significant role in the digestive process, prior to being digested themselves.
- That raw foods have higher nutrient and antioxidants values than foods that have been cooked. In reality, whether cooking degrades nutrients or increases their availability, or both, depends on the food and how it is cooked.
- That cooked foods, and especially meat, contain harmful toxins, which can cause chronic disease and other problems, including trans fatty acids produced by heating oil, acrylamide produced by frying, advanced glycation end products (AGEs), and polycyclic aromatic hydrocarbons. While it is true that a healthy diet minimizes fried food and red meat, not all cooked food contains harmful chemicals (a serving of french fries has 200 times the AGEs of a bowl of cooked oatmeal), and a diet containing a normal mix of cooked and raw food does not shorten life. High rates of some of these compounds formed by cooking meat can cause cancer in other animals; whether such an exposure causes cancer in humans remains unclear. According to the American Cancer Society it is not clear, as of 2013, whether acrylamide consumption affects people's risk of getting cancer.

Health Effects

A meta-analysis clinical trials and epidemiological studies published in 2004, and covering a broad range of cancers, found that it appears that there is an inverse relationship between the risk of developing certain types of cancer and eating both raw and cooked vegetables. Consumption of raw vegetables tended to be associated with decreased cancer risks somewhat more often than consumption of cooked vegetables. On the other hand, a raw food diet is likely to impair the development of children and infants.

Care is required in planning a raw vegan diet, especially for children. Dr. Joel Fuhrman, author of *Disease-Proof Your Child*, says there may not be enough vitamin B_{12}, enough vitamin D, and enough calories for a growing child on a totally raw vegan diet. Fuhrman fed his own four children raw and cooked vegetables, fruits, nuts, grains, beans, and occasionally eggs.

Food poisoning is a health risk for all people eating raw foods, and increased demand for raw foods is associated with greater incidence of foodborne illness, especially for raw meat, fish, and shellfish. Outbreaks of gastroenteritis among consumers of raw and undercooked animal products (including smoked, pickled or dried animal products) are well-documented, and include raw meat, raw organ meat, raw fish (whether ocean-going or freshwater), shellfish, raw milk and products made from raw milk, and raw eggs.

In his book *Health or Hoax*, nutritionist Arnold E. Bender has written that "Many raw foods are toxic and only become safe after they have been cooked. Some raw foods contain substances that destroy vitamins, interfere with digestive enzymes or damage the walls of the intestine. Raw meat can be contaminated with bacteria which would be destroyed by cooking; raw fish can contain substances that interfere with vitamin B1 (anti-thiaminases)"

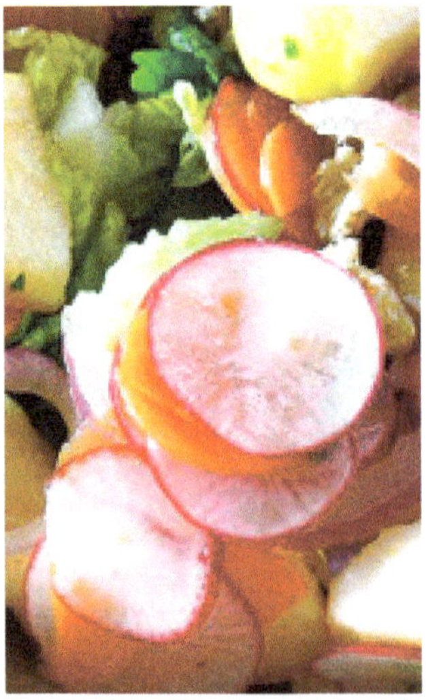

A close-up of a raw food dish

Cooking and Global Warming

It has also been pointed out that cooking food, directly or indirectly, requires energy and may thus release gases associated with global warming. Raw diets mitigate the use of non-renewable resources, which results in raw diets being less environmentally deleterious than cooked food diets in this respect.

Role of Cooking in Human Evolution

Richard Wrangham, professor of biological anthropology at Harvard University, proposes that cooked food played a pivotal role in human evolution. Evidence of a cooked diet, according to Wrangham, can be seen as far back as 1.8 million years ago in the anatomical adaptations of *Homo erectus*. Reduction in the size of teeth and jaw in *H. erectus* indicate a softer diet, requiring less chewing time. This combined with a smaller gut and larger brain indicate to Wrangham that *H. erectus* was eating a higher quality diet than its predecessors. To explain a decreased gut providing the amount of energy required for an increased brain size, Wrangham links his research on the digestive effects of cooked versus raw foods with the lower reproductive abilities of female raw foodists, and BMI in both sexes, to support his hypothesis that cooked starches provided the energy necessary to fuel evolution from *H. erectus* to *H. sapiens*.

Theories opposed to Wrangham's include that of Leslie Aiello, professor of biological anthropology at University College London, and physiologist Peter Wheeler. Aiello and Wheeler believe it was soft animal foods, including bone marrow and brains, which contributed to humans developing the characteristics Wrangham attributes to cooked foods. Further, archaeological evidence suggests that cooking fires began in earnest only around 250 kya, when ancient hearths, earth ovens, burnt animal bones, and flint appear regularly across Europe and the Middle East. Two million years ago, the only sign of fire is burnt earth with human remains, which many anthropologists consider coincidence rather than evidence of intentional fire. Many anthropologists believe the increases in human brain-size occurred well before the advent of cooking, due to a shift away from the consumption of nuts and berries to the consumption of raw meat.

References

- De Smet, PA (Aug 1995). "Health risks of herbal remedies.". Drug safety : an international journal of medical toxicology and drug experience. 13 (2): 81–93. PMID 7576267. doi:10.2165/00002018-199513020-00003
- Robert S. Goodhart; Maurice E. Shils (1980). Modern Nutrition in Health and Disease (6th ed.). Philadelphia: Lea and Febinger. pp. 134–138. ISBN 0-8121-0645-8
- Food and Drug Administration (20 March 2014). "Q&A on Dietary Supplements". fda.gov. Archived from the original on 27 May 2014. Retrieved 26 June 2014
- Katz DL, Meller S (2014). "Can we say what diet is best for health?". Annu Rev Public Health. 35: 83–103. PMID 24641555. doi:10.1146/annurev-publhealth-032013-182351
- Palermo, M; Pellegrini, N; Fogliano, V (April 2014). "Review: The effect of cooking on the phytochemical content of vegetables.". Journal of the science of food and agriculture. 94 (6): 1057–70. PMID 24227349. doi:10.1002/jsfa.6478

- Fitzgerald M (2014). Diet Cults: The Surprising Fallacy at the Core of Nutrition Fads and a Guide to Healthy Eating for the Rest of US. Pegasus Books. ISBN 978-1-60598-560-2
- Griffith-Greene, Megan (November 13, 2015). "Marketplace: Some protein powders fail fitness test". CBC News. Retrieved December 11, 2015
- Macpherson, CN (2005). "Human behaviour and the epidemiology of parasitic zoonoses". International Journal for Parasitology. 35 (11–12): 1319–31. PMID 16102769. doi:10.1016/j.ijpara.2005.06.004
- Gazzaniga, Michael S. (2006). The Ethical Brain: The Science of Our Moral Dilemmas (P.S.). New York, N.Y: Harper Perennial. p. 184. ISBN 0-06-088473-8
- O'CONNOR, ANAHAD. "Herbal Supplements Are Often Not What They Seem". New York Times. Retrieved 12 November 2013
- Cox, JM (1995). "Salmonella enteritidis: the egg and I". Australian Veterinary Journal. 72 (3): 108–15. PMID 7611983. doi:10.1111/j.1751-0813.1995.tb15022.x
- Malenka RC, Nestler EJ, Hyman SE (2009). Sydor A, Brown RY, eds. Molecular Neuropharmacology: A Foundation for Clinical Neuroscience (2nd ed.). New York: McGraw-Hill Medical. p. 454. ISBN 9780071481274
- Kiefer, I. (2007). "Brain Food". Scientific American Mind. 18 (5): 58–63. doi:10.1038/scientificamericanmind1007-58. Retrieved November 1, 2009
- Malykh AG, Sadaie MR (February 2010). "Piracetam and piracetam-like drugs: from basic science to novel clinical applications to CNS disorders". Drugs. 70 (3): 287–312. PMID 20166767. doi:10.2165/11319230-000000000-00000

Permissions

All chapters in this book are published with permission under the Creative Commons Attribution Share Alike License or equivalent. Every chapter published in this book has been scrutinized by our experts. Their significance has been extensively debated. The topics covered herein carry significant information for a comprehensive understanding. They may even be implemented as practical applications or may be referred to as a beginning point for further studies.

We would like to thank the editorial team for lending their expertise to make the book truly unique. They have played a crucial role in the development of this book. Without their invaluable contributions this book wouldn't have been possible. They have made vital efforts to compile up to date information on the varied aspects of this subject to make this book a valuable addition to the collection of many professionals and students.

This book was conceptualized with the vision of imparting up-to-date and integrated information in this field. To ensure the same, a matchless editorial board was set up. Every individual on the board went through rigorous rounds of assessment to prove their worth. After which they invested a large part of their time researching and compiling the most relevant data for our readers.

The editorial board has been involved in producing this book since its inception. They have spent rigorous hours researching and exploring the diverse topics which have resulted in the successful publishing of this book. They have passed on their knowledge of decades through this book. To expedite this challenging task, the publisher supported the team at every step. A small team of assistant editors was also appointed to further simplify the editing procedure and attain best results for the readers.

Apart from the editorial board, the designing team has also invested a significant amount of their time in understanding the subject and creating the most relevant covers. They scrutinized every image to scout for the most suitable representation of the subject and create an appropriate cover for the book.

The publishing team has been an ardent support to the editorial, designing and production team. Their endless efforts to recruit the best for this project, has resulted in the accomplishment of this book. They are a veteran in the field of academics and their pool of knowledge is as vast as their experience in printing. Their expertise and guidance has proved useful at every step. Their uncompromising quality standards have made this book an exceptional effort. Their encouragement from time to time has been an inspiration for everyone.

The publisher and the editorial board hope that this book will prove to be a valuable piece of knowledge for students, practitioners and scholars across the globe.

Index

A
Adipose Tissue, 101-102, 119
Amino Acid Composition, 8
Anaerobic Exercise, 53-54
Animal Nutrition, 32, 93, 203
Anti-vitamins, 166
Antinutrient, 41
Auto-oxidation, 121

B
Biochemistry, 68, 71, 83, 88, 98, 108, 113, 123-124, 152, 163, 203
Biodegradable Plastics, 84
Bioinformatics, 79, 151
Biosynthesis, 29, 69, 81, 83, 92, 96, 127, 184-186, 189
Breast Cancer, 106, 109, 152, 182

C
Cancer Research, 46, 66
Carbohydrate Chemistry, 126, 131
Cardiovascular Disease, 14, 37-38, 45, 48, 55, 102, 104-105, 109, 111, 144, 146, 182
Carotenoids, 157, 163, 167-168, 172
Catabolism, 16, 23, 90, 97, 131, 142, 189
Cell Signaling, 14, 75
Cellular Functions, 11, 73
Cellular Localization, 77-79
Chemical Synthesis, 71, 95
Cholesterol Metabolism, 141-142
Colorectal Cancer, 24, 106, 112, 144, 182
Common Cold, 180, 182
Conditionally Essential Nutrients, 5-6

D
Dermatology, 177, 203
Dietary Deficiency, 5
Dietary Fiber, 4, 22, 24, 67, 123, 129-130, 133-135, 137-145, 147
Disaccharides, 2, 23, 123, 125, 127-130
Docosahexaenoic Acid, 11-13, 15, 39, 111
Double-fortified Salt, 154-155
Dyslipidemia, 105

E
Environmental Nutrition, 33
Enzymes, 24-25, 29, 52, 68, 72, 75-76, 78, 81-82, 89-90, 96, 99, 129, 131, 133, 137, 140, 144, 148-149, 156-157, 166, 180, 184, 189, 199, 202, 219, 221-222
Essential Amino Acid, 5-6, 10
Essential Fatty Acid, 10-11, 13-15, 25, 209

F
Fat Profiles, 103
Fatty Acid, 6, 10-15, 23-25, 39, 67, 98-101, 104-105, 107-108, 110, 113-114, 116-118, 120-121, 141, 147, 209
Fiber Intake, 138, 143-146
Food Sources, 7, 14, 25, 41, 112, 133, 144, 167

G
Gene Transcription, 175-176
Genetic Code, 67, 70, 83-84, 89-90, 93, 97

H
Healthy Diet, 16, 32, 43, 46-48, 184, 206
High Birth Weight, 62, 65
Hydrogenation, 24, 94, 99-100, 121
Hypertension, 38, 43, 47-48, 55, 112, 147
Hyponatremia, 38, 41

I
Interchangeability, 9
Intestinal Bacterial Flora, 32
Isoelectric Point, 87-88
Isomerism, 85, 126

L
Lavoisier, 19
Ligand Binding, 75

M
Macrominerals, 2, 29, 38, 153
Macronutrients, 1-3, 23, 37, 48, 67, 98
Malnutrition, 10, 33, 35-36, 56, 155, 204

Mental Agility, 38
Mental Disorders, 39
Metabolic Syndrome, 16, 40-41
Metabolism, 1, 3, 5, 19, 30, 32, 51, 56, 66, 68, 75, 92, 102, 106, 118, 122, 127, 130-132, 137-138, 141-142, 157, 168, 175, 179, 189, 201
Monosaccharides, 23, 123-129, 131, 186
Monounsaturated Fat, 104, 109-110

N
Non-essential Nutrients, 4-5
Non-standard Amino Acids, 90, 92
Nullomers, 93
Nutrient Intake, 1, 5-6
Nutrition Literacy, 34-36

O
Oat Bran, 146, 151
Obese Women, 60-61, 65
Ovarian Cancer, 106
Ozonolysis, 121

P
Peptide Bond Formation, 95
Performance Enhancing Supplements, 50
Pharmacology, 161
Physicochemical Properties, 97, 138-139
Phytochemicals, 22, 31, 42
Plant Nutrition, 32-33
Polyunsaturated Fat, 104, 110, 112
Prenatal Nutrition, 54
Prostate Cancer, 106, 181
Protein Disorder, 80
Protein Per Calorie, 8
Protein Purification, 77
Protein Sources, 8, 26
Proteomics, 79
Public Health, 44, 46, 49, 66, 102, 153-154, 211-212, 223

R
Rancidity, 25, 109
Recovery Supplements, 51
Reference Intake Values, 15
Retinoids, 170, 172, 177
Ring-straight Chain Isomerism, 126

S
Salt Iodization, 153-154
Saturated Fat, 31, 37, 99, 102-107, 109-111, 150-151
Side Chains, 68, 71, 74, 83, 85-86, 88, 94, 98
Sports Nutrition, 50
Structural Proteins, 74, 76
Structure Prediction, 73, 79-80, 82

T
Toxicity, 5, 33, 43, 158, 170-171, 178, 180, 184, 202, 210, 214
Trace Minerals, 29, 38, 153, 201

U
Underweight Women, 60-61, 65
Unhealthy Diets, 48
Upper Gastrointestinal Tract, 139

V
Vitamin A Supplementation, 154, 169-170, 204

Z
Zinc Deficiencies, 155
Zinc Fertilization, 155
Zwitterions, 87-88